HANDBOOK OF THE

ASSISTED REPRODUCTION
LABORATORY

HANDBOOK OF THE
ASSISTED REPRODUCTION LABORATORY

edited by
Brooks A. Keel, Ph.D., HCLD
Jeffrey V. May, Ph.D., HCLD
Christopher J. De Jonge, Ph.D., HCLD

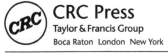

CRC Press
Taylor & Francis Group
Boca Raton London New York

CRC Press is an imprint of the
Taylor & Francis Group, an **informa** business

CRC Press
Taylor & Francis Group
6000 Broken Sound Parkway NW, Suite 300
Boca Raton, FL 33487-2742

First issued in paperback 2019

© 2000 by Taylor & Francis Group, LLC
CRC Press is an imprint of Taylor & Francis Group, an Informa business

No claim to original U.S. Government works

ISBN-13: 978-0-8493-1677-7 (hbk)
ISBN-13: 978-0-367-39867-5 (pbk)
Library of Congress Card Number 99-086572

Library of Congress Cataloging-in-Publication Data

Handbook of the assisted reproduction laboratory / edited by Brooks A. Keel, Jeffrey V. May, Christopher J. De Jonge.
    p. cm.
    Includes bibliographical references and index.
    ISBN 0-8493-1677-4 (alk. paper)
    1. Infertility—Diagnosis—Handbooks, manuals, etc. 2. Diagnosis,
Laboratory—Handbooks, manuals, etc. I. Keel, Brooks A. II. May, Jeffrey Verner.
III. Jonge, Christopher J. De
RC889 . H258 2000
616.6′92—dc21   99-086572
                                                   CIP

Visit the Taylor & Francis Web site at
http://www.taylorandfrancis.com

and the CRC Press Web site at
http://www.crcpress.com

Preface

The field of reproductive biology and medicine has exploded over the past decade. With the advent of *in vitro* fertilization and other associated technologies (now termed collectively Assisted Reproductive Technologies, or ART), our understanding of the reproductive system in both men and women has progressed exponentially. Along with this increase in knowledge, new and advanced laboratories have emerged to perform techniques aimed at diagnosing and treating infertility problems. As these laboratories multiply, so does the need for properly trained clinical laboratorians. In many cases, the ART laboratories are staffed with biologists well trained in reproductive research techniques, but lacking the necessary clinical laboratory technical and administrative skills to manage these laboratories. An earlier CRC Press publication, *Handbook of the Laboratory Diagnosis and Treatment of Infertility* (1990), edited by Brooks Keel and Bobby Webster, was aimed at the technical component of the ART laboratories and at the technologists performing these procedures. It contained descriptions of the technical procedures for the diagnosis and treatment of infertility and served as a procedure manual as well as a reference. It was directed primarily toward the technologists working at the bench. It did not, however, provide the laboratorian staffing and directing these ART labs with adequate management information and background information on reproductive biology and medicine. It is the goal of the current handbook to fill these gaps, to provide updated information, and to serve as a companion edition to the 1990 *Handbook*. It will complement and extend the *Handbook of the Laboratory Diagnosis and Treatment of Infertility*, rather than replace it.

In general, the current *Handbook* will (1) review male and female reproductive systems and processes, (2) discuss the clinical diagnosis and management of male and female infertility, (3) provide new information on the state-of-the-art techniques of egg and embryo culture, micromanipulation, and biopsy, and (4) present various aspects of quality control, quality assurance, and clinical laboratory management. It is intended that this *Handbook* will be used by laboratory directors as a management tool, by technologists and bench personnel (especially new hires) as a training guide, and by students as a resource for study. Laboratory personnel preparing for professional board and certification examinations will find it a useful review.

This *Handbook* was designed by inviting a group of internationally recognized experts in the field of ART to discuss these topics. We have allowed these experts freedom in terms of the organization and presentation of their information, which has resulted in a blend of presentation styles. Like the 1990 *Handbook*, we hope this current edition will serve as a guide for current investigation and as a stimulus for future developments in the field.

About the Editors

Brooks A. Keel, Ph.D., HCLD, is the Daniel K. Roberts Professor of Obstetrics and Gynecology, Professor of Pediatrics, and Associate Dean for Research at the University of Kansas School of Medicine, Wichita. Dr. Keel serves as the President and CEO of the Women's Research Institute and is the President and Director of the Reproductive Medicine Laboratories in Wichita, Kansas. Dr. Keel received his Ph.D. in reproductive endocrinology from the Medical College of Georgia in 1982. After three years of postdoctoral training at the University of Texas Health Science Center in Houston and the University of South Dakota School of Medicine, Dr. Keel moved to the University of Kansas School of Medicine, Wichita in 1985 where he helped establish the laboratory components of the Center for Reproductive Medicine, including an infertility clinic, andrology laboratory (Reproductive Medicine Laboratories), assisted reproductive technology (ART) program, and laboratory and basic science research program (Women's Research Institute). Nationally, Dr. Keel serves on the Board of Directors of the American Board of Bioanalysis (ABB) and the American Association of Bioanalysts (AAB) and is a Past President of the AAB. He played an instrumental role in establishing the certification requirements for High-Complexity Clinical Laboratory Directors in the specialities of Embryology and Andrology through the ABB and in founding the College of Reproductive Biology of the AAB. Dr. Keel is a member of numerous professional societies. He has authored more than 60 peer-reviewed scientific publications, written 15 book chapters, and edited 4 books in the area of reproductive medicine and biology. His basic science research on the control of cellular growth and development of the reproductive tissues has been funded by the National Institutes of Health and other private foundations.

Christopher De Jonge, Ph.D., HCLD, is Professor in the Department of Obstetrics and Gynecology and Women's Health Center at the University of Minnesota and Director of Laboratories at the Reproductive Medicine Center, University of Minnesota Physicians in Minneapolis, Minnesota. Dr. De Jonge most recently was an Associate Professor in the Department of Ob/Gyn and the Graduate College at the University of Nebraska Medical Center, and he was the Director of the Center for Reproductive Medicine Laboratories and Scientific Director of the Center for Reproductive Medicine. Dr. De Jonge was responsible for the design and implementation of the laboratories in Nebraska and Minneapolis. Dr. De Jonge is board-certified as a High-Complexity Clinical Laboratory Director. He received his Ph.D. and the Graduate College Award for excellence in research among graduate students from Rush University in 1989. Dr. De Jonge was the recipient of the 1995 American Society of Andrology Young Andrologist Award and first runner-up for the 1995 Hamilton Thorn Outstanding Original Research Award and The University of Nebraska Medical Center 1993–94 Outstanding Professional Achievement Award.

He has served as an ad hoc reviewer for a number of granting agencies, including the NIH, NSF, Swiss National Science Foundation, The Israel Science Foundation, United States–Israel Binational Science Foundation, and the Wellbeing Programme. Dr. De Jonge is an Editor for *Human Reproduction*, an Associate Editor for the *Journal of Andrology*, Section Editor of the "Andrology Laboratory Corner" in the *Journal of Andrology*, and is on the Editorial Committee for the *World Health Organization Laboratory Manual for the Examination of Human Semen and Sperm-Cervical Mucus Interaction*. He has authored more than 35 peer-reviewed scientific publications and 12 book chapters and has edited several books in the area of reproductive medicine and biology. His varied research interests focus primarily on aspects of reproductive biology.

Jeffrey V. May, Ph.D., HCLD, is Associate Professor of Obstetrics and Gynecology at the University of Kansas School of Medicine, Wichita, Scientific Director for the Women's Research Institute, and Adjunct Associate Professor of Biological Sciences at the Wichita State University. Dr. May received a Ph.D. degree in Biochemistry from the University of Rhode Island in 1979. He completed four years of postdoctoral training in Reproductive Endocrinology at Duke University and then served as Assistant Professor in the departments of Obstetrics and Gynecology and Physiology for four additional years at Duke. In 1987, Dr. May moved to Wichita as one of the initial scientists at the Women's Research Institute and in 1988 assumed the directorship of the assisted reproductive technology (ART) laboratory associated with the Center for Reproductive Medicine, a position he held for nine years. Dr. May was active in the development of the Reproductive Biology Professional Group within the American Society for Reproductive Medicine and was instrumental in developing the initial examinations for embryology laboratory certification for the American Board of Bioanalysis. Dr. May's research interests are centered upon the intraovarian regulation of folliculogenesis, reproductive consequences associated with exposure to endocrine disruptors, and reproductive aging. Dr. May has served on numerous NIH study sections including a four-year term on the Reproductive Biology Study Section. Dr. May also serves as a consultant to the Ob/Gyn Devices Panel of the Food and Drug Administration.

Contributors

Christopher L. R. Barratt, Ph.D.
Reproductive Biology and Genetics
  Group
University Department of Medicine and
  Obstetrics and Gynecology
Birmingham Women's Hospital
Edgbaston, Birmingham, U.K.

J. Michael Bedford, Vet. M.B., Ph.D.
The Center for Reproductive Medicine
  and Infertility
The New York Hospital
Cornell Medical Center
New York, New York

Jeffrey P. Boldt, Ph.D., HCLD
Midwest Reproductive Medicine
Indianapolis, Indiana

Roy A. Brandell, M.D.
James Buchanan Brady Foundation
Department of Urology
The New York Presbyterian Hospital
Weill Medical College of Cornell
  University
The Population Council, Center for
  Biomedical Research, New York

Grace M. Centola, Ph.D., HCLD
Rochester Regional Cryobank and
  Andrology Laboratory
University of Rochester
  Medical Center
Rochester, New York

Christopher J. De Jonge, Ph.D., HCLD
Department of Obstetrics and
  Gynecology
Reproductive Medicine Center
  Laboratories
University of Minnesota
Minneapolis, Minnesota

D. M. de Kretser, Ph.D.
Monash Institute of Reproduction and
  Development
Monash University
Clayton, Victoria, Australia

M. Esposito, M.D.
Department of Obstetrics and
  Gynecology
University of Pennsylvania Medical
  Center
Philadelphia, Pennsylvania

Norbert Gleicher, M.D.
The Center for Human
  Reproduction—Illinois
Chicago, Illinois

Kathryn J. Go, Ph.D., HCLD
Pennsylvania Reproductive Associates
Pennsylvania Hospital
Philadelphia, Pennsylvania

Chad A. Johnson, Ph.D., HCLD
Reproductive Studies Laboratory
Cincinnati, Ohio

Brooks A. Keel, Ph.D., HCLD
The Women's Research Institute
Reproductive Medicine
 Laboratories
Department of Obstetrics and
 Gynecology
University of Kansas School of
 Medicine
Wichita, Kansas

Theresa A. Kellom, Ph.D., HCLD
Embryology Network
Albany, New York

O. Khorram, M.D., Ph.D.
Department of Obstetrics and
 Gynecology
University of Wisconsin
Madison, Wisconsin

S. Kulshrestha, M.D.
Department of Obstetrics and
 Gynecology
University of Pennsylvania Medical
 Center
Philadelphia, Pennsylvania

Bruce A. Lessey, Ph.D., M.D.
Department of Obstetrics and
 Gynecology
Division of Reproductive
 Endocrinology and Infertility
University of North Carolina
Chapel Hill, North Carolina

Laurie P. Lovely, M.D.
Travis Air Force Base
Vallejo, California

Victoria M. Maclin, M.D.
Department of Obstetrics and
 Gynecology
University of Nebraska Medical Center
Omaha, Nebraska

Jeffrey V. May, Ph.D., HCLD
The Women's Research Institute
University of Kansas School of
 Medicine
Wichita, Kansas

Gianpiero D. Palermo, M.D.
The Center for Reproductive Medicine
 and Infertility
The New York Hospital
Cornell Medical Center
New York

Pasquale Patrizio, M.D.
Department of Obstetrics and
 Gynecology
University of Pennsylvania Medical
 Center
Philadelphia, Pennsylvania

Peter N. Schlegel, M.D.
James Buchanan Brady Foundation
Department of Urology
The New York Presbyterian Hospital
Weill Medical College of Cornell
 University
The Population Council, Center for
 Biomedical Research, New York

Lynette A. Scott, Ph.D.
Reproductive Science Center
Walter Reed Army Medical Center
Washington, D.C.

Kathy L. Sharpe-Timms, Ph.D., HCLD
Department of Obstetrics and
  Gynecology
University of Missouri
Columbia, Missouri

Matthew J. Tomlinson, Ph.D.
Reproductive Biology and Genetics
  Group
University Department of Medicine and
  Obstetrics and Gynecology
Birmingham Women's Hospital
Edgbaston, Birmingham, U.K.

Randall L. Zimmer, M.D.
Department of Obstetrics and
  Gynecology
University of Missouri
Columbia, Missouri

Contents

1 Human Fertilization

Christopher J. De Jonge

CONTENTS

I. INTRODUCTION

The fertilization process can be imagined as an elegant pas de deux, with fertilization success dependent upon the precise timing and accuracy of a well-choreographed series of steps between male (spermatozoa) and female (oocytes) gametes. Perhaps the greatest performer in the fertilization process is the spermatozoon. The spermatozoon must overcome numerous obstacles and undergo dynamic changes in order to achieve its destiny, while the oocyte assumes a fairly passive role in events leading to and culminating in fertilization. Some of the prefertilization processes that a mammalian spermatozoon must undergo have been revealed only in the last 10 to 15 years,[1,2] while other aspects still remain as somewhat of an enigma. This chapter will summarize what is presently known about prefertilization processes occurring in humans with primary attention on the spermatozoon. Aspects related to fertilization in nonhuman mammalian and nonmammalian species can be found in the many review articles cited herein.

II. CAPACITATION

Until ejaculated human spermatozoa are removed from seminal plasma, they cannot fertilize a fully invested human oocyte. The first step in separation from seminal plasma *in vivo* occurs through the dissolution of sperm-coagulating proteins, termed liquefaction, which allows sperm to have unrestricted movement and subsequently to gain access to the cervix. At the moment sperm enter into cervical mucus they become isolated from the seminal plasma, and capacitation begins. One reason sperm must be removed from seminal plasma is because proteins in the seminal plasma biochemically restrict the sperm plasma membrane, at least as it relates to fertilizing ability. A number of terms have been applied to these proteins, e.g., decapacitation factor, acrosome-stabilizing factor. As sperm swim through the cervical mucus, proteins adsorbed to the plasma membrane begin to be removed. Once these proteins are removed, changes occur, in crescendo-like fashion, that prepare the spermatozoon for fertilization. These unique changes collectively have been termed capacitation and were first described by Chang and Austin.[3,4] Since those landmark publications, additional reports addressing the biochemical and physiological aspects of capacitation have been published, the results of which can be found in a number of review articles.[5-22]

Capacitation is a requisite preparatory process for fertilization. Certain events leading up to capacitation characterize this process: (1) an increase in membrane fluidity,[1] (2) a decrease in net surface charge,[1] (3) increases in oxidative processes and cAMP production,[1,9,23] (4) a decrease in the plasma membrane cholesterol to phospholipid ratio,[1,24,25] (5) expression of mannose binding sites as a consequence of cholesterol removal,[25] (6) an increase in tyrosine phosphorylation,[9,23] (7) an increase in reactive oxygen species,[9] and (8) changes in sperm swimming patterns, termed hyperactivation.[1,26] The only clear indicator as to the progress of capacitation is susceptibility to acrosome reaction induction (see below), but its occurrence merely signifies that a sperm cell has become fully capacitated.

To study capacitation one typically must rely on *in vitro* assays. Thus, when studying capacitation one must consider composition of culture medium and incubation conditions. The media most commonly used for *in vitro* incubation of human sperm are based on those used for nonhuman sperm, and they have a combination of balanced salts as their basic components, e.g., Tyrode's; Krebs-Ringer's; and Biggers, Whitten, and Whittingham medium.[1] Protein is typically added to the media since it has been shown to support capacitation, the acrosome reaction, and fertilization *in vitro*.[1,27-31] The protein supplements most commonly used are serum albumin (typically human or bovine) and fetal cord serum. When human spermatozoa are incubated *in vitro* at 37°C in balanced saline containing 0.3 to 3.5% human serum albumin, capacitation time is typically 2 to 4 hours.[1,27-31]

Data from several recent studies on capacitation suggest that protein supplementation helps remove cholesterol from the sperm membranes resulting in a change in the cholesterol to phospholipid ratio and an increase in membrane fluidity.[24,25] A possible consequence of increased membrane fluidity is the localization and expression of membrane receptors that upon interaction with an appropriate ligand will initiate the signaling sequence(s) that culminate in the acrosome reaction. For example, in the human sperm plasma membrane is a receptor that binds mannose-containing ligands.[25] Expression of this receptor depends on capacitation time. The capacitation-dependent localization of the mannose lectin on the sperm plasma membrane overlying the acrosomal cap complies with the requirement that a receptor be present in that region in order to coordinate exocytosis.[25]

Along with changes in plasma membrane fluidity and composition come changes that will prepare and sensitize the spermatozoon for acrosome reaction stimulation. One change that has been shown to occur during the time course to induce capacitation involves an influx of calcium.[32] Apparently, sperm must be exposed to extracellular calcium during the time course to induce capacitation, but the same is not true for the time during which sperm undergo the acrosome reaction (see below).[33]

Another recently described change that may assist in or control capacitation and that can be related, in part, to cholesterol removal is an increase in phosphorylation on tyrosine residue-containing proteins.[2,9,23,26] Tyrosine phosphorylation appears to be regulated by two effector molecules/pathways. The first mechanism involves a change in the oxidation-reduction (redox) state of the cell that is induced by an increase in reactive oxygen species (ROS), specifically hydrogen peroxide.[2] The second route for tyrosine phosphorylation increases seems to occur through the activity of cyclic AMP (cAMP) as the effector molecule.[23] The specific metabolic sequence(s) leading to the production of cAMP and subsequent tyrosine phosphorylation has not been clarified but likely involves a pathway that has calcium, a bicarbonate-sensitive adenylate cyclase, and cAMP-dependent kinase as its components.[23]

The time to induce capacitation depends on incubation conditions, e.g., *in vivo* versus *in vitro*. When sufficient time has elapsed, sperm become susceptible to stimuli that will induce a process called the acrosome reaction.[27-31,34-38]

III. ACROSOME REACTION

The acrosome reaction is an exocytotic process occurring in the sperm head that is essential for successful penetration of the oocyte zona pellucida. Sperm that do not undergo an acrosome reaction on, or in extremely close proximity to, the zona pellucida cannot fertilize the oocyte without assistance.[1] Many believe that the acrosome reaction cannot be induced unless sperm have completed the capacitative process. While this principle certainly holds true for the "physiological" acrosome reaction, recent data suggest that the reaction can be biochemically induced without the spermatozoa first having been capacitated, presumably by bypassing membrane-mediated event(s).[39,40] These and other data indicate that the processes of capacitation and acrosomal exocytosis are distinct and separable in human spermatozoa.

In order to appreciate the role of the acrosome reaction in fertilization, one must understand the structure of the sperm head and the components of the acrosome reaction. Contained within the anterior portion of the sperm head and immediately underlying the plasma membrane is a membrane-bound cap-like structure called the acrosome. The acrosomal membrane comprises the outer acrosomal membrane, i.e., facing the overlying plasma membrane, and the inner acrosomal membrane, i.e., facing the nucleus. With these landmarks identified morphologically the acrosome reaction can be characterized as point fusions occurring between the plasma and outer acrosomal membranes. The formation of fenestrations and hybrid vesicles (consisting of both plasma and outer acrosomal membranes) immediately follows membrane fusion. As a consequence, the interior of the acrosome, termed the acrosomal matrix, becomes exposed and solubilized, allowing for the activation of enzymes (see below) that will play a key role in the fertilization process.[41,42]

The acrosome is a unique organelle that is analogous to both a lysosome and a regulated secretory vesicle.[41,42] Contained within the acrosomal vesicle are several lytic enzymes that are released as a part or consequence of the acrosome reaction.

One of the principal enzymes, a serine glycoproteinase called acrosin, exists in a proenzyme form called proacrosin. Approximately 93% of acrosin exists as proacrosin. Proacrosin has been found to be localized on the acrosomal membranes and in the acrosomal matrix. However, the latter has not been proven conclusively. While the precise *in vivo* mechanism(s) by which proacrosin (inactive form) is converted to acrosin (active form) is ill-defined, a change in acrosomal pH is thought to be involved. The earliest time at which acrosin has been detected as being activated is immediately before membrane vesiculation. Thus, we can reason that proacrosin already has been almost entirely converted to the functional form of acrosin by the early stages of the acrosome reaction, i.e., fusion and fenestration of the outer acrosomal and plasma membranes.[43,44] The following section relays the significance of the early onset of acrosin activation.

Evidence demonstrates that acrosin plays an important role in the fertilization process:[41,42] (1) acrosin appears to become functional during the acrosome reaction;[44,45] (2) active and liberated acrosin plays an important role in sperm-oocyte fusion, specifically at the level of zona binding and penetration;[44,46,47] and (3) residual acrosin remains associated with the outer acrosomal membrane possibly to facilitate sperm binding with the oolemma.[43,44]

Thus, if one considers the temporal and spatial aspects of fertilization, one recognizes that the capacitative process must situate and prime sperm receptors for zona ligands so that the subsequent ligand-receptor induced signaling events that culminate in the acrosome reaction and the localized activation and release of acrosomal enzymes will occur in immediate proximity to the oocyte. In fact, an increasing amount of evidence supports that human spermatozoa must be acrosome-intact when they contact, bind, and acrosome react to the zona pellucida glycoproteins.[48,49] Thus, prematurity or disorganization in the aforementioned sequence of events likely will lead to reduced fertilization potential.

IV. SIGNAL TRANSDUCTION AND THE ACROSOME REACTION

All the molecular events required for the acrosome reaction have not been characterized definitively. Unlike the somatic cell, the sperm cell does not have the machinery in place to recapitulate exocytosis. Thus, many of the methods used to study exocytosis in somatic cells simply cannot be applied to the sperm cell. Regardless, the process of exocytosis in the somatic cell remains an effective model for studying the acrosome reaction. As a result, some of the membrane-associated and intracellular processes that constitute the acrosome reaction have been described.[37,38,50]

A species-selective barrier to fertilization surrounds the mammalian oocyte and is called the zona pellucida. The zona pellucida is an acellular matrix consisting of three glycoproteins ZP1, ZP2, and ZP3.[51] Experiments have shown that the zona pellucida initiates sperm-zona binding.[47,52–55] In addition, both solubilized[40,56,57] and intact[47–49,52–55] zonae stimulate the acrosome reaction, and the former does so in a dose-dependent manner.[56] Recombinant technology revealed the role(s) of ZP3 in the fertilization process. Specifically, ZP3 appears to be the primary ligand for sperm-zona binding and acrosome reaction induction.[58,59] While ZP3 has been fairly well characterized as a ligand for sperm,[58,59,60] such is not the case for ZP3 receptor(s) on the sperm plasma membrane.

The majority of current data concerning sperm receptors for zona glycoproteins is restricted to nonhuman mammalian and nonmammalian species. In humans, one of the best described ZP3 receptor candidates is a lectin that binds mannose-containing ligands.[25] Expression of this receptor depends on the capacitation time, as capacitation time increases so does receptor expression. The capacitation-dependent localization of the mannose lectin on the sperm plasma membrane overlying the acrosomal cap complies with the requirement that a receptor be present in that region in order to coordinate exocytosis. Data demonstrating a correlation between mannose lectin expression and acrosomal status supports this latter aspect.[25]

Another ZP3 receptor candidate on human sperm is a 95kDa receptor tyrosine kinase (RTK).[61] This receptor is thought to initiate intracellular pH changes that culminate in the acrosome reaction. Interestingly, both intact zona pellucida and progesterone stimulate tyrosine phosphorylation.[62] Whether these two agonists act via the same RTK is questionable. Further, some controversy exists over whether the 95kDa RTK has a unique and defined role in sperm-zona recognition as a receptor specifically responsible for sperm binding and acrosome reaction initiation.

Guanine nucleotide-binding proteins (G-proteins) are typically involved in communicating the consequence of ligand-receptor binding to an effector molecule. The effector molecule then initiates a cascade of molecular events that culminates in a cellular response, e.g., exocytosis.[63,64] Some evidence supports the role of G-proteins in communicating the consequence of zona pellucida ligand(s) to receptor(s) on the sperm plasma membrane and induction of the acrosome reaction.[55,65–67] However, no specific G-protein class (Gs, Gi, Go) or link between G-protein(s) and effector molecule(s) has been demonstrated clearly. In contrast, much work identifies and characterizes downstream molecules, i.e., occurring after effector molecule activation, that might play a role in the acrosome reaction.

Some reason that since calcium plays an important role in somatic cell exocytosis, calcium must play a similar role in spermatozoa exocytosis. In fact, it has long been suggested that an influx of calcium must occur for the acrosome reaction to take place. While a large amount of data support a role for calcium in certain aspects of human sperm function, e.g., capacitation and motility, its absolute requirement for the human sperm acrosome reaction is a matter for debate.

Unlike in some mammalian species, the addition of excess calcium ions to a culture medium containing capacitated human spermatozoa does not induce the acrosome reaction. However, if a calcium mobilizing agent that transports calcium from the extracellular to intracellular space is used, such as calcium ionophore A23187, then a significant stimulation of the reaction is induced.[28,37,38] In contrast, if extracellular calcium is removed, then A23187 fails to induce the reaction.[28] These data, while produced under pharmacological conditions, implicate a role for Ca^{2+} ions in the acrosome reaction process.

Experiments that tested biologically relevant agents provide further support for a role of calcium in the acrosome reaction. The addition of periovulatory follicular fluid or progesterone to capacitated spermatozoa causes an influx of calcium ions that is coincident with the acrosome reaction.[67–71] The mechanism by which progesterone stimulates the acrosome reaction has been investigated intensively and appears to involve a nongenomic steroid receptor/chloride channel in which binding of progesterone to the receptor results in calcium influx and simultaneous chloride efflux.[72] Since periovulatory follicular fluid contains progesterone one may conclude that the mechanism by which follicular fluid stimulates a calcium transient and the acrosome reaction is as a result of the progesterone; however, other acrosome reaction-stimulating factors, e.g., atrial natriuretic peptide (see below), have been detected in this complex fluid, and their role in fertilization cannot be discounted.[73]

Calcium channels represent an additional route for calcium entry. Recent investigations report that, similar to nonhuman mammals, the human sperm plasma membrane appears to contain a voltage-dependent calcium channel that becomes activated as a result of ligand binding.[67] However, specific characterization of the activating ligand(s) and control mechanism(s) for regulating the putative voltage-dependent calcium channel requires additional investigation.

Inhibition or a breakdown in the Ca^{2+}-ATPase may also contribute to the acrosome reaction process. Supportive evidence comes from experiments in which exposure of capacitated spermatozoa to the Ca^{2+}-ATPase inhibitor thapsigargin resulted in acrosome reaction induction.[74] This initial result has since been extended. Experiments revealed that the sperm plasma membrane contains a thapsigargin-insensitive calcium pump, and the acrosomal membrane contains a thapsigargin-sensitive calcium pump.[75] While these data are preliminary, they suggest that the acrosome itself may serve as a storage site for calcium and that concomitant with the acrosome reaction it becomes mobilized.

These combined data support a critical role for calcium in the acrosome reaction. However, other data suggest a less important role for this ion. Recent studies demonstrate that the acrosome reaction can occur in the absence of extracellular calcium using either solubilized human zona pellucida or stimulators of either cAMP-, Ca^{2+}, phospholipid-, or cGMP-dependent kinase pathways.[33,39,40,57] The percentage acrosome reaction induced by kinase stimulators was similar whether spermatozoa were incubated under calcium rich or poor conditions. However, the same was not true when sperm were treated with solubilized zonae. The percentage of sperm stimulated to undergo the acrosome reaction in calcium poor conditions was roughly half that of sperm incubated in a medium containing calcium. Thus, we conclude that while calcium may contribute to the overall acrosome reaction response it may not be required to complete the reaction.

Experiments that tested the influence of biological and chemical stimulators and inhibitors suggest that several protein kinases and the second messengers responsible for their activation are involved in the acrosome reaction.[28,34,37,38] Adenosine 3':5'-cyclic monophosphate (cAMP) is a second messenger that has a number of different functions, e.g., activation of cAMP-dependent kinase and calcium channels.[63] Treatment of somatic cells with analogues of cAMP, e.g., dibutyryl cAMP, results in an artificial increase in intracellular cAMP. When these same compounds are added to capacitated spermatozoa a dose-dependent stimulation of the acrosome reaction occurs.[50,76] If the phosphodiesterase responsible for cAMP breakdown is inhibited then the positive effects of elevated cAMP levels on cell function will persist. Adding phosphodiesterase inhibitors, such as caffeine and pentoxifylline, to capacitated sperm stimulates the acrosome reaction.[50,76] These data show that the intracellular second messenger cAMP plays a positive role in the acrosome reaction.

Adenylate cyclase is a membrane-bound enzyme responsible for hydrolyzing ATP to cAMP. Therefore, activation or inhibition of adenylate cyclase will regulate cAMP production. Forskolin, *coleum forskoli*, has been shown to activate adenylate cyclase in isolated cell membranes and in intact cells from a variety of mammalian tissues.[77] Forskolin stimulates a dose-dependent acrosome reaction in capacitated human spermatozoa. In addition, treatment of capacitated spermatozoa with inhibitors of adenylate cyclase prevents the forskolin-induced reaction, but that inhibition can be bypassed and the acrosome reaction induced with the addition of cAMP analogues. These results along with those previously mentioned confirm the participation of adenylate cyclase and cAMP in the acrosome reaction.[50,76]

The activation of cAMP-dependent protein kinase A (PKA) by cAMP results in protein phosphorylation. Inhibitors with good specificity for PKA have been shown to prevent stimulation of the acrosome reaction by dbcAMP and forskolin and in a dose-response fashion.[50,76] Further, PKA inhibitors prevent the follicular fluid and solubilized zona pellucida-induced acrosome reaction.[76] While the target(s) of cAMP-dependent kinase activity remains elusive, the aforementioned data provide convincing evidence for the role of the cAMP-dependent kinase pathway in the human sperm acrosome reaction.

Phosphatidylinositol 4,5-bisphosphate (PIP$_2$) is hydrolyzed through the activity of the membrane-bound enzyme phospholipase C (PLC). The result is the production of two second messengers, diacylglycerol (DAG) and inositol 1,4,5-trisphosphate (InsP$_3$). DAG, along with the required cofactors of Ca^{2+} (presumably resting intracellular levels are sufficient) and phospholipid, activates Ca^{2+}, phospholipid-dependent protein kinase C (PKC). The other second messenger, InsP$_3$, primarily stimulates the release of intracellular Ca^{2+} stores.

Involvement of the PIP$_2$ pathway in human sperm prefertilization processes was first demonstrated by evidence of PLC activity and the subsequent generation of DAG and inositol phosphates.[78,79] Additional evidence comes from data showing that the treatment of sperm with inhibitors of PLC prevents the acrosome reaction. However, the mechanism by which PLC might become activated is not yet known.[75,80]

Another indication that the PIP$_2$ pathway might have a role in the acrosome reaction comes from data that show the activation of PLC, the subsequent hydrolysis of PIP$_2$, and generation of second messengers, i.e., DAG and InsP$_3$, after sperm were treated with acrosome reaction-inducing agents.[81] In addition, the formation of InsP$_3$ occurs as a consequence of the progesterone-stimulated acrosome reaction and its formation is dependent on an influx of extracellular calcium.[68]

Information concerning a role for the PLC/PIP$_2$/PKC pathway, and specifically Ca^{2+}, phospholipid-dependent kinase, in the acrosome reaction comes from data that show a dose-dependent acrosome reaction in capacitated spermatozoa after treatment with PKC stimulators. Additional support comes from data showing that the reaction can be prevented in a dose-dependent manner by using PKC inhibitors.[33,50,82,83] The aforementioned studies support a significant role for the PLC/PIP$_2$/PKC pathway in the human sperm acrosome reaction. However, no receptor has been clearly identified that would communicate the consequence of ligand binding and initiate the subsequent cascade of events.

Lastly, data implicates an atrial natriuretic peptide receptor-mediated guanylyl cyclase pathway in the occurrence of the human sperm acrosome reaction.[57,73] However, the role of this messenger in the human sperm acrosome reaction remains speculative since no recent data confirms those initial reports.

Solubilized human zonae have been used to understand what signaling pathways might participate in the acrosome reaction. While the reports are few, they suggest that treating capacitated spermatozoa with solubilized zonae results in activation of multiple signal transduction pathways, specifically the cAMP-dependent, cGMP-dependent, and Ca^{2+}, phospholipid-dependent kinase pathways. This activation culminates in the acrosome reaction.[57]

Based on the cited data, the possibility exists that one or more signaling/second messenger pathways might interact or communicate in the sequence of events that terminates in the acrosome reaction. Indeed, this might endow the spermatozoon with sensitive control mechanisms for regulating cellular response(s) as it swims through the varied and changing environment of the female reproductive tract. In fact, this arrangement could enable these cells to sense and respond to molecules/ligands present in the female reproductive tract that have been shown to initiate the acrosome reaction, e.g., follicular and oviductal fluids, and cumulus oophorus.

Based on results indicating that the cAMP-dependent and Ca^{2+}, phospholipid-dependent kinase pathways participate in the acrosome reaction, several studies examined whether these two pathways might interact or communicate to elicit the reaction.[50] The results from one study suggested that a convergent mechanism of crosstalk might occur between the two pathways, with the possibility that each pathway kinase has the same target protein.[50] However, these data are preliminary and the conclusions drawn should be regarded similarly.

V. SPERM-EGG FUSION AND OOCYTE ACTIVATION

After a spermatozoon goes through the acrosome reaction and its zona-penetrating enzymes are activated, it can then pass through the zona. Enzymatic degradation of zona proteins and vigorous flagellar motion facilitate entry and passage through the zonae, leaving in its wake a penetration slit. In order to gain access into the oocyte interior, the spermatozoon must contact, bind to, and fuse with the oocyte plasma membrane. At some point during or after the fusion process the oocyte is activated. Activation involves a calcium-dependent release of cortical granules into the perivitelline space, followed by the resumption of meiosis, as evidenced by the extrusion of the second polar body. The cortical granules modify the zona glycoproteins, specifically ZP2 and ZP3, on the inner aspect of the zona pellucida. This modification inhibits the glycoproteins' ability to stimulate the acrosome reaction and tight binding so as to prevent penetration by other sperm. Failure of the oocyte to synthesize or exocytose the cortical granules, and to do so in a timely fashion, will result in polyspermic fertilization.

Scholars are only beginning to understand the process of sperm-egg fusion. However, they have identified several features of the process. The acrosome reaction not only culminates in the release of enzymes, but also brings about a remodeling of the plasma membrane. As discussed earlier, plasma and outer acrosomal membranes fuse and the acrosomal matrix disappears. In order for the spermatozoon to maintain a patent enveloping membrane, the inner acrosomal and plasma membranes must fuse. As a result, new sperm membrane proteins become exposed—a process integral for sperm-egg fusion success.

Recent data indicate that sperm-egg fusion begins with signal transduction processes that involve adhesion molecules, in the form of ligands and receptors, on both sperm and egg plasma membranes. In fact current research shows that adhesion of human spermatozoa to the oolemma is mediated by integrins.[84–86] Integrins are a class of heterodimeric adhesion receptor molecules that participate in cell-to-cell and cell-to-substratum interactions and are present on essentially all human cells. Further, all mammalian eggs express integrins on their plasma membrane surface.

Integrins that recognize the Arg-Gly-Asp sequence RGD have been detected on the plasma membrane of human oocytes. Fibronectin and vitronectin, glycoproteins that contain functional RGD sequences, are present on human spermatozoa.[84–87] When oligopeptides specifically designed to block fibronectin or vitronectin receptors were tested on human spermatozoa in a zona-free hamster oocyte assay, the peptide for blocking cell attachment to fibronectin exhibited no effect while the other peptide which blocks both fibronectin and vitronectin receptors inhibited sperm-egg binding. These data suggest that a possible mechanism for sperm-egg adhesion and fusion involves an integrin-vitronectin receptor-ligand interaction.[88]

Another potential ligand for oolemmal integrin is human fertilin β.[89] Fertilin, formerly PH30, is a heterodimeric sperm surface protein with binding and fusion domains compatible for interacting with integrin receptors on the oocyte. Because of its domains, human fertilin β can be identified as a member of the ADAM family—membrane-anchored proteins having A Disintegrin And Metalloprotease domain.[89] While fertilin has been relatively well described in nonhuman mammalian systems, its precise role in human sperm-egg adhesion and fusion requires more investigation. The possibility exists that fertilin and vitronectin act in tandem during gamete interaction.

The start of this section explained that at or around the time of sperm-egg fusion the oocyte becomes activated to resume meiosis and extrude cortical granules through a calcium-dependent process. The mechanism(s) by which the spermatozoon activates the oocyte has not been clearly defined. However, two hypotheses emerge: the first involves a ligand-receptor mediated interaction and the second involves a soluble sperm-derived factor that enters the oocyte at the time of fusion.

Evidence for a receptor-mediated mechanism in oocyte activation largely comes from nonhuman mammalian systems and involves G-protein activation of phospholipase C, hydrolysis of PIP_2, and the formation of $InsP_3$ and DAG. A combination of experimental approaches confirms each component's participation of this pathway in the stimulation of Ca^{2+} transients, cortical granule secretion, and zona modifications.[90]

The sperm factor hypothesis hinges on the "latent period," that is the time between sperm and egg plasma membrane's fusion and prior to oocyte activation. It is during this time that a soluble sperm messenger is alleged to diffuse from sperm to egg. Evidence to support this hypothesis largely comes from nonhuman mammal and nonmammalian species experiments.[91] In mammals, this factor tentatively has been identified as a protein (Mr 33,000 to 100,000) that when injected into oocytes stimulates Ca^{2+} transients and oocyte activation. Additionally, sperm factor isolated from one species can activate oocytes from other species and from other phyla. One problem with the plausibility of the sperm factor hypothesis relates to effective concentration. In a majority of the experiments, the concentration is in units of sperm, i.e., number of sperm cell units. No convincing evidence shows that the contents from a single spermatozoon can activate a single oocyte. Thus, this intriguing hypothesis requires further investigation.

Once the spermatozoon has entered and activated the oocyte, a number of additional critical events must occur: sperm nuclear decondensation, microtubule organization by the sperm centrosome, pronuclear migration, and syngamy. These events also may be considered as a part of fertilization, but are beyond the scope of this review.

VI. CONCLUSIONS

Based on information presented, the following conditions must be satisfied in order to optimize the potential for successful fertilization:

1. The seminal fluid should promote sperm viability.
2. Seminal fluid should stabilize the sperm plasma membrane to prevent premature activation.
3. Seminal fluid elements should protect sperm from the hostile environment of the vagina.
4. Binding of seminal coating proteins should be reversible in order for sperm membrane modifications to occur (capacitation) that will allow for expression of integral proteins (receptors) necessary for initiation of events (acrosome reaction) required for fertilization.
5. The ejaculate must contain a sufficient number of mature viable spermatozoa.
6. A good percentage of the mature spermatozoa must be normally-shaped.
7. These sperm must have forwardly progressive motion to propel them from the seminal plasma, through the cervical mucus, into the uterine cavity and the fallopian tube for ultimate encounter with the cumulus-oocyte complex.
8. Sperm motion should change to a hyperactivated state, presumably close to or at the time of acrosome reaction and zona penetration.
9. All components of signaling pathways integral to sperm-zona recognition, binding, and penetration must be appropriately situated, primed, and functional.
10. All components of signaling pathways integral to sperm-egg adhesion and fusion must be appropriately situated, primed, and functional.
11. All post-fusion molecular and genetic events must be coordinated and compatible with producing a viable, metabolically active zygote.

REFERENCES

1. Yanagimachi, R., Mammalian fertilization, in *The Physiology of Reproduction*, Vol. 1, Knobil, E. and Neill, J., Eds., Raven Press, New York, 1994, 189.
2. Aitken, R. J., Molecular mechanisms regulating human sperm function, *Mol. Hum. Reprod.*, 3, 169, 1997.
3. Chang, M. C., Fertilizing capacity of spermatozoa deposited in fallopian tubes, *Nature*, 168, 997, 1951.
4. Austin, C. R., The "capacitation" of the mammalian sperm, *Nature*, 170, 326, 1952.
5. Austin, C. R., Sperm maturation in the male and female genital tracts, in *Biology of Fertilization*, Vol. 2, Metz, C. B. and Monroy, A., Eds., Academic Press, New York, 1985, 121.
6. Bedford, J. M. and Hoskins, D. D., The mammalian spermatozoa. morphology, biochemistry and physiology, in *Physiology of Reproduction*, Vol. 2, Lamming, G. E., Ed., Churchill Livingston, Edinburgh, 1990, 379.
7. Chang, M. C., Meaning of sperm capacitation, *J. Androl.*, 5, 45, 1984.
8. Clegg, E. D., Mechanisms of mammalian sperm capacitation, in *Mechanism and Control of Animal Fertilization*, Hartman, J. F., Ed., Academic Press, New York, 1983, 177.
9. de Lamirande, E., Leclerc, P., and Gagnon, C., Capacitation as a regulatory event that primes spermatozoa for the acrosome reaction and fertilization, *Mol. Hum. Reprod.*, 3, 175, 1997.
10. Drobnis, E., Capacitation and acrosome reaction, in *Reproductive Toxicology and Infertility*, Scialli, A. R. and Zinaman, M. J., Eds., McGraw-Hill, New York, 1993, 77.
11. Florman, H. M. and Babcock, D. F., Progress toward understanding the molecular basis of capacitation, in *Elements of Mammalian Fertilization*, Vol. 1, Wassarman, P. M., Ed., CRC Press, Boca Raton, FL, 1991, 105.
12. Fraser, L. R., Requirements for successful mammalian sperm capacitation and fertilization, *Arch. Path. Lab. Med.*, 116, 345, 1992.
13. Hinrichsen-Kohane, A. C., Hinrichsen, M. J., and Schill, W. B., Molecular events leading to fertilization, *Andrologia*, 16, 321, 1984.
14. Langlais, J. and Roberts, K. D., A molecular membrane model of sperm capacitation and the acrosome reaction of mammalian spermatozoa. *Gamete Res.*, 12, 183, 1985.
15. O'Rand, M. G., Changes in sperm surface properties correlated with capacitation, in *The Spermatozoa*, Fawcett, D. W. and Bedford, J. M., Eds., Urban and Schwarzenberg, Baltimore, MD, 1979, 195.
16. O'Rand, M. G., Modification of the sperm membrane during capacitation, *Ann. NY Acad. Sci.*, 383, 392, 1982.
17. Rogers, B. J. and Bentwood, B. J., Capacitation, acrosome reaction and fertilization, in *Biochemistry of Mammalian Fertilization*, Zaneveld, L. J. D. and Chatterton, R. T., John Wiley & Sons, New York, 1982, 203.
18. Bedford, J. M., Sperm capacitation and fertilization in mammals, *Biol. Reprod.*, 2 (Suppl.), 128, 1970.
19. Rogers, B. J., Mammalian sperm capacitation and fertilization *in vitro*: a critique of methodology, *Gamete Res.*, 1, 165, 1978.
20. Sidhu K. S. and Guraya, S. S., Cellular and molecular biology of capacitation and acrosome reaction in mammalian spermatozoa, *Int. Rev. Cytol.*, 118, 231, 1989.
21. Storey, B. T., Sperm capacitation and the acrosome reaction, *Ann. NY Acad. Sci.*, 637, 457, 1991.

22. Zaneveld, L. J. D., De Jonge, C. J., Anderson, R. A., and Mack, S. R., Human sperm capacitation and the acrosome reaction, *Hum. Reprod.*, 6, 1265, 1991.
23. Carrera, A., Moos, J., Gerton, G. L., Tesarik, J., Kopf, G. S., and Moss, S. B., Regulation of protein tyrosin phosphorylation in human sperm by a calcium/calmodulin dependent mechanism: Identification of A Kinase Anchor Proteins as major substrates for tyrosine phosphorylation, *Dev. Biol.*, 180, 284, 1996.
24. Hamamah, S., Grizard, G., Gadella, B. M., Barthelemy, C., and Royere, D., Lipid composition of sperm plasma membrane: alteration during the fertilization process, in *Male Gametes, Production and Quality*, Hamamah, S. and Mieusset, R., Eds., INSERM, Paris, 1996, 187.
25. Benoff, S., Carbohydrates and fertilization: an overview, *Mol. Hum. Reprod.*, 3, 599, 1997.
26. Kopf, G. S., Visconti, P. E., Moos, J., Galantino-Homer, H., and Ning, X. P., Integration of tyrosine kinase- and G-protein-mediated signal transduction pathways in the regulation of mammalian sperm function, in *Human Sperm Acrosome Reaction*, Fenichel, P. and Parinaud, J., Eds., John Libbey Eurotext, Ltd., Colloque INSERM, 1995, 236, 191.
27. Mortimer, D., *Practical Laboratory Andrology*. Oxford University Press, Oxford, 1994, 267.
28. De Jonge, C. J., Diagnostic significance of the induced acrosome reaction, *Reprod. Med. Rev.*, 3, 159, 1994.
29. Stock, C. E. and Fraser, L. R., Divalent cations, capacitation, and the acrosome reaction in human spermatozoa, *J. Reprod. Fertil.*, 87, 463, 1992.
30. Fraser, L. R., Mechanisms regulating capacitation and the acrosome reaction, in *Human Sperm Acrosome Reaction*, Fenichel, P. and Parinaud, J., Eds., John Libbey Eurotext, Ltd., Colloque INSERM, 1995, 236, 17.
31. Aitken, R. J., Wang, Y-F., Liu, J., Best, F., and Richardson, D. W., The influence of medium composition, osmolarity and albumin content on the acrosome reaction and fertilizing capacity of human spermatozoa: development of an improved zona-free hamster egg penetration test, *Int. J. Androl.*, 6, 180, 1983.
32. Baldi, E., Casano, R., Flasetti, C., Krausz, C., Maggi, M., and Forti, G., Intracellular calcium accumulation and responsiveness to progesterone in capacitating human spermatozoa, *J. Androl.*, 12, 323, 1991.
33. De Jonge, C. J., Han, H-L., Mack, S. R., and Zaneveld, L. J. D., Effect of phorbol diesters, synthetic diacylglycerols, and a protein kinase inhibitor on the human sperm acrosome reaction, *J. Androl.*, 12, 62, 1991.
34. Zaneveld, L. J. D., Anderson, R. A., Mack, S. R., and De Jonge, C. J., Mechanism and control of the human sperm acrosome reaction, *Hum. Reprod.*, 8, 2006, 1994.
35. Kopf, G. S. and Gerton, G. L., The mammalian sperm acrosome and the acrosome reaction, in *Elements of Mammalian Fertilization*, Vol. 1, Wassarman, P. M., Ed., CRC Press, Boca Raton, FL, 1991, 153.
36. Meizel, S., Molecules that initiate or help stimulate the acrosome reaction by their interaction with the mammalian sperm surface, *Am. J. Anat.*, 174, 285, 1985.
37. Brucker, C. and Lipford, G. B., The human sperm acrosome reaction: physiology and regulatory mechanisms: an update, *Hum. Reprod. Update*, 1, 51, 1995.
38. Breitbart, H. and Spungin, B., The biochemistry of the acrosome reaction, *Mol. Hum. Reprod.*, 3, 195, 1997.
39. Anderson, R. A., Feathergill, K. A., De Jonge, C. J., Mack, S. R., and Zaneveld, L. J. D., Facilitative effect of pulsed addition of dibutyryl cAMP on the acrosome reaction of uncapacitated human spermatozoa, *J. Androl.*, 13, 398, 1992.

40. Bielfeld, P., Anderson, R. A., Mack, S. R., De Jonge, C. J., and Zaneveld, L. J. D., Are capacitation or calcium ion influx required for the human sperm acrosome reaction?, *Fertil. Steril.*, 62, 1255, 1994.
41. Zaneveld, L. J. D. and De Jonge, C. J., Mammalian sperm acrosomal enzymes and the acrosome reaction, in *A Comparative Overview of Mammalian Fertilization*, Dunbar, B. S. and O'Rand, M. G., Eds., Plenum Press, New York, 1991, 63.
42. Eddy, E. M. and O'Brien, D. A., The spermatozoon, in *The Physiology of Reproduction*, Vol. 1, Knobil, E. and Neill, J., Eds., Raven Press, New York, 1994, 29.
43. Tesarik, J., Drahorad, J., Testart, J., and Mendoza, C., Acrosin activation follows its surface exposure and precedes membrane fusion in human sperm acrosome reaction, *Development*, 110, 391, 1990.
44. Tesarik, J., Drahorad, J., and Peknicova, J., Subcellular immunochemical localization of acrosin in human spermatozoa during the acrosome reaction and the zona pellucida penetration, *Fertil. Steril.*, 50, 133, 1988.
45. De Jonge, C. J., Mack, S. R., and Zaneveld, L. J. D., Inhibition of the human sperm acrosome reaction by proteinase inhibitors, *Gamete Res.*, 23, 387, 1989.
46. Tesarik, J., Appropriate timing of the acrosome reaction is a major requirement for the fertilizing spermatozoon, *Hum. Reprod.*, 4, 957, 1989.
47. Oehninger, S., Coddington, C. C., Scott, R., Franken, D. A., Burkman, L. J., Acosta, A. A., and Hodgen, G. D., Hemizona assay: assessment of sperm dysfunction and prediction of *in vitro* fertilization outcome, *Fertil. Steril.*, 51, 665, 1989.
48. Liu, D. Y. and Baker, H. W. G., Inducing the human acrosome reaction with a calcium ionophore A23187 decreases sperm-ZP binding with oocytes that failed to fertilize *in vitro*, *J. Reprod. Fertil.*, 89, 127, 1990.
49. Liu, D. Y. and Baker, H. W. G., Acrosome status and morphology of human sperm bound to the zona pellucida and oolemma determined using oocytes that failed to fertilize *in vitro*, *Hum. Reprod.*, 9, 673, 1994.
50. Doherty, C. M., Tarchala, S. M., Radwanska, E., and De Jonge, C. J., Characterization of two second messenger pathways and their interactions in eliciting the human sperm acrosome reaction, *J. Androl.*, 16, 36, 1995.
51. Bleil, J. D., Sperm receptors of mammalian eggs, in *Elements of Mammalian Fertilization*, Vol. 1, Wassarman, P. M., Ed., CRC Press, Boca Raton, FL, 1991, 133.
52. Coddington, C., Fulgham, D. L., Alexander, N. J., Johnson, D. J., Herr, J. C., and Hodgen, G. D., Sperm bound to zona pellucida in hemizona assay demonstrate acrosome reaction when stained with T-6 antibody, *Fertil. Steril.*, 54, 504, 1990.
53. Hoshi, K., Sugano, T., Endo, C., Yoshimatsu, N., Yanagida, K., and Sato, A., Induction of the acrosome reaction in human spermatozoa by human zona pellucida and effect of cervical mucus on zona-induced acrosome reaction, *Fertil. Steril.*, 60, 149, 1993.
54. Burkman, L. J., Coddington, C. C., Franken, D. R., Kruger, T. F., Rosenwaks, Z., and Hodgen, G. D., The hemizona assay (HZA): development of a diagnostic test for the binding of human spermatozoa to the human hemizona pellucida to predict fertilization potential, *Fertil. Steril.*, 49, 688, 1988.
55. Franken, D. R., Morales, P. J., and Habenicht, U. F., Inhibition of G protein in human sperm and its influence on acrosome reaction and zona pellucida binding, *Fertil. Steril.*, 66, 1009, 1996.
56. Cross, N. L., Morales, P., Overstreet, J. W., and Hanson, F. W., Induction of acrosome reactions by the human zona pellucida, *Biol. Reprod.*, 38, 235, 1988.
57. Bielfeld, P., Zaneveld, L. J. D., and De Jonge, C. J., The zona pellucida-induced acrosome reaction of human spermatozoa is mediated by protein kinases, *Fertil. Steril.*, 61, 536, 1994.

58. Van Duin, M., Ploman, J. E. M., De Breet, I. T. M., Van Ginneken, K., Bunschoten, H., Grootenhuis, A., Brindle, J., and Aitken, R. J., Recombinent human zona pellucida protein ZP3 produced by Chinese hamster ovary cells induces the human sperm acrosome reaction and promotes sperm-egg fusion, *Biol. Reprod.*, 51, 607, 1994.

59. Barratt, C. L. R. and Hornby, D. P., Induction of the human acrosome reaction by rhuZP3, in *Human Sperm Acrosome Reaction*, Fenichel, P. and Parinaud, J., Eds., John Libbey Eurotext, Ltd., Colloque INSERM, 1995, 236, 105.

60. Moos, J., Faundes, D., Kopf, G. S., and Schultz, R. M., Composition of the human zona pellucida and modifications following fertilization, *Hum. Reprod.*, 10, 2467, 1995.

61. Burks, D. J., Carballada, R., Moore, H. D. M., and Saling, P. M., Interaction of a tyrosine kinase from human sperm with the zona pellucida at fertilization, *Science*, 269, 83, 1995.

62. Tesarik, J., Moos, J., and Mendoza, C., Stimulation of protein tyrosine phosphorylation by a progesterone receptor on the cell surface of human sperm, *Endocrinology*, 133, 328, 1993.

63. Berridge, M. J., The molecular basis of communication in the cell, *Sci. Am.*, 253, 142, 1985.

64. Birnbaumer, L., Abramowitz, J., and Brown, A. M., Signal trasnduction by G proteins, *Biochim. Biophys. Acta*, 919, 255, 1990.

65. Lee, M. A., Check, L. H., and Kopf, G. S., Guanine nucleotide-binding regulatory protein in human sperm mediates acrosomal exocytosis induced by the human zona pellucida, *Mol. Reprod. Dev.*, 31, 78, 1992.

66. Tesarik, J., Carreras, A., and Mendoza, C., Differential sensitivity of progesterone- and zona pellucida-induced acrosome reactions to pertussis toxin, *Mol. Reprod. Dev.*, 34, 183, 1993.

67. Brandelli, A., Miranda, P. V., and Tezon, J. G., Voltage-dependent calcium channels and Gi regulatory protein mediate the human sperm acrosomal exocytosis induced by N-acetylglucosaminyl/mannosyl neoglycoproteins, *J. Androl.*, 17, 522, 1996.

68. Thomas, P. and Meizel, S., Phosphatidylinositol 4,5-bisphosphate hydrolysis in human sperm stimulated with follicular fluid or progesterone is dependent upon Ca^{2+} influx, *Biochem. J.*, 264, 539, 1989.

69. Blackmore, P. F., Beebe, S. J., Danforth, D. R., and Alexander, N., Progesterone and 17a-hydroxyprogesterone novel stimulators of calcium influx in human sperm, *J. Biol. Chem.*, 265, 1376, 1990.

70. Baldi, E., Casano, R., Flasetti, C., Krausz, C., Maggi, M., and Forti, G., Intracellular calcium accumulation and responsiveness to progesterone in capacitating human spermatozoa, *J. Androl.*, 12, 323, 1991.

71. Tesarik, J., Carreras, A., and Mendoza, C., Single cell analysis of tyrosine kinase dependent and independent Ca^{2+} fluxes in progesterone induced acrosome reaction, *Mol. Hum. Reprod.*, 2, 225, 1996.

72. Meizel, S., Amino acid neurotransmitter receptor/chloride channels of mammalian sperm and the acrosome reaction, *Biol. Reprod.*, 56, 571, 1997.

73. Anderson, R. A., Feathergill, K. A., Drisdel, R. C., Rawlins, R. G., Mack, S. R., and Zaneveld, L. J. D., Atrial natriuretic peptide (ANP) as a stimulus of the human acrosome reaction and a component of ovarian follicular fluid: correlation of follicular ANP content with *in vitro* fertilization outcome, *J. Androl.*, 15, 61, 1994.

74. Meizel, S. and Turner, K. O., Initiation of the human sperm acrosome reaction by thapsigargin, *J. Exp. Zool.*, 267, 350, 1993.

75. Spungin, B. and Breitbart, H., Calcium mobilization and influx during sperm exocytosis, *J. Cell Sci.*, 109, 1947, 1996.

76. De Jonge, C. J., Role of cAMP pathways: cross-talk mechanisms for the acrosome reaction, in *Human Sperm Acrosome Reaction*, Fenichel, P. and Parinaud, J., Eds., John Libbey Eurotext, Ltd., Colloque INSERM, 1995, 236, 257.

77. Seamon, K. B. and Daly, J. W., Forskolin: its biological and chemical properties, in *Advances in Cyclic Nucleotide and Protein Phosphorylation Research*, Greengard, P. and Robison, G. A., Eds., Raven Press, New York, 1986, 1.

78. Ribbes, H., Plantavid, M., Bennet, P. J., Chap, H., and Douste-Blazy, L., Phospholipase C from human sperm specific for phosphoinositides, *Biochim. Biophys. Acta*, 919, 245, 1987.

79. Bennet, P. J., Moatti, J.-P., Mansat, A., Ribbes, H., Cayrac, J.-C., Pontonnier, F., Chap, H., and Douste-Blazy, L., Evidence for the activation of phospholipases during acrosome reaction of human sperm elicited by calcium ionophore A23187, *Biochim. Biophys. Acta*, 919, 255, 1987.

80. Spungin, B., Margalit, I., and Breitbart, H., Sperm exocytosis reconstructed in a cell-free system. Evidence for the involvement of phospholipase C and actin filaments in membrane fusion, *J. Cell Sci.*, 108, 2525, 1995.

81. Thomas, P. and Meizel, S., An influx of extracellular calcium is required for initiation of the human sperm acrosome reaction induced by human follicular fluid, *Gamete Res.*, 20, 397, 1988.

82. Breitbart, H., Lax, Y., Rotem, R., and Naor, Z., Role of protein kinase C in the acrosome reaction of mammalian spermatozoa, *Biochem. J.*, 281, 473, 1992.

83. Rotem, R., Paz, G. F., Homonnai, Z. T. et al., Calcium-independent induction of acrosome reaction by protein kinase C in human sperm, *Endocrinology*, 131, 2235, 1992.

84. Bronson, R. A. and Fusi, F. M., Integrins and human reproduction, *Mol. Hum. Reprod.*, 2, 153, 1996.

85. Allen, C. A. and Green, D. P., The mammalian acrosome reaction: gateway to sperm fusion with the oocyte?, *Bioessays*, 19, 241, 1997.

86. Snell, W. J. and White, J. M., The molecules of mammalian fertilization, *Cell*, 85, 629, 1996.

87. Fusi, F. M., Vignali, M., Gailit, J., and Bronson, R. A., Mammalian oocytes exhibit specific recognition of the RGD (Arg-Gly-Asp) tripeptide and express oolemmal integrins, *Mol. Reprod. Dev.*, 36, 212, 1993.

88. Fusi, F. M., Bernocchi, N., Ferrari, A., and Bronson, R. A., Is vitronectin the velcro that binds the gametes together?, *Mol. Hum. Reprod.*, 2, 859, 1996.

89. Vidaeus, C. M., von Kapp, Herr-C., Golden, W. L., Eddy, R. L., Shows, T. B., and Herr, J. C., Human fertilin beta: identification, characterization, and chromosomal mapping of an ADAM gene family member, *Mol. Reprod. Dev.*, 46, 363, 1997.

90. Schultz, R. M. and Kopf, G. S., Molecular basis of mammalian egg activation, *Curr. Top. Dev. Biol.*, 30, 21, 1995.

91. Wilding, M. and Dale, B., Sperm factor: what is it and what does it do?, *Mol. Hum. Reprod.*, 3, 269, 1997.

2 Overview of Spermatogenesis and Ejaculation

D. M. de Kretser

CONTENTS

I. INTRODUCTION

The production of sperm in the ejaculate of the human male involves a complex process called spermatogenesis, the transport and storage of sperm in the epididymis, and the movement of the mature sperm to mix with the secretions of the prostate and seminal vesicles in the process of ejaculation.

The cytological events that constitute spermatogenesis can be divided into several phases: (1) replication of the stem cells called spermatogonia, (2) the progression through meiosis in which the chromosomal complement is reduced from the diploid to the haploid number, and (3) a complex series of cytological changes, known as spermiogenesis, resulting in the transformation of a round cell into a spermatozoon.[1]

In the human, this entire process of spermatogenesis takes a period of about 70 days, and available data indicate that this duration cannot be altered by such agents as hormones.[2]

17

A. SPERMATOGONIAL REPLICATION

In the human testis three types of spermatogonia can be identified and are called type A pale, type A dark, and type B. The A pale have a round nucleus, a peripherally placed nucleolus, and mitochondria that are clumped in a perinuclear aggregation. The principal feature distinguishing the A dark spermatogonia is the presence of a pale area within the nucleus, sometimes called a nuclear vacuole, in which there is a lack of chromatin granulation. In contrast, the type B have a variable contact with the basement membrane, show peripheral clumping of chromatin, contain several noncompact nucleoli, and have dispersed mitochondria. The type B spermatogonia begin meiosis without further cell division and remain joined, like other germ cells, by cytoplasmic bridges, which represent incomplete cytokinesis.

B. MEIOSIS

The entry of type B spermatogonia into meiosis is marked by the loss of contact with the basement membrane and the appearance of chromosomal threads. During the first meiotic division these cells are called primary spermatocytes and can be divided into several subclasses representing defined stages of the long prophase. These stages represent the leptotene, zygotene, pachytene, and diplotene primary spermatocytes and are best characterized by the features of the chromosomes, initially appearing as unpaired structures in the leptotene stage. Pairing, thickening, and shortening of homologous chromosomes denotes the pachytene stage. At an electron microscopic level, structures termed synaptinemal complexes can be seen in the nucleus and represent the pairing mechanism. In the diplotene stage, the paired homologous chromosomes begin to separate as a prelude to the initiation of metaphase. The completion of the first meiotic division results in the formation of two secondary spermatocytes that have the haploid number of chromosomes, each of which is comprised of two chromatids. The secondary spermatocytes enter the second meiotic division within 6 hours of their formation. As a consequence, they are sparsely represented in the seminiferous epithelium in terms of numbers.

C. SPERMIOGENESIS

The conversion of the round spermatid, formed by the division of the secondary spermatocyte, into the mature spermatozoon involves a complex series of changes termed spermiogenesis[3,4] (Figure 2.1). These changes can be subdivided into the following processes:

1. Changes in the nucleus: As spermiogenesis progresses, the nucleus of the spermatid becomes eccentrically placed and comes to lie adjacent to the cell membrane at one pole. A progressive condensation in the size of the nucleus alters its shape during this phase. These changes are associated with the compaction and cross-linking of the DNA in the nucleus and are linked to the removal of histones and their replacement with protamines. In the human spermatid, this process results in a marked increase in the

electron density of the nucleus, more commonly known as the head of the spermatid at this stage.

2. Formation of the acrosome: In the round spermatid, the Golgi complex gives rise to a large secretory vesicle that migrates to one pole of the nucleus and is applied as a cap-like structure termed the acrosome. In essence, the acrosome is a modified lysosome that contains enzymes essential to enable the sperm to penetrate the zona pellucida of the oocyte during fertilization. The acrosomal pole of the nucleus is the region that becomes applied to the spermatid cell membrane during the nuclear-cytoplasmic reorganization, which results in eccentric placement of the nucleus.

3. Development of the sperm tail: The tail develops from one of the pair of centrioles in the round spermatid as these structures lie adjacent to the Golgi region. The core of the sperm tail is a structure termed the axial filament, which comprises nine doublet microtubules arranged equally spaced around the periphery of a circle at the center of which are two single microtubules. When it initially appears from the centriole, the axial filament lies free in the cytoplasm but then migrates to lodge in a slight depression in the nucleus at the opposite pole to the acrosome. As it lengthens, the axial filament protrudes from the developing spermatid, but it is surrounded by a sleeve of cytoplasm enclosed by the spermatid cell membrane. At the point where the tail protrudes from the spermatid, a ring-like structure called the annulus appears and marks the terminal end of the future mid-piece of the sperm.

A series of accessory structures surrounds the axial filament. One represents the outer dense fibers of which there are nine, each closely applied to each of the nine doublet microtubules of the axial filament. The outer dense fibers extend from the neck of the sperm throughout the mid-piece, terminating at varying points along the region of the sperm tail known as the principal piece. The second accessory structure is the fibrous sheath, which surrounds the axial filament from the annulus throughout the length of the principal piece. The precise function of this structure and the outer dense fibers is still unknown, but they are thought to modify the motility generated by the axial filament into the wave form observed during the movements of the sperm tail.

4. Reorganization of the cytoplasm and cell organelles: Significant changes in the arrangement of the cytoplasm, nucleus, and other organelles occur during spermiogenesis. As discussed above the nucleus takes up an eccentric position in the spermatid. This most likely is achieved by a redistribution of the cytoplasm relative to the nucleus, probably resulting from microtubular and microfilamentous mechanisms. The mitochondria of the spermatid initially are distributed around the periphery of the cell, but in the terminal stages of spermiogenesis, these mitochondria coalesce and form a helix surrounding the region of the sperm tail known as the mid-piece and defined above by the neck and distally by the annulus. Toward the final stages of spermiogenesis, the cytoplasm, which surrounds

the tail, develops vacuoles that appear to be invaginated by fine processes of Sertoli cell cytoplasm. The latter, in effect, enable the Sertoli cell to "pull" the remaining cytoplasm from the spermatid as it is released from the epithelium during spermiation. This cytoplasm is engulfed by the Sertoli cell and the structure is known as the residual body, which migrates towards the base of the Sertoli cell and is destroyed by lysosomal activity.

5. Terminology: Because this text is a handbook for the assisted reproduction laboratory, it must convey the importance of using appropriate terminology. This usage is particularly crucial with spermatids as many laboratories strive to achieve fertilization using immature spermatids. No accepted terminology for the stages of spermiogenesis exists. However, the classification of the spermatid stages proposed by Clermont[5] and illustrated in Figure 2.1 represents a very useful nomenclature which, if used widely, would assist greatly in comparing the outcome of studies using spermatids obtained by testicular sperm retrieval.

D. SERTOLI CELLS

Consideration of spermatogenesis is not possible without an understanding of the Sertoli cells. These cells represent the supporting cells within the seminiferous epithelium and extend from the basement membrane of the tubule to the lumen along the radial axis. The base of the Sertoli cell could represent a cylinder abutting the basement membrane with prolongations extending between the surrounding germ cells. These prolongations are not visible by light microscopy and are best appreciated by electron microscopy. Further, as these projections extend in many directions, the luminal regions of the Sertoli cell take on the appearance of the branches of a tree (Figure 2.2). Because these processes surround all germ cells other than spermatogonia, one can see that the Sertoli cell is placed strategically to influence the function and viability of all the centrally placed germ cells. This concept achieves further importance in view of the involvement of the Sertoli cells in the formation of the blood-testis barrier. This functional barrier has a morphological counterpart in the tight inter-Sertoli cell junctions formed where two adjacent Sertoli cells abut.[6,7] These occur central to the position of the spermatogonia in the epithelium and effectively divide it into a basal and adluminal compartment; the former contains the spermatogonia and the bases of the Sertoli cells and the latter all other germ cells. Because the barrier prevents intercellular transport, all the cells in the adluminal compartment are dependent on the Sertoli cells for transport of their metabolic requirements.[8] Data demonstrating that the sperm output of the testis in a mammal is governed by the number of Sertoli cells in the testis illustrates the dependence of the germ cells on the Sertoli cells.[9] The Sertoli cell complement in adults is fixed since these cells do not divide after the completion of puberty. Therefore, factors affecting Sertoli cell development may modify adult sperm output. This concept emerges from a number of studies of the rat testis, but some data also comes from the induction of spermatogenesis in hypogonadotrophic men by the use of gonadotropins or gonadotropin releasing hormone. Research indicates that in such men sperm output rarely reaches the levels found in normal men, and pregnancies are

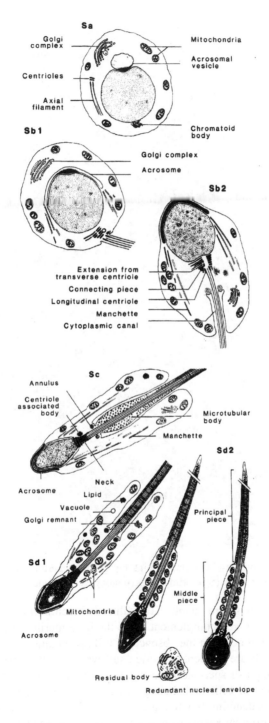

FIGURE 2.1 The structural changes that occur during spermiogenesis as seen at the electron microscopic level. The stages of spermiogenesis as classified by Clermont[5] are identified.

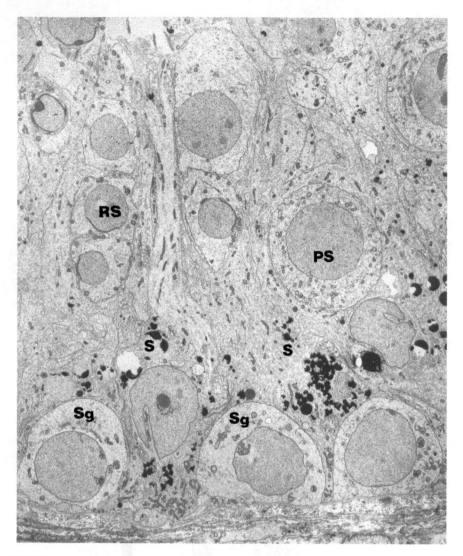

FIGURE 2.2 The complex interrelationships between the Sertoli cell (S) and germ cells consisting of spermatogonia (Sg), primary spermatocytes (PS), and round spermatids (RS).

often achieved at low sperm counts. The failure to reach normal sperm output may reflect a lower Sertoli cell complement since the intra-uterine period of Sertoli cell multiplication would occur in the absence of FSH stimulation.[10]

The Sertoli cells are resilient and often survive a variety of pathological insults that cause disruption of spermatogenesis and destruction of germ cells. Often the survival of the Sertoli cells and their persistence in the seminiferous tubules has been interpreted as denoting functional normality of these cells. However, in experiments in which different agents were used to induce spermatogenic damage, lower testicular inhibin and fluid production indicated functional disruption.[11,12] The recent demonstration that inhibin B represents the principal circulating form of inhibin in men[13] and the availability of specific assays for this hormone open the prospect that measurement of this protein in the blood will provide a functional assessment of the Sertoli cell complement of the testis.

E. TRANSPORT OF SPERM FROM THE TUBULE

Following spermiation, the testicular sperm are transported toward the rete testis by the Sertoli cells' production of fluid and the irregular contractile movements of the seminiferous tubules. The latter result from the contractions of the peritubular cells that surround the seminiferous tubules. These cells are flattened plate-like cells that are apposed to the outside of the tubules being separated from the basement membrane of the tubule by a narrow gap. In man, two or three layers of these cells, when cut in cross-section, appear as spindle-shaped elongated structures. Electron microscopic studies indicate that these cells are modified smooth muscle cells sometimes known as myoid cells.

II. THE INTER-TUBULAR TISSUE OF THE TESTIS

One cannot consider the control of the testis without knowledge of the structural features of the inter-tubular tissue. The seminiferous tubules are avascular structures and receive their blood supply from vessels that branch in the inter-tubular tissue forming capillary networks that surround the tubules but do not enter them. Consequently, diffusion from these capillaries through the basement membrane of the tubule supports the metabolic requirements of the seminiferous epithelium. Thereafter, facilitated transport mechanisms operative within the Sertoli cells handle the metabolic requirements. Increased peritubular fibrosis, which sometimes occurs in various types of damage to the seminiferous epithelium, clearly would increase the distance across which the tubules' metabolic requirements must pass. In the human testis, a network of lymphatic vessels accompanies the blood vessels, whereas in some species such as rodents, a large lymphatic sinusoidal network occupies a large part of the inter-tubular tissue.[14]

Within the inter-tubular tissue lie the testosterone producing cells known as Leydig cells. Human Leydig cells exhibit a marked variability, but in general they are large irregularly shaped cells with a nucleus containing a prominent nucleolus. The cytoplasm of many Leydig cells appears to be vacuolated, and these cells sometimes contain crystalloid bodies called the crystals of Reinke. The Leydig cells collect in small clumps surrounding the capillary network, and in a damaged testis sometimes they collect into larger groups. The secreted testosterone diffuses through the inter-tubular tissue bathing the seminiferous tubules in a higher concentration of testosterone. The capillaries and lymphatics carry androgens from the testis.

The testes of mammalian species, including man, contain many macrophages that appear to reside within the testis.[15] These macrophages can be augmented by monocytic infiltration from the bloodstream during periods of inflammation. Increasing data support the view that the response of the testicular macrophages to inflammatory stimuli is dampened, and this process may have a role in modulating the immune response thereby protecting sperm from the production of anti-sperm antibodies.[15]

III. THE CONTROL OF SPERMATOGENESIS

A. HORMONAL CONTROL

Scholars generally agree that spermatogenesis depends on the production of FSH and LH by the pituitary gland under the control of the hypothalamic peptide gonadotropin releasing hormone. In response to the pulsatile secretion of GnRH, LH and FSH exude from the pituitary in an episodic pattern and act through specific receptors found on the Leydig cells and Sertoli cells respectively.[16,17] To date, no receptors for gonadotropins have been found on germ cells.

LH acts through the presence of receptors on Leydig cells to stimulate testosterone production. Testosterone is a specific requirement for spermatogenesis to proceed normally. This view is supported by the failure of spermatogenesis in men with major mutations in the androgen receptor and the demonstration in rodents that high doses of testosterone can support spermatogenesis in hypophysectomised animals wherein FSH levels are low or absent.[18,19] However, it is important to note that in intact rats or in rats following GnRH immunization, high doses of testosterone can stimulate FSH levels, an action yet to be demonstrated in men. Furthermore, the demonstration that complete spermatogenesis could be achieved in the gonadotropin-deficient hpg mice by high doses of testosterone adds further support to the essential requirement of this hormone and questions the need for FSH[20] and following targeted disruption of the FSH β subunit gene.[21]

Although no one would question that testosterone is essential for spermatogenesis, some data suggests that supra-physiological concentrations of testosterone may limit spermatogonial number in rodent models of spermatogenic disruption[22,23] and in man.[24] Like gonadotropin receptors, germ cells do not contain receptors for testosterone, and the androgenic signal must be transduced through androgen receptors present on peritubular cells and Sertoli cells. The nature of the molecules that are involved in transmitting the androgenic signal from the Sertoli cells to the germ cells remains unknown. Increasing data indicates that while the extremely high levels of testosterone found within the testis are not absolutely required for full spermatogenesis, levels at least 5- to 10-fold above those in the circulation are required for normal spermatogenesis.[18,19] Given that to date, only one androgen receptor has been identified, it is difficult to understand why the testis requires high testosterone levels to facilitate spermatogenesis when the function of other androgenic tissues is well maintained by the normal circulating levels of testosterone.

The debate concerning the requirement of FSH for spermatogenesis has been further augmented by the demonstration that in mice, in which the gene encoding the β subunit of FSH has been "knocked out," spermatogenesis proceeds to completion, albeit in smaller testes, and the mice are fertile.[21] The observation that the spermatogenic process is complete but occurs in smaller testes suggests that the number of Sertoli cells in these testes are smaller because of the absence of FSH, a known stimulus to cell multiplication during fetal and pubertal development.

Whether spermatogenesis in primates and in man can proceed to completion and be quantitatively normal in the absence of FSH remains undetermined.

B. OTHER REGULATORY PROCESSES

In a complex process such as spermatogenesis, many regulatory events must occur in sequence to enable a normal sperm output. While some of these events are hormonally regulated, others involve growth factors, cytokines, and other regulatory molecules. Increasing numbers of gene knock outs are being published that identify the genes, and the molecules they encode, crucial to spermatogenesis. These include chaperones such as heat shock protein 70-2,[25] which prevents the completion of meiosis and cell survival molecules such as *bcl w*.[26] Progressively, the molecular mechanisms regulating the proliferation of spermatogonia, the entry and completion of meiosis, and the successful completion of spermiogenesis will be elucidated. This understanding of the regulatory processes is required before appropriate diagnostic and therapeutic modalities can be developed to improve the management of the infertile man.

IV. DISORDERS OF SPERMATOGENESIS

This discussion is included in this chapter to help the reader understand the types of pathology found in the testis in infertile men. Increasingly, physicians use assisted reproductive technology, and in particular intracytoplasmic sperm injection, to achieve pregnancies in the partners of men with low or zero sperm counts in their ejaculates.[27] Further, the approach of using testicular sperm retrieval in men with both obstructive and nonobstructive azoospermia has expanded the horizons for the assisted reproductive technology laboratory.[28] Further attempts are in progress to use immature spermatids from the testis to achieve fertilization in men in whom the testis contains no mature spermatids.

For proper examination, testicular tissue must be fixated using Bouins or Cleland's fixatives rather than the routinely used formalin fixation. This is particularly important since formalin causes gross distortion and shrinkage of the seminiferous epithelium and loss of the chromatin patterns so crucial in identifying differing germ cells. Scientists and clinicians also must be able to identify each of the germ cell types described earlier in this chapter. By careful analysis of the size of the seminiferous tubules, the presence or absence of each germ cell type in the seminiferous epithelium, and a crude assessment of their numbers, physicians can reasonably assess this process.

Classification of the disorders of spermatogenesis (Figures 2.3 and 2.4) are usually made into the following categories:[29]

1. **Normal**.
2. **Hypospermatogenesis**. In this category all stages of the spermatogenic process are present, but the numbers of germ cells occupying the epithelium are reduced to varying degrees. This may be mild, moderate, or severe. In the latter condition, spermatogenesis ceases at different stages

as evidenced in tubules, e.g., spermatogonia, primary spermatocyte, or where spermatids are found in lesser numbers than normal. Should any tubule in the biopsy show the presence of elongating spermatids of the Sd stage of the Clermont classification, then the diagnosis should be hypospermatogenesis.

3. **Germ cell arrest**. This category is reserved for biopsy appearances wherein spermatogenesis ceases completely at a specific stage of spermatogenesis. Most commonly this is at the primary spermatocyte stage, but may occur at the spermatogonial level or, rarely, at the round spermatid stage. Again this diagnosis is made if all of the tubules show the cessation of spermatogenesis at the specific stage identified.

4. **Sertoli cell only syndrome**. This diagnosis is used when all of the tubules in the entire specimen contain only Sertoli cells and no germ cells. Because of the heterogeneity of some spermatogenic lesions, in small biopsies, all tubules may show Sertoli cells only, but in an adjacent region, obtained by a second biopsy, foci of spermatogenesis may be present.

5. **Seminiferous tubule hyalinization**. This category is reserved for those testicular biopsies wherein the entire seminiferous epithelium has been lost and all that remains of the seminiferous tubule is a hyalinized fibrotic remnant. Again in certain pathological conditions, foci of seminiferous tubule hyalinization may coexist with areas of spermatogenesis, which maybe identified on a larger biopsy.

6. **Immature testis**. This diagnosis is usually reserved for patients with seminiferous cords and gonocytes rather than spermatogonia. The Sertoli cells in these men are usually immature, and their nuclei do not show the typical large nucleolus that characterizes the adult Sertoli cell. In such men, hypogonadotrophic hypogonadism is the etiological factor.

V. SPERM STORAGE AND MATURATION

Sperm pass through the testis to enter the efferent ductules which, in man, constitute part of the head of the epididymis. These ductules empty into the duct of the epididymis, which is markedly coiled and forms part of the head, body, and tail of the epididymis. Contraction of the smooth muscle layer of the epididymis causes spermatozoa to pass through the epididymis.[30] This layer becomes progressively organized distally so that the contractile activities exhibit a peristaltic action. Thus, in the caudal region of the epididymis, the peristaltic activity is coordinated with the contractions of the vas that occur during the process of ejaculation.

In the head of the epididymis, a progressive reabsorption of approximately 90% of the fluid emanating from the testis occurs. Recent studies suggest that the fluid reabsorptive process is under the influence of estradiol.[31] In the majority of mammalian species, spermatozoa mature progressively as they pass through the epididymis such that they acquire the capacity for fertilization and motility in the cauda epididymis. However, studies utilizing the anastomosis of the vas to differing levels of the epididymis in man have suggested that bypass of a significant part of the epididymis does not prevent fertility. It should be noted that attempts to use

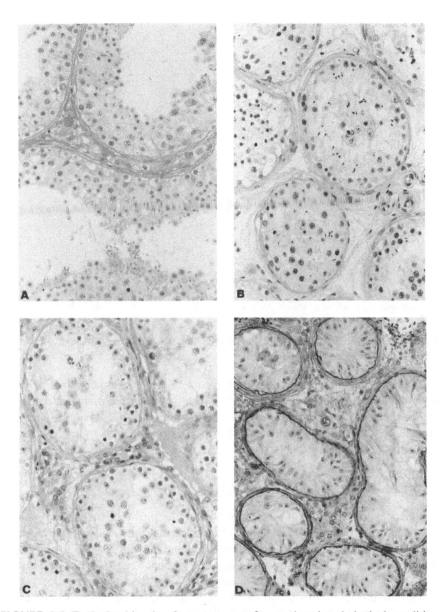

FIGURE 2.3 Testicular biopsies from a range of normal and pathological conditions. (A) Normal, (B) hypospermatogenesis, (C) germ cell arrest at primary spermatocyte stage, (D) Sertoli cell only syndrome.

epididymal spermatozoa in IVF achieve poor fertilization,[32] and it has only been since the use of intracytoplasmic sperm injection that good fertilization rates have been achieved using epididymal and testicular sperm. These results point to the importance of sperm maturation in the epididymis to enable natural fertility, which may be dependent upon changes to the surface of the spermatozoa that occur during epididymal transit and that facilitate sperm oocyte interactions.

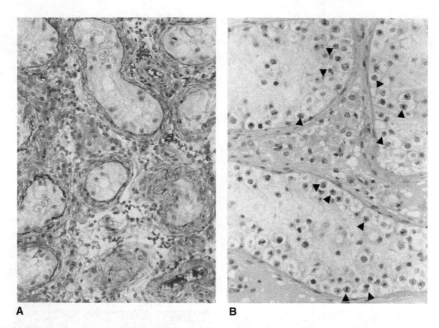

FIGURE 2.4 (A) Sertoli cell only syndrome and seminiferous tubule hyalinization. (B) Carcinoma *in situ* of testis. Note the large abnormal cells indicated by arrow heads.

Epididymal transit time ranges from 1 to 12 days, and in some infertile men, the epididymal storage area becomes hostile resulting in degradation of spermatozoa (epididymal necrozoospermia). In such individuals, diminishing sperm storage time through the use of frequent ejaculation programs, may result in an improvement of the quality of spermatozoa obtained.[33]

VI. EJACULATION

To understand the process of ejaculation, the reader must understand the anatomy of the terminal end of the vas deferens. In this region, the vas lies posterior to the bladder and shows a dilatation known as the ampulla of the vas. At its distal end, the ampulla is joined by the duct draining the seminal vesicles and together these structures form the ejaculatory duct. On each side, the ejaculatory duct passes through the prostate to open into the prostatic urethra at the region known as the vera montanum. In the prostatic urethra, the secretions of the seminal vesicle and the accompanying testicular component containing the spermatozoa meet the prostatic secretions entering the prostatic urethra through multiple ducts. For semen to be expelled into the penile urethra, the internal sphincter of the bladder must contract, otherwise the contractions of the vas and ejaculatory duct may result in retrograde ejaculation into the bladder. The process of ejaculation results from a coordinated series of contractions wherein the seminal vesicular component, accompanied by the spermatozoa, precedes the secretion of the prostate which usually completes the ejaculatory process. Consequently, in a split ejaculate where the seminal fluid is collected temporally into different containers, varying concentrations of the major components of seminal fluid appear such that the seminal vesicular components occur in the earlier fraction. These fractions usually have an alkaline pH whereas the prostatic component has a pH of less than 7.2. Thus, in patients who have congenital absence of the vas and the accompanying seminal vesicles, the semen volume is reduced to less than 1 ml and is acidic (pH less than 7) due to the absence of the alkaline component contributed by the seminal vesicles. In patients with ejaculatory duct obstruction, a similar feature is noted.

REFERENCES

1. de Kretser, D. M. and Kerr, J. B., The cytology of the testis, in, *The Physiology of Reproduction*, Knobil, E. and Neill, J. D., Eds., Raven Press, New York, 1177–1290, 1994.
2. Clermont, Y., Kinetics of spermatogenesis in mammals: seminiferous epithelium cycle and spermatogonial renewal, *Physiol. Rev.*, 52:198, 1972.
3. de Kretser, D. M., Ultrastructural features of human spermiogenesis, *Z Zellforsch*, 98:477, 1969.
4. Holstein, A. F. and Roosen-Runge, E. C., *Atlas of Human Spermatogenesis*. Grosse Verlag, Berlin, 1981.
5. Clermont, Y., The cycle of the seminiferous epithelium in man, *Am. J. Anat.*, 112:35, 1963.
6. Dym, M. and Fawcett, D. W., The blood-testis barrier in the rat and the physiological compartmentation of the seminiferous epithelium, *Biol. Reprod.*, 3:308, 1970.
7. Setchell, B. P. and Waites, G. M. H., The blood-testis barrier, in Hamilton, D. W. and Greep, R. O., Eds., *Handbook of Physiology*, section 7, vol 5. William & Wilkins, Baltimore, 1975, 143.
8. Jutte, N. H. P. M., Jansen, R., Grootegoed, A. J. et al., Regulation of survival of rat pachytene spermatocytes by lactate supply from Sertoli cells, *J. Reprod. Fertil.*, 65:431, 1982.
9. Orth, J. M., Gunsalus, G. L., and Lamperti, A. A., Evidence from Sertoli cell-depleted rats indicates that spermatid number in adults depends on numbers of Sertoli cells, *Endocrinology*, 787, 1988.
10. Sheckter, C. B., McLachlan, R. I., Tenover, J. S., Matsumoto, A. M., Burger, H. G., de Kretser, D. M., and Bremner, W. J., Serum inhibin concentrations rise during GnRH treatment of men with idiopathic hypogonadotrophic hypogonadism, *J. Clin. Endocr. Metab.*, 67:1221–1224, 1988.
11. Au, C. L., Robertson, D. M., and de Kretser, D. M., An *in vivo* method for estimating inhibin production by adult rat testes, *J. Reprod. Fertil.*, 71:259, 1985.
12. Au, C. L., Robertson, D. M., and de Kretser, D. M., Changes in testicular inhibin following a single episode of heating of rat testes, *Endocrinology*, 120:973–977, 1987.
13. Anawalt, B. D., Bebb, R. A., Matsumoto, A. M., Groome, N. P., Illingworth, P. J., McNeilly, A. S., and Bremner, W. J., Serum inhibin B levels reflect Sertoli cell function in normal men and men with testicular dysfunction, *J. Clin. Endocrinol. Metab.*, 81:3341–3345, 1996.
14. Fawcett, D. W., Neaves, W. B., and Flores, M. N., Comparative observations on intertubular tissue of the mammalian testis, *Biol. Reprod.*, 9:500, 1973.

15. Hedger, M. P., Testicular leucocytes: what are they doing? *Reviews of Reprod.*, 2:38–47, 1997.
16. de Kretser, D. M., Catt, K. J., and Paulsen, C. A., Studies on the *in vitro* testicular binding of iodinated luteinizing hormone in rats, *Endocrinology*, 88:332–337, 1971.
17. Means, A. R. and Vaitukaitis, J. L., Peptide hormone "receptors": specific binding of 3 H-FSH to testis, *Endocrinology*, 90:39–46, 1972.
18. Cunningham, G. R. and Huckins, C., Persistence of complete spermatogenesis in the presence of low intra-testicular concentration of testosterone, *Endocrinology*, 105:177–186, 1979.
19. Sun, Y. T., Wreford, N. G., Robertson, D. M., and de Kretser, D. M., Quantitative cytological studies of spermatogenesis in intact and hypophysectomised rats: identification of androgen-dependent stages, *Endocrinology*, 127:1215, 1990.
20. Singh, J., O'Neill, C., and Handlesman, D. J., Induction of spermatogenesis by androgens in gonadotropin deficient (hpg) mice, *Endocrinology*, 136:5311–5321, 1995.
21. Kumar, T. R., Wang, Y., Lu, N., and Matzuk, M., Follicle stimulating hormone is required for ovarian follicle maturation but not male fertility, *Nature Genet.*, 15:201–204, 1997.
22. Meachem, S. J., Wreford, N. G., Robertson, D. M., and McLachlan, R. I., Androgen action on the restoration of spermatogenesis in adult rats: effects of human chorionic gonadotrophin, testosterone and flutamide administration on germ cell number, *Int. J. Andrology*, 20, 70, 1997.
23. Meachem, S. J., Wreford, N. G., Stanton, P. G., Robertson, D. M., and McLachlan, R. I., Follide stimulating hormone is required for the initial phase of spermatogenic restoration in adult rats following gonadotrophin suppression, *J. Andrology*, 19, 725, 1998.
24. Zhengwei, Y., Wreford, N. G., Royce, P., de Kretser, D. M., and McLachlan, R. I., Stereological evaluation of human spermatogenesis following suppression by testosterone treatment: heterogeneous pattern of spermatogenic impairment, *J. Clin. Endocrin. Metab.*, 83:1284–1291, 1998.
25. Dix, D. J., Allen, J. W., Collins, B. W., Mori, C., Nakamura, N., Poorman-Allen, P., Goulding, E. H., and Eddy, E. M., Targetted disruption of Hsp 70–2 results in failed meiosis, germ cell apoptosis and male infertility, *Proc. Natl. Acad. Sci. USA*, 93:3264–3268, 1996.
26. Print, C. G., Loveland, K., Gibson, L., Meehan, T., Stylianou, A., Wreford, N. G., de Kretser, D. M., Metcalf, D., Köntgen, F., Adams, J. M., and Cory, S., Apoptosis regulator Bcl-w is essential for spermatogenesis but is otherwise dispensable, *Proc. Natl. Acad. Sci. USA*, 95:12424–12431, 1998.
27. Van Steirteghem, A. C., Nagy, Z., Joris, H. et al., High fertilization and implantation rates after intracytoplasmic sperm injection, *Hum. Reprod.*, 8:1061–1066, 1993.
28. Silber, S. J., Devroey, P., Tournaye, H., and Van Steirteghem, A., Fertilizing capacity of epididymal and testicular sperm using intracytoplasmic sperm injection (ICSI), in Intracytoplasmic sperm injection: the revolution in male infertility, *Reprod. Fertil. Develop.*, 7:147–160, 1995.
29. de Kretser, D. M., Burger, H. G., Fortune, D., Hudson, B., Long, A. R., Paulsen, C. A., and Taft, H. P., Hormonal, histological and chromosomal studies in adult males with testicular disorders, *J. Clin. Endocr. Metab.*, 35:392–401, 1972.
30. de Kretser, D. M., Temple-Smith, P. D., and Kerr J. B., Anatomical and functional aspects of the male reproductive organs, in Bandhauer, K. and Frick, J., Eds., *Handbuch der Urologie*, vol. XVI, Springer-Verlag, Berlin, 1982, 1.

31. Hess, R. A., Bunick, D., Lee, K. H., Bahr, J., Taylor, J. A., Korach, K. S., and Lubahn, D. B., A role for oestrogens in the male reproductive tract, *Nature*, 390:509–512, 1997.
32. Temple-Smith, P. D., Southwick, G. J., Yates, C. A., Trounson, A. O., and de Kretser, D. M., Human pregnancy by IVF using sperm aspirated from the epididymis, *J. In Vitro Fert. Embryo Transfer*, 2:119–122, 1985.
33. Wilton, L. J., Temple-Smith, P. D., Baker, H. W. G. et al., Human male infertility caused by degeneration and death of sperm in the epididymis, *Fertil. Steril.*, 49:1052–1058, 1988.

3 Implantation

Bruce A. Lessey and Laurie P. Lovely

CONTENTS

I. INTRODUCTION

Despite years of research and interest, we are only now beginning to understand the biochemical basis for one of the most interesting events in reproductive biology. The joining of the nascent embryo with the maternal circulation is a continuation of the developmental strategy of the blastocyst leading to the establishment of the mature placenta. While the stages and events vary between species, in most, synchronous development of the endometrium and embryo occurs as a prerequisite for successful implantation. Alterations in the temporal relationship between embryonic and maternal environment can disrupt this process and lead to infertility or recurrent pregnancy loss.

Early descriptions of implantation focused on the morphologic changes within the endometrium. Modern molecular biology techniques have shifted the attention to the determination of the cellular proteins and their interactions that orchestrate the cascade of events that mediate implantation. These highly coordinated events are tightly regulated and involve endocrine, paracrine, juxtacrine, and autocrine mechanisms of cellular communication. Increasingly, researchers direct efforts to understand the involvement of the extracellular matrix (ECM) and enzymes or receptors for ECM in implantation. The adhesion molecules and ligands that promote cell-cell attachments, invasion, and apoptosis and the proteases that digest the extracellular matrix have been found to be active during the key events of implantation. Differences in the regulation of such molecules and interactions among them may account for the surprising variety of placentation strategies that occur in various mammal species. It is not surprising that the invasive behavior of the early embryo mirrors that of cancer cells and suggests that malignancies display a regressive phenotype using common biochemical paradigms used by the trophoblast. Conversely, we can learn about implantation mechanisms by studying normal and abnormal examples of invasion, such as that seen in preeclampsia or recurrent pregnancy loss. The purpose of this review of implantation is to emphasize what is currently known about these developmental pathways and outline future goals for understanding this important and complex physiologic process.

II. TIMING AND STAGES OF IMPLANTATION

Implantation can be divided into distinct stages relating to the developmental progression of the nascent embryo and its interaction with maternal cell types. Implantation has been viewed as a stepwise progression involving apposition, attachment or adhesion, and finally invasion with eventual penetration into the maternal vasculature. Apposition and adhesion appear common to all species,[1] though the timing and characteristics of invasion are quite variable.

The earliest aspects of implantation in the human encompass the sequence of events leading from fertilization to blastocyst attachment and invasion. The entire process is driven by ovarian steroids. Follicular development leading to maturation and ovulation of the oocyte increases serum estradiol levels that begin the preparation of the endometrium. As a mitogen, estrogen acts through the estrogen receptor (ER) to induce growth of the epithelial glands and a thickening of the endometrium. As shown in Figure 3.1, the nascent oocyte is transported through the Fallopian tube where fertilization occurs, defining Stage I of implantation. With entry into the uterine cavity the embryo continues cell division, which marks the initiation of Stage II. At Stage III, the ball of embryonic cells, now called a morula, enters the uterine cavity where further divisions result in formation of the blastocyst.

These events occur within a narrow time frame. In humans, the embryo enters the uterine cavity at 72 to 96 hours after fertilization.[2,3] In a natural menstrual cycle, endometrial growth begun in response to rising estrogen stimulation from the developing follicle undergoes a secretory transformation in response to serum progesterone and peptide hormones from the newly formed corpus luteum.[4] The first secretory changes appear in the glandular epithelium by cycle day 15 to 16.[5] As below, the

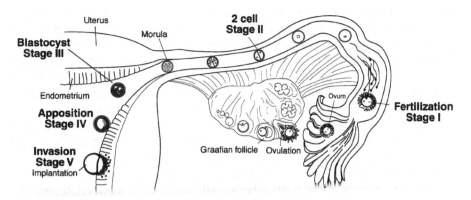

FIGURE 3.1 Schematic showing the different stages of implantation (I to V). Ovulation begins the process at mid cycle. Stage I begins with fertilization in the Fallopian tube. Transport through the Fallopian tube and the first cell division marks Stage II. At Stage III, the blastocyst enters the uterine cavity and with the onset of uterine receptivity, adheres to the uterine lining (Stage IV). Invasion of the embryo into the endometrium signals the beginning of Stage V.

hormonal and paracrine milieu ultimately leads to a defined period of uterine receptivity that is critical for successful nidation. Hatching of the embryo with dissolution of the zona pellucida occurs by day 5 (about 110 to 120 hours after ovulation).[3]

Stage IV corresponds to the time of apposition. In the human, it has been difficult to study these early stages of implantation directly and much uncertainty remains about the precise timing of this event. Based primarily on early studies by Hertig and colleagues, apposition is now thought to occur in the mid-secretory phase.[6] These observations were based on secretory phase hysterectomies in fertile women and careful identification of early embryos found in their uteris or fallopian tubes. In this landmark study, the stage of identified embryos was correlated with the time from the last menstrual cycle. Of the 34 cases in which embryos were found, 8 were free floating (all prior to day 19 of the menstrual cycle) and 26 were found already attached (all after day 21). These data suggest that in the human, initial apposition and attachment occurs around cycle day 20, or 6 days after ovulation occurs.

Appostion is followed quickly by epithelial penetration and invasion (Stage V).[7] What triggers these orderly cells lining the blastocyst to suddenly intrude through the surface epithelium is unknown, but likely involves cellular receptors and critical signaling pathways. A number of cellular components including extracellular matrix, cell adhesion molecules, growth factors and their receptors, and matrix metalloproteinases hatch from the zona pellucida and likely orchestrate this process of invasion. Studies describe the changes in the ECM that occur on both trophoblast[8] and endometrium[9] around the time of implantation, and the importance of ECM on cell surface proteolysis has been reviewed recently.[10] Evidence suggests that upon invasion, cell migration and the acquisition of an invasive phenotype may be stimulated by exposed ECM and digested fragments of the endometrial or trophoblast ECM mediated in large measure by activation of specific MMPs.[11–13] Despite the role of digestive enzymes, little evidence suggests that this is a destructive process; rather the syncytial trophoblast sends out processes and moves the luminal epithelium out of its way, implying a weakening of the cell-cell contacts between the surface epithelial cells. The intruding trophoblast appears to adhere to the lateral surfaces of the luminal epithelium with formation of junctional complexes. After establishing an expanded "trophoblastic plate" there may be a brief pause before the nascent trophoblast invades through the basement membrane into the underlying stroma.[14]

With time, invasion into the maternal circulation becomes a priority as the growing embryo will require increasing quantities of nutrients and oxygen and better management of cellular waste for its survival. The stage of implantation is marked by rapid expansion of both cytotrophoblast and synctial trophoblast (Figure 3.2A and B). At Stage 5a, the maternal vasculature remains intact, but becomes surrounded by the expanding syncytium. With further growth, the syncytium and cytotrophoblast invade the maternal vasculature, and the cytotrophoblast is incorporated into the wall of maternal vessels. As detailed later in the chapter, this ability to mimic endothelial cell characteristics is critical to this invasion; using stealth and deception, the trophoblast establishes a blood supply and a presence within the maternal tissues that will remain intact for the remainder of pregnancy.

As shown in Figure 3.2 C and D, Stage 5b is characterized by expansion of the syncytium and cytotrophoblast and establishment of lacunae as a result of vasculature invasion. By Stage 5c, the embryo is fully below the luminal surface, the circumference of the embryo is surrounded by a layer of cytotrophoblast that will soon bud

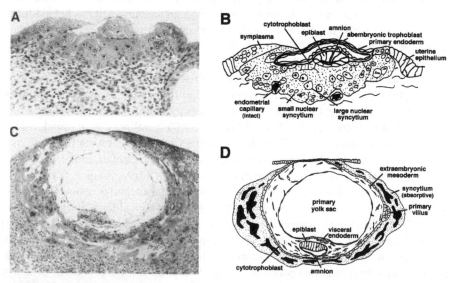

FIGURE 3.2 Photomicrograph (A) and schematic drawing (B) of a human implantation site during early implantation (stage 5a). At this stage the maternal vasculature remains intact, but becomes surrounded by the expanding syncytium. By stage 5c, (C and D) the embryo is fully below the luminal surface. A layer of cytotrophoblast that will soon bud to form villi surrounds the embryo, and lacunae have formed as a result of maternal vascular invasion. Development of the placenta and Stage V ends about 11 to 12 days after ovulation with the development of primary villi. (Courtesy of Dr. Allen Enders, University of California.)

to form villi. Development of the placenta and Stage 5 ends 11 to 12 days after ovulation with the development of primary villi.

III. MATERNAL RECOGNITION OF PREGNANCY

The endometrium of many species, including humans, undergoes cyclic development in preparation for pregnancy. Unlike induced ovulators, such as the rabbit, humans shed the endometrium once a month if conception does not occur. If pregnancy does occur, this menstrual breakdown of the endometrium is avoided. Recent studies demonstrate that programmed cell death (apoptosis) has already begun by cycle day 25 to 26 in nonconception cycles,[15] and a repertoire of molecules have assembled for the purpose of remodeling the endometrial lining.[16-18] The corpus luteum (CL), which also undergoes a process of apoptosis, must be rescued by signals from the nascent pregnancy and its function maintained until the placenta takes over hormonal support of the pregnancy at about 8 to 10 weeks.[19] Removal of the CL prior to the 5 weeks after implantation leads to a decrease in progesterone and a loss of the pregnancy.[20] These relationships were demonstrated in the classical experiments of Knobil and co-workers during the 1970s.[21]

Signals for the recognition of pregnancy determine the success of the pregnancy.[22] In primates, the embryo provides an early signal in the form of chorionic gonadotropin. This is a member of a closely related glycoprotein family of hormones consisting of identical *a* subunits with different *b* subunits, and including luteinizing hormone (LH), follicle stimulating hormone (FSH), thyroid stimulating hormone (TSH), and chorionic gonadotropin (CG). Chorionic gonadotropin is unique to primates, and due to its similarity to LH is capable of maintaining corpus luteal function beyond that which ordinarily occurs in a nonconception cycle. Mechanisms in ruminants, for example, are quite different. Unlike the human, in which the signal for the CL to regress (luteolysis) is unknown, the sheep must actively turn off a luteolytic signal in the form of prostaglandin F2α which arises from the nonpregnant uterus late in the estrus cycle. Secretion of interferon tau (INFt) by the mononuclear cells of the trophoblast prevent uterine secretion of PGF2α and stimulate new protein secretion by the endometrium.[23,24] In the rodent, there is no known signal arising from the embryo that signals its presence. Coitus-stimulated prolactin maintains early CL function in this species, and researchers believe that placental steroidogenesis acts synergistically with prolactin to maintain the pregnancy.[25]

The timing of CG production by the human embryo is thought to begin after hatching, but maternal serum levels begin to rise only after embryo attaches to maternal tissues. Using hypersensitive hCG measurements, Bergh and Navot concluded that implantation occurs between days 20 to 24,[26] in keeping with the early data from Hertig, Rock, and Adams,[27] Croxotto et al.,[2] and Buster et al.[3] *In vitro* assessment of CG in primate embryos corroborates these data.[28] Regulation of CG production also may depend on other molecular signals as recently reviewed by Jameson and Hollenborg.[29] It is interesting to note that hCG isoform changes occur early in pregnancy, suggesting a more active hCG is present initially.[30] Such differences may be important in cases of recurrent pregnancy failure.

Finally, the viability of the pregnancy also depends on keeping the maternal immune cells from recognizing and destroying the early pregnancy. The human placenta expresses HLA-G, a nonclassical (class Ib) MHC molecule that appears to play a role in maternal tolerance. This molecule is expressed by the invading cytotrophoblast cells, which may allow these cells to penetrate unnoticed. In addition, endometrial peptides such as glycodelin (formally known as PP14) may have immunomodulatory effects during pregnancy.[31]

IV. MODELS TO STUDY IMPLANTATION

Historically, animal models have served as the major method to study implantation. A window of implantation was suggested by Psychoyos,[32] McLaren,[33] and Finn and Martin.[34] Studies in animal models helped to refine this concept.[35-37] We have learned much from the studies on comparative placentation[1] and gained information about the differences between species.[38] Nevertheless, limitations arise from the differences in timing and mechanism of implantation that exist between species. While it is beyond the scope of this chapter to review all the *in vivo* models of implantation, rodents and primates are discussed as they constitute the mainstay of this research.

In mice, implantation occurs on the evening of the fourth day following coitus and occurs in response to estrogen. Further, as estrogen is required for implantation in this species, it is possible to suspend embryos within the uterus in what is called the "delayed implantation" model, using daily injections of progesterone in mice that are ovariectomized soon after mating has occurred. Implantation can then be triggered conveniently by the administration of exogenous estradiol. This model helps investigate the relative contributions of embryonic as well as uterine development in the implantation reaction.[39,40] Significant advances in our understanding of implantation have also come from mice with targeted mutations of specific genes.[41-45] In many cases, researchers found that factors considered critical had no effect while other factors were critical for implantation.[5,44] Other mammals also show promise for implantation research. As induced ovulators, rabbits provide a useful model for implantation.[46] Primates, which are more similar to humans, also have been employed with good success to investigate the mechanism and regulation of implantation.[36,47]

Several *in vitro* methods to study implantation have been proposed in the last several years. These include the use of purified endometrial epithelium[48] and cytotrophoblast.[49,50] Recombinant studies using intact villi or dissociated cytotrophoblast have been reported.[51,52] The ability to achieve appropriate epithelial/stromal interaction and establishment of a polarized phenotype[53,54] remains the limiting factor in these models. Endometrial explants have been advocated for this reason and appear to offer some advantages over other models for study of the endometrium.[55]

V. REGULATION OF IMPLANTATION

With the discovery of new bioregulatory molecules, the factors that regulate implantation become increasingly complex. Appreciation grows for the complex interactions that occur between ovarian steroids, growth factors, cytokines, and the extracellular matrix (ECM) and their respective roles in the cascade of events leading to successful implantation. Our understanding of this process is made more difficult by the spatial and temporal relationships between such signals and by the large number of receptors for these signals that are highly regulated and cell-type specific, e.g., receptors for prostaglandins[56] or the EGF family.[57] Over the past 10 years, the focus of implantation research has shifted from the study of its endocrinology to that of paracrinology and autocrine signaling. As outlined below, highly coordinated events, involving cell-adhesion molecules coupled with regulation of synthesis and secretion of the ECM and the enzymes that degrade this material, control implantation. We hope this chapter serves as an overview of these relationships and identifies the underlying principals of this important physiologic process.

A. STEROID HORMONES AND UTERINE RECEPTIVITY

Ultimately, implantation and its progression is regulated by the ovary and the sex steroids from the developing follicle and later by the corpus luteum.[4] As a developmental process, the initial factors that control implantation can be divided into those that participate in *embryonic* receptivity and those that render the *endometrium* receptive during the putative implantation window. Estradiol from the developing follicle stimulates endometrial growth and cell division to increase the epithelial and vascular components of the endometrium. Progesterone transforms this interval of epithelial growth following ovulation from the newly formed corpus luteum, which turns the proliferative endometrium into a secretory structure capable of supporting implantation and the ensuing pregnancy. Progesterone is essential for the success of the pregnancy.[58]

The steroid hormone receptors, primarily estrogen receptor (ER) and the progesterone receptor (PR), dictate the action of steroid hormones.[59] It has long been known that estrogen up regulates both ER and PR in human endometria[60,61] as well as in primates and other mammals.[4,62] Likewise, these studies have shown that progesterone down regulates ER and PR during the secretory phase of the cycle.[63] In 1988, several laboratories demonstrated that the down regulation of ER and PR was not uniform within the cells of the endometrium, but rather differentially down regulated in epithelial cells.[64,65] Interestingly, the loss of epithelial PR in the endometrium correlates with the establishment of uterine receptivity in humans as well as in most mammals studied.[66–68] In the endometrium of women, a delay in the opening of the window of implantation corresponds to a delay in the down regulation of epithelial PR, which is correctable with exogenous progesterone treatment.[69] From a practical standpoint, this lack of direct ovarian influence on the epithelium of the endometrium after cycle day 20 mandates a greater regulatory role for the stroma and implanting embryo on epithelial function. The possibility also exists that certain genes are repressed by progesterone or estrogen and thereby activated with the down regulation of ER and PR at the time of implantation.[70] Whatever the case, the loss of epithelial ER and PR seems critical for the initiation of uterine receptivity towards embryonic implantation, as blockage of progesterone's action by anti-progestins maintains PR and leads to atrophic changes in the endometrium.[71]

Another major role for progesterone is the induction of specific secretory phase endometrial proteins that facilitate endometrial and embryonic receptivity. These include growth factors, glycoproteins, ECM molecules and their receptors, enzymes, binding proteins, and secreted products that likely influence both embryonic and endometrial physiology.[72-74] Many of these proteins mark uterine receptivity in the human endometrium[75] as outlined later in this chapter. Two of the major secretory products of the endometrium originally were designated placental protein-12[76] and placental protein-14.[77] These two major endometrial proteins now represent IGF binding protein 1(IGFBP-1)[78] and glycodelin,[31] respectively. In a recent review,[79] IGFBP-1 appeared to play dual roles in modulation of insulin-like growth factor (IGF) activity and in interaction with the integrin a5β1 through its arg-gly-asp (RGD) site.[80] This interaction may play a role in limiting the trophoblast and serves as one of many examples of stromal protective mechanisms against uncontrolled invasiveness.[79] Glycodelin, previously referred to as PP14 or PEP, appears to have a contraceptive potential given its ability to inhibit binding of human spermatozoa to the human zona pellucida *in vitro*[81] and may have immunosuppressive functions as well.[31] Regulation of each of these major secretory proteins is complex involving both steroid and peptide signals.[79,82]

The importance of steroid hormones in the regulation of endometrial function is perhaps highlighted best by the clinical sequela of inadequate progesterone secretion commonly known as luteal phase deficiency (LPD). This topic has recently been reviewed in detail.[83] The clinical diagnosis is based on a demonstrated delay in the dating criteria of Noyes et al.,[5] that established criteria for the histologic assessment of the endometrium. Inadequate progesterone levels (or inadequate response to progesterone) results in a histologic lag that delays the interval of uterine receptivity. As shown in animal models,[84] histologic delay leading to uterine asynchrony shifts the window of implantation and results in embryonic loss, shown to occur in human pregnancies as well.[85] This asynchronous development of the endometrium corresponds to a delay in the down regulation of the epithelial PR. A delay or diminution of other secretory products has also been documented in women with inadequate progesterone secretion[6,86-88] and suggests the LPD is primarily an endometrial defect. Should implantation occur in this setting, the delay in uterine receptivity may result in late or ineffectual rescue of the corpus luteum and contribute to the observed association between LPD and recurrent pregnancy loss or infertility.

B. CYTOKINES AND GROWTH FACTORS IN IMPLANTATION

Many of the endometrial peptides that are synthesized and secreted in support of implantation are cytokines or growth factors that mediate autocrine, paracrine, and juxtacrine signaling. Several recent reviews cover this topic in detail.[89-91] While the list of biological signals in the endometrium and implanting embryo is long and continues to grow, studies point to several "key" factors that seem essential for normal implantation.

1. CSF-1

Colony Stimulating Factor-1 (CSF-1) is a growth factor expressed by fibroblasts, monocytes, macrophages, and endothelial cells.[92,93] CSF-1 is a 50–70 kDa glyco-protein initially shown to be involved in proliferation and differentiation of cells of the monocyte lineage. The receptor for CSF-1 is the proto-oncogene c-fms, which is abundantly expressed by trophoblast cells[94] and on pre- and post-implantation embryos in the human.[95] Interest in CSF-1 increased with the discovery that osteo-petrotic (op/op) mutant mice that lacked CSF-1 were infertile. Evidence based on cross-mating suggested that this was due to implantation failure.[96] Immunostaining in the human endometrium localized to the glandular epithelium in the first trimester of pregnancy and levels appear to drop with increasing gestational age.[95] Kauma et al. examined CSF-1 through the menstrual cycle and noted some increase around day 22, but found dramatic increases in CSF-1 and c-fms in the late secretory phase and early pregnancy.[97] Several investigators have examined the function of CSF-1 in implantation. Haimovici and Anderson demonstrated that CSF-1 stimulated mouse trophoblast outgrowth,[98] and Garcia-Lloret et al. showed that both CSF-1 and GM-CSF stimulated cytotrophoblast aggregation into large patches of syncytium.[99] Hence, the temporal and spatial expression of this cytokine and its receptor, coupled with the data from the CSF-1 null mutants, suggest that this cytokine is essential for the process of implantation.

2. Leukemia Inhibitory Factor (LIF)

The second essential cytokine is leukemia inhibitory factor (LIF). A recent review examined the importance of LIF in implantation.[100] LIF originally was shown to induce differentiation of a myeloid leukemia cell line, M1,[101] though interest in this factor was heightened significantly when Bhatt, Brunet, and Stewart observed that LIF transcripts were present in the mouse uterus with maximal expression on the day of implantation (day 4 of pregnancy).[102] Using the delayed implantation model, researchers showed that uterine receptivity, associated with an injection of estradiol, correlated with an increase in LIF expression. More conclusive was the finding that female homozygotes lacking a functional LIF gene were infertile while homozygous males were fertile. When examined closely, the female homozygotes had normal appearing blastocytes within the uterus that failed to undergo implantation.[41] Adding exogenous LIF resulted in a partial reversal of defect, and embryos taken from LIF-deficient females and placed into normal female surrogates implanted normally. These data demonstrated the failure of implantation was maternal in origin and not due to abnormalities associated with the blastocyst.

Further human studies demonstrate that LIF appears in the endometrium at the time of implantation.[103–105] Nachtigall et al. demonstrated that LIF markedly decreased trophoblast production of hCG and increased the expression of the fetal fibronectin mRNA and protein, suggesting that LIF is an important modulator of human embryonic implantation through direct effects on trophoblast differentia-tion.[106] Cullinan et al. noted that LIF was present during the window of implantation and may be decreased in the endometria of some women with infertility.[105]

Danielsson et al. showed reduced immunostaining for LIF after treatment with the anti-progestin mifepristone.[107] LIF also appears essential for decidualization as attempts to induce decidualization in LIF-deficient females were unsuccessful.[100] Other null mutants including Hoxa-10 deficient mice[43] and COX-2 deficient mice[108] share this defect of decidualization. Hoxa-10 is a developmental homeobox gene that is also expressed during the window of implantation while COX-2 is a rate limiting enzyme in the prostaglandin synthesis pathway. LIF appears to be an essential endometrial product that plays a role in implantation in both mice and in humans. Its expression is associated with the window of implantation, and factors that prevent or delay its expression are associated with defects in uterine receptivity.

3. IL-1 Family

Interleukin-1 (IL-1) represents a family of peptides composed of IL-1α (159 amino acids), IL-1β (153 amino acids), and an inhibitor called IL-1 receptor antagonist (IL-1ra; 152 amino acids).[109] IL-1β has been shown to be produced by macrophages,[110] in oocytes and embryos,[93,111] and the endometrial stroma.[112] Kauma et al. noted very high levels of IL-1β in both first trimester and term placenta membranes.[113] The IL-1 system also has been examined in implantation sites.[114] IL-1β, IL-1ra and IL-1 receptor type 1 (IL-1R tI) were localized to macrophages in the villus trophoblast, the maternal-trophoblast interface, and the maternal decidual during early pregnancy.

In the endometrium, IL-1 modulates epithelial cell function supporting the theory that the embryo may facilitate its own implantation[115] and modulate decidualization.[112] De los Santos et al. have shown that all embryos do not all share the capacity to produce this cytokine.[115] IL-1β, IL-1ra, and IL-1R tI were present in oocytes and embryos cultured with endometrial epithelial cell conditioned media, but not present in embryos cultured with endometrial stromal cells or in stromal cell conditioned media. Two populations of embryos were observed: those that produced IL-1 and those that did not. Such studies suggest that embryonic competency relates to the presence or absence of cytokine signals.

The receptors for IL-1β comprise 2 subtypes termed type I (IL-1R tI)[116] and type II (IL-1R tII).[117] These receptors for IL-1 occur in the epithelial component of the human endometrium.[118] Simón et al. measured IL-1R tI throughout the menstrual cycle in human endometria with significantly elevated expression during the mid and late secretory phase.[119] The same group demonstrated that the IL-1R tI increases upon exposure to IL-1β.[120]

The IL-1 receptor antagonist also has been studied in the human endometrium. Sahakian et. al. identified IL-1 receptor antagonist in the glandular epithelium of 7 out of 8 endometrial samples studies.[121] Simón et al. found IL-1ra present throughout the menstrual cycle, localized primarily to the endometrial epithelium, but present at significantly higher levels during the follicular phase compared to the earlier and mid secretory phases.[122] In mice, IL-1ra has been used successfully to block implantation suggesting a critical role for IL-1 in this process.[123] Implantation rates in female mice injected with IL-1ra were low, independent of toxic effects of this compound to the embryo. These data are at odds, however, with IL-1 receptor null mutant studies that demonstrate normal implantation with or without the addition of IL-1 receptor antagonist. This lack of effect may indicate that developmental loss of this cytokine leads to compensatory mechanisms that overcomes the deficit observed in the setting of acute perturbation. Other postulated functions of IL-1 during implantation include its stimulatory effect of prostaglandin E2[118–124] and the stimulatory effect of IL1 on hCG release by human trophoblast.[125,126] IL-1β also inhibits stromal cell growth[127] and inhibits attachment of blastocytes to fibronectin while enhancing blastocyst outgrowth.[128] IL-1β[129] and IL-1α[130] have been reported to be toxic to early embryos. The precise role and essential nature of this cytokine awaits further investigation.

1. EGF and EGF-Like Molecules

Epidermal growth factor (EGF) is a 6 kD growth factor long known for its biological role as a potent mitogen that stimulates proliferation of a variety of cell types.[131] EGF has gained attention in the area of reproduction because of its potential role in growth and development of the endometrium. Nelson et al. showed that EGF acts as an "estromedin," able to replace the action of estradiol in stimulating the growth differentiation of the murine genital track *in vivo*.[132] In addition, recent evidence points to complex roles for EGF and various EGF-like molecules during the implantation window in rodents and humans.

The EGF family of growth factors has expanded dramatically in recent years and now encompasses both EGF and TGFα as well as amphiregulin, heparin binding EGF (Hb-EGF), and betacellulen.[57,131,133–136] EGF acts through a specific receptor, ErbB. Several epidermal growth factor-related peptide members of the ErbB family of receptor kinases have been described. Four members include ErbB receptor 1 (ErbB-1), ErbB-2, ErbB-3, and ErbB-4, each with specificity for the various ligands thus far described.[137] EGF has been immunolocalized during the menstrual cycle in human endometrium, decidua, and placenta.[138,139] Hofmann and co-workers noted that EGF was localized in endometrial stromal cells in the proliferative phase of the menstrual cycle with a shift to luminal and glandular epithelial staining during the secretory phase.[138] Intense staining for EGF occurred in the decidua, suggesting a role for EGF in the implantation process. Chegini et al. reported no significant difference in the secretory and proliferative phase for EGF or another endometrial mitogen platelet derived growth factor (PDGF).[140] In the primate model, Fazleabas and colleagues found IGF-I and EGF in the glandular epithelium of the endometrium and observed changes at the implantation site of this species, suggesting a role in trophoblast invasion and/or decidualization.[74] Others did not find either TGFα or EGF in the normal cycling endometrium, but noted increased expression in the decidua of pregnancy.[141,142] By immunohistochemistry and PCR, Imai et al. reported an increase in EGF, TGFα, and EGF receptor in the late follicular phase and luteal phase compared to early follicular phase, again suggesting that these growth factors are regulated during the menstrual cycle. These data contradict the work of Ace and Okulicz who saw a down regulation of EGF in progesterone dominate tissue using PCR in the primate model.[143]

One function of EGF appears be the stimulation of embryo development. Machida et al. demonstrated that EGF and TGFα significantly stimulated trophoblast outgrowth *in vitro*.[144] The EGF receptor increases after the 4 cell preimplantation stage in the mouse[145] and on the syncytiotrophoblast of early and term placenta.[146] Paria and Dey observed that TGFα and EGF produced higher hatching rates in mouse embryos.[150] Taga et al. suggested a role for EGF in decidualization and the establishment of uterine receptivity,[147] in agreement with the immunohistochemical localization of EGF.[138,148]

The importance of EGF and EGF-like molecules in implantation has been well demonstrated in the mouse model. Huet-Hudson et al. indicated that mouse uterine EGF is estrogen dependent in uterine epithelial cells.[149] EGF receptors are present in the blastocyst,[150] and the EGF receptor gene is regulated in mouse blastocyst by estrogen in the delayed implantation mouse model.[151] Such studies suggest that activation of the dormant blastocyst and its competence for implantation depends on EGF action. Furthermore, cross talk between the uterus and the blastocyst appears to define the window of implantation.[39] Das et al. studied TGFα and the other EGF-like ligands in the mouse uterus during implantation.[152] TGFα occurred primarily in the luminal and glandular epithelial cells on day 1 of pregnancy and again on day 4 of pregnancy, the day of implantation in this species.[153] Inappropriate expression of TGFα in the uterus of transgenic mice resulted in down regulation of TGFβ receptor subtypes and delayed the initiation of implantation.[154] EGF could induce implantation like estradiol in the delayed implantation model.[155] Heparin binding EGF was found to localize temporally and spatially to the mouse uterine epithelium surrounding the blastocyst 6 to 7 hours before the attachment reaction[156] and has recently been shown to be expressed during the window of implantation in the porcine[157] and human uterus as well.[158] Mouse blastocytes adhere to those cells expressing the transmembrane form of the heparin binding EGF-like growth factor.[159] This growth factor, like EGF, enhances the development of human embryos *in vitro*.[160] Hb-EGF is regulated differentially in the endometrial epithelium and stroma by estrogen and progesterone, respectively,[161,162] and decidual expression can be blocked by anti-progestins.[163] Other EGF-like molecules, including amphiregulin and betacellulin, also appeared in the mouse uterine epithelium on day 4 of pregnancy at the time of blastocyst attachment and are expressed exclusively in the luminal epithelium at the site of blastocyst attachment.[152,164]

5. IGF Family of Growth Factors

The IGF family of growth factors encompasses not only IGF-I and IGF-II hormones, but two distinct receptors and at least six different binding proteins that modulate IGF's activity.[165,166] IGF-I and IGF-II are mitogenic growth factors that bear structural similarities to insulin and are present in the mouse uterus and throughout the menstrual cycle in women.[167-171] Both hormones are present in the stroma, though the receptors are present in both epithelial and stromal cells.[168] IGF-I is more abundant in the proliferative phase and may assist epithelial proliferation, while IGF-II is expressed in a more robust fashion in secretory phase and is thought to be a mitogen for the stroma and decidua of pregnancy. IGF-I binds to both the Type I

IGF receptor (IGF-I receptor), which is structurally similar to the insulin receptor, and the Type II receptor (IGF-II receptor), with high affinity. IGF-II binds the latter with high affinity but does not bind well to the former receptor. IGF-II is also produced by the cytotrophoblast cells and may be important to the invasiveness of these cells during implantation.[79]

Six binding proteins exist for IGF growth factors, which bind to and modulate the activity of IGF I and II.[172,173] Each of the six binding proteins is present in the cycling endometrium.[167] IGF binding protein-1 (IGFBP-1), formerly known as PP12 or α1-PEG, is a major secretory protein of the stroma and is made by both epithelial and stromal cells.[78] Progesterone regulates IGFBP-1[174] and anti-progestins inhibit its expression.[175] The endometrial vasculature cells produce IGFBP-3 while IGFBP-5 is made primarily by the proliferative phase stroma. The remainder are produced by secretory stroma. IGFBP-2 and 3 increase in early to mid secretory phase while IGFBP-4 and 6 increase in the late secretory phase.

Because insulin, IGF-I, and IGF-II all inhibit decidualization, the presence of IGFBP-1 probably counteracts the effect of trophoblast IGF-II.[176] IGFBP-1 appears to have dual functions: to bind and mitigate the effect of IGFs and to influence cell motility or invasive potential of target cells. This latter function requires binding to the integrins in the cellular membrane using a three amino acid integrin recognition sequence arg-gly-asp (RGD).[177] While several integrins recognize this binding motif, IGFBP-1 is recognized specifically by α5β1 present on the cytotrophoblast cells[178] and on endometrial stroma and decidua.[179] One function of IGFBP-1 may be to limit invasion of the cytotrophoblast, though the mechanism of this effect is unknown.[79]

VI. MEDIATORS OF ATTACHMENT AND INVASION

Since the mid 1980s, discoveries abound involving the ECM, cell adhesion molecules, and the enzymes that degrade the ECM. Implantation is an example of these concepts applied to a dynamic rapidly changing system in which cells are directed through developmental and migratory cascades leading to predictable and controlled cell-cell interactions. As outlined above, steroid hormones, growth factors, and cytokines orchestrate this process as do the ECM and the molecules that degrade this matrix. Within this miraculous process, cells divide, migrate, and even die on command to allow interactions that are necessary for survival of the nascent embryo.

A. EXTRACELLULAR MATRIX OF THE ENDOMETRIUM AND EMBRYO

The ECM comprises secreted proteins and glycoproteins that form the "ground substance" outside of cells and yet play a vital role in cellular function. Researchers examine the ECM of the endometrium using immunohistochemical staining and the changes described throughout the menstrual cycle and in early pregnancy.[9] Fibronectin and type III and V collagen occur throughout the menstrual cycle and into pregnancy, primarily in the stroma. Type VI collagen appears primarily in the proliferative phase and becomes less abundant in the secretory phase and in the decidua. Epithelial cells, which sit on basement membrane, are surrounded by type IV collagen and laminin, as well as heparin sulphate proteoglycan. An epithelialization of the stroma includes basement membrane constituents in early pregnancy. Expression of epithelial cell adhesion molecules accompanies this conversion.[179,180] Differences also exist between the endometrial ECM components of fertile and infertile women,[181] though the significance of these findings remains unclear. At implantation, changes in the fine structure of the luminal epithelial surface take place.[182,183] The extracellular coating of the luminal glycocalyx surface thins[184,185] and an associated reduction in negative charge occurs.[186,187] Using lectins, Chavez noted changes in the molecular complement of carbohydrates at the interface between maternal and embryonic epithelia.[188] Other molecules have been described that may limit embryonic attachment, namely MUC-1. The disappearance of MUC-1 at the time of implantation in the rodent is timed to the establishment of uterine receptivity[189,190] and may account for the thinning in the glycocalyx that has been described. Studies in the human have been less conclusive and the role of MUC-1 in human implantation remains unresolved.[191,192] A reduction in two major components of basement membrane, namely laminin and type IV collagen, have been described for the luminal surface.

Complementary changes in embryonic ECM also occur. Embryonic elaboration of a specialized type of fibronectin has been described[193,194] and suggested to be the "glue" used by the embryo during implantation.[195] Such theories support the observation that known recognition sequences for integrins, such as arg-gly-asp (RGD), will block attachment and outgrowth of mouse embryos *in vitro*.[196] Fibronectin fragments containing the central cell-binding domain and the RGD site supported trophoblast outgrowth as well as native fibronectin[197] The shorter heparin-binding domain and an alternative non-RGD site did not support adhesion. Plasminogen activator (PA) activity in mouse embryos increased upon exposure to fibronectin, an effect that was blocked by RGD peptides.[198] Added fibronectin also enhanced embryonic matrix metalloproteinase secretion (see below),[194] and it has been shown that the MMP and fetal fibronectin secretion depend on integrins.[199]

B. MATRIX METALLOPROTEINASES AND THEIR INHIBITORS

Matrix metalloproteinases (MMPs) are zinc-containing endopeptidases that enzymatically digest certain extracellular matrix proteins and therefore play an important role in tissue remodeling processes.[200,201] The highly regulated expression and interaction of MMPs with other key endometrial and trophoblast enzymes, receptors, and growth factors suggest their singular importance in endometrial and embryonic physiology leading to successful implantation. In lieu of pregnancy, these molecules regulate the timely degradation and remodeling of the endometrial lining as part of menstruation.[202,203]

MMP nomenclature is not straightforward, as most of these enzymes have more than one name. The MMPs may be divided into three groups, based the enzymes' preferred substrates. A current list of MMPs is shown in Table 3.1. The gelatinases, gelatinase A (MMP-2) and gelatinase B (MMP-9), degrade type IV collagen and denatured collagens (gelatins). In addition, several collagenases exist, notably interstitial collagenase (MMP-1), neutrophil collagenase (MMP-8), collagenase 3 (MMP-13), and collagenase 4 (MMP-18, human). The collagenases degrade types

I, II, III, VII, and X collagen of the interstitial extracellular matrix. A third group consists of the stromelysins, made up of stromelysin-1 (MMP-3), matrilysin (MMP-7), stromelysin-2 (MMP-10), and stromelysin-3 (MMP-11). This group has the broadest specificity for their substrates, degrading types IV, V, and VII collagen, and laminin, fibronectin, gelatins, elastin, and proteoglycans.

The MMPs initially are secreted as inactive, pre-forms that must be activated by either proteases, denaturants, or heat.[204] Four different membrane-type MMPs, known as MT-MMPs, have been identified and are known to be effective activators of some MMPs such as MMP-2. Because many of these MMPs activate themselves or other members of this family, the possibility exists for a complex cascade of enzyme activation that might lead to uncontrolled degradation of the surrounding matrix were it not for the inhibitors of this process. Regulation of activity can occur via differential activation of the MMP or by the tissue inhibitors of metalloproteinases (TIMPs).

TABLE 3.1
Matrix Metalloproteinases

Class	Name	Substrate	Comments	Cell Source
Collagenases	MMP-1	Collagen I, II and III, VII, VIII, X	57 kDA	Endometrial stroma, invading cytotrophoblast
	MMP-8	Similar to MMP-1	85 kDA	
Gelatinases	MMP-2 (gelantinase A)	Type collagen IV gelatin	72 kDa	Endometrial stroma, invading cytotrophoblast
	MMP-9 (gelantinase B)	Type collagen IV gelatin	92 kDa	Endometrial stroma, invading cytotrophoblast
Stromelysin	MMP-3 (stromelysin-1)	Fibronectins, laminin, collagens III, IV, V, elastin, proteoglycan core proteins	60 kDa	Endometrial stroma
	MMP-10 (stromolysin-2)	Similar to MMP3	53 kDa	Endometrial stroma
	MMP-11 (stromolysin-3)	?	51 kDa	Endometrial epithelium
	MMP-7 (matrilysin)	Collagen IV, gelatin, fibronectin, proteoglycans	28 kDa	Proliferative endometrial epithelium
Membrane-type MMPs	MT-MMP-1 MT-MMP-2 MT-MMP-3	?	Activates MMP-2; transmembrane segments	?

Inhibition occurs per one of the three known tissue inhibitors of metalloproteinases (TIMPs).[205] These enzymes are tightly regulated, thus establishing a balance of MMP activity and inhibition in normal tissues. TIMP-1 inhibits all MMPs in active form and gelatinase B (MMP-9) in both latent and active forms. TIMP-2 binds to both forms of gelatinase A (MMP-2) and its activity on other MMPs is much lower. TIMP-3, expressed in both mouse and human, also inhibits MMPs.

The activities of MMPs include the regulation of cellular function through modification of the surrounding ECM. The term coined by Bissell, "dynamic reciprocity," describes the concept that a cell produces the ECM and then is altered by it through specific receptors on its cell surface. The signal generated by this interaction modifies the cell's phenotype including cell shape and gene expression.[206,207] Degradation of this material is another mechanism by which ECM and, therefore, cellular phenotype can be altered. Lochter and colleagues recently illustrated this with the over-expression of stromelysin-1 in mammary epithelial cells.[208] The activity of this MMP converted epithelial cells to a more mesenchymal phenotype. The researchers noted cleavage of E-cadherin-1, down regulation of cellular cytokeratins, up regulation of vimentin, induction of keratinocyte growth factor expression, up regulation of endogenous MMPs, and adoption of invasive behavior. Degradation of the surrounding ECM can also trigger cell migration[12] or even apoptosis.[209,210]

Important functional interactions occur between MMPs and other molecules in the embryo-endometrial complex that likely facilitate implantation. Perhaps the best example is the observation that engagement of a placental integrin with fibronectin induces MMP expression.[211] This is one of the earliest studies demonstrating a signal transduction role for integrins. Many of the behaviors of malignant cells that are considered abnormal mimic the invasive behavior of the early blastocyst. These include the activity of MMPs, growth factors, and integrin expression that occurs during the invasive phases of implantation. Membrane bound, polarized MMP or uPA activity that orchestrates invasion in cancer cells is used by the embryo during early implantation. Not surprisingly, many of the mechanisms of implantation have already been described first in cancer. These include the observation that MMPs interact with integrins, as major receptors for the ECM. MMP-2 binds to and is activated by the $\alpha v \beta 3$ integrin.[13] Surface MMP-2 allows cells to invade in the direction of their migration.[212] Neutralization of the $\alpha 3 \beta 1$ integrin increases MMP-2 production[213] and activation.[214] Matrilysin (MMP-7) specifically cleaves $\alpha 6 \beta 4$ integrin,[215] which may play a role in embryonic invasion through BM of the luminal epithelium. MMP-3 recently has been shown to cleave and release Hb-EGF from the membrane,[216] with possible relevance to embryo-endometrial interaction. Recent evidence shows that this growth factor improves embryo quality *in vitro*.[217]

The distribution of MMPs during trophoblast invasion has been well characterized.[218] MMP-1 appears in the basal lamina between proximal cell columns and in the villous stroma of the placenta. Invading cytotrophoblast exhibited uniform extracellular staining. MMP-2 was most active in the distal invasive areas of the cell columns, whereas MMP-3 is expressed uniformly throughout pregnancy in extravillous trophoblast cells along the entire invasive pathway, both intra and extracellularly. Decidual cells do not express MMP-3. MMP-9 appeared to have only faint staining but occurred within the entire invasive pathway. These studies have been corroborated with *in vitro* of trophoblast invasion as well.[219] Tissue inhibitors of matrix metalloproteinases also reside in the placenta.[220] The cytotrophoblasts that expressed MMPs are also those that exhibited the strongest cytoplasmic staining for TIMP-2. Thus, TIMP-2 may be involved in autoregulation of the invasive behavior of the trophoblast. As discussed below, decidual cells share in the expression of these inhibitors and provide a barrier to uncontrolled invasion of the embryo.[221] Studies demonstrate that both rodents and human placental invasiveness depends on production of MMP-9 (gelatinase B).[222] Increased MMP-9 expression in human trophoblast corresponds to an increase in TIMP-3.[223]

Distribution of MMPs in the endometrium points strongly to a role in endometrial remodeling, with maximal expression during the proliferative and the late secretory phase and with menstrual shedding.[203] Studies demonstrate that mRNA for pro-MMP-1 and 3 were detectable only during the perimenstrual part of the cycle. MMP-3 and 11 are suppressed by progesterone in stromal cells *in vitro*.[224,225] Production of all but MMP-2 could be stimulated by IL-1 and TNFα.[226] The cytotrophoblast collagenases exhibit similar regulation.[227] MMP-1, 3, and 9 are associated with degraded tissue in menstrual endometrium. Only 72-kD gelatinase (MMP-2) and tissue inhibitor of metalloproteinases-1 were detected throughout the cycle.[225] All of the MMPs were stromal in origin except MMP-7[225] and MMP-9.[228]

The invasive pathway involves molecular interactions that are both complex and elegant. Plasminogen, its activators, and its inhibitors participate in this process.[90] Plasmin derived from plasminogen is a protease that requires serine for its catalytic activity. In addition to activity in fibrinolysis, plasmin activates certain MMPs by cleaving pro-collagenase or pro-gelatinase B to their active forms leading eventually to degradation of the ECM. This process is tightly regulated with many of the controlling enzymes produced by the embryo, trophoblast, or syncytium. Regulation of plasminogen to plasmin conversion is stimulated by urokinase type plasminogen activator (uPA) and inhibited by alpha 2 macroglobulin (α2MG). uPA activity occurs in rodent and human endometria[229,230] and on human embryos,[231] and the receptor for uPA on the embryo and trophoblast directs its activity. Both mouse and human trophoblast express uPA[235,236] and uPA receptors are present on the trophoblast.[237] Mutations associated with reduced PA cause implantation failure.[238] α2MG has been described in the human endometrium as well, present in the stroma throughout the menstrual cycle.[232] Activity of PAs is tightly regulated by specific inhibitors of PAs (PAI and PAI2), which bind and inactivate PAs.[233,234] Plasmin also activates TGFβ from its latent to active form which in turn stimulates TIMP and PAI production, which inhibit plasmin activation. These pathways are illustrated in Figure 3.3.

C. INTEGRIN CELL ADHESION MOLECULES

Research interest in ECM receptors as modulators of endometrial and embryonic function has increased. Damsky, Fisher, and others finally established integrins' role in implantation by defining the developmental progression of integrins on the early embryo[239] and placenta.[240,178] Noninvasive epithelial trophoblast stem cells express α6 integrins whereas invasive cytotrophoblast up regulate α1 and α5 integrin subunits. Recently, the invasive phenotype of the cytotrophoblast has been shown to

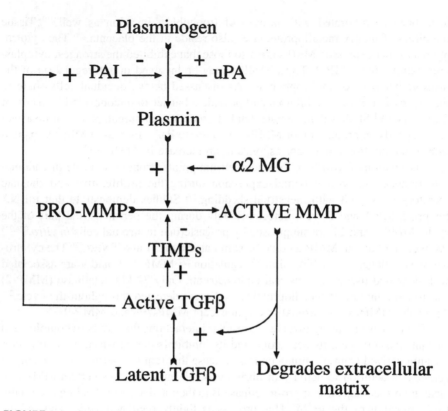

FIGURE 3.3 Schematic of plasmin/matrix metalloproteinase-mediated degradation pathways during implantation and the factors that regulate their activity. The conversion of plasminogen to plasmin is tightly controlled by activators and inhibitors, many of which come from the trophoblast. PAI = plasminogen activator inhibitor; uPA = urokinase plasminogen activator; α2MG = alpha 2 macroglobulin; MMP = matrix metalloproteinases, TIMPs = tissue inhibitors of metalloproteinases; TGFβ = transforming growth factor β.

express a series of endothelial integrins (α1β1, α4β1, and αvβ3) along with VCAM. This shift in integrin expression allows the invading embryonic cells to blend in with the maternal endothelial cells as invasion of the maternal vessels progresses.[241] This invasive phenotype is disrupted by the clinical situation of preeclampsia, in which placentation is shallow and associated with maternal hypertension, proteinuria, and poor fetal growth. Researchers now recognize this condition as a failure of the placenta to adopt the vascular and invasive phenotype[242,243] and suggest that it may result from placental hypoxia.[244]

The endometrium is also a site of integrin expression that may correspond to the establishment of uterine receptivity towards implantation.[6,179,245–248] The window of implantation first suggested by Finn[249] has been studied in animal models.[35,36] Hertig and colleagues suggested that in the human this window occurs around the mid-secretory phase. These researchers performed secretory phase hysterectomies on women who were thought to be pregnant. They demonstrated that embryos found in uteri obtained prior to cycle day 20 were all free floating in the tubes or uterus while embryos from day 21 and beyond had all attached to the uterine lining.[250] These data and more recent studies utilizing donor/recipient cycles[26,251] suggest that attachment occurs around cycle day 20 of an idealized 28 day cycle and that there are temporal limits on the embryo's ability to implant.

While many molecular markers have been proposed to identify this period of receptivity,[75] the most intensively studied are the integrins.[6,179,245] Like the tropho-blast, endometrial cells display alteration of integrins in the epithelium and decidua during and after implantation.[179,180] Three integrins appear to frame the window of implantation, being co-expressed only during cycle days 20 to 24, the putative window of implantation (Figure 3.4). The luminal epithelium expresses both $\alpha v \beta 3$ and $\alpha v \beta 5$ on the apical pole, suggesting a role for these integrins in embryo-endometrial interaction.[252,253] These integrins recognize the three amino acid sequence arg-gly-asp (RDG) which has been implicated in trophoblast attachment and outgrowth.[196,197] Researchers find the pattern of integrin expression, as potential markers of the receptive endometrium, to be quite interesting. Such patterns provide clues about the factors that favor the establishment of receptivity and potential mechanisms of endometrial-mediated trophoblast invasion. Conversely, examining the failure of normal endometrial integrin expression may help diagnose and treat implantation failure[6,246,254] and assist in the diagnosis of unexplained infertility.[247]

The study of endometrial integrins also may provide clues to better understand the molecular regulation of uterine receptivity. The secretory phase pattern of three epithelial integrins, including $\alpha 1 \beta 1$, $\alpha 4 \beta 1$, and $\alpha v \beta 3$ suggests that steroid hormones may participate in their expression. We know that estrogen and progesterone play a major role in preparation of the endometrium. With the discovery of the $\alpha 1 \beta 1$ collagen/laminin receptor (VLA-1) and its expression on secretory phase endometrium, Tabibzadeh and Satyaswaroop demonstrated that progesterone could up regulate this integrin directly in endometrial explants in vitro.[255] This has since been confirmed using the well-differentiated cell line, Ishikawa cells.[256] Researchers suspect that $\alpha 4 \beta 1$ will also turn out to be regulated by progesterone in the endometrium.

The expression of $\alpha v \beta 3$ integrin on cycle day 20, 6 to 8 days after ovulation, is more difficult to explain, as it appears well after the rise in serum progesterone has begun. In 1988, researchers demonstrated that endometrial epithelial cells selec-tively lose progesterone receptor (PR) while stromal cells maintain expression of this receptor.[64,65,257] PR is lost because of rising serum progesterone levels, driving down its own receptor as well as the estrogen receptor. This shift in receptor content occurs immediately before the onset of uterine receptivity on cycle day 19 to 20 (post LH surge day 5 to 6) and occurs at the time of implantation in other mammals.[66] Based on this observation, scientists believe that $\alpha n \beta 3$ (and uterine receptivity in general) is inhibited by the sex steroids. Loss of their receptors may signal a loss of inhibitory control at the time of implantation. In addition to the down regulation by sex steroids, TGFα and EGF significantly enhance the expression of epithelial $\alpha v \beta 3$ integrin expression, suggesting that the loss of epithelial steroid receptors signals a shift from endocrine to paracrine control and advancing a role for the stroma in directing changes in the overlying epithelium.[70,258] Because the early blastocyst also expresses a rich pattern of integrins,[239,259] including αv-containing

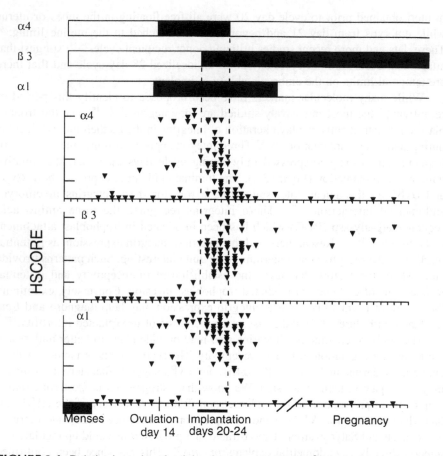

FIGURE 3.4 Relative intensity of staining for the epithelial α4, β3, and α1 integrin subunits throughout the menstrual cycle and in early pregnancy. Immunohistochemical staining was assessed by a blinded observer using the semi-quantitative HSCORE (ranging from 0 to 4) and correlated to the estimate of histological dating based on pathologic criteria or by LMP in patients undergoing therapeutic pregnancy termination. The negative staining (open bars) was shown for immunostaining of an HSCORE 0.7, for each of the three integrin subunits. Positive staining for all three integrin subunits was seen only during a four day interval corresponding to cycle day 20 to 24, based on histologic dating criteria of Noyes et al.[5] This interval of integrin co-expression corresponds to the putative window of implantation. Of the three, only the αvβ3 integrin was seen in the epithelium of pregnant endometrium. (From Lessey, B. A. et al., *Fertility and Sterility*, 62, 497, 1994. With permission.)

integrins such as αvβ1, αvβ3, and αvβ5 on the outer exposed apical surfaces, questions remain as to whether these cell adhesion molecules interact to adhere embryonic and maternal surfaces.

D. OTHER MARKERS OF UTERINE RECEPTIVITY

A structural feature of receptive endometrium that is also used as a marker of receptive endometrium is the pinopod, first described by Psychoyos and Mandon.[260]

These striking modifications of the luminal epithelium are visible by electron microscopy and appear to be involved in absorption of luminal fluid and thinning of the glycocalyx.[261] The value of pinopods lies in the correlation between their expression and the putative window of implantation.[262,263] Like other markers, pinopod absence may portend poor reproductive outcome[264] or enhancement of receptivity in artificial cycle.[265]

A growing number of proteins are candidate markers for uterine receptivity in the endometrium.[75] Besides the integrins, mucins were suggested early on as detectable markers for both LPD and unexplained infertility.[87,266] MUC-1 is a large membrane-bound glycoprotein that appears to barr implantation when the endometrium is nonreceptive and must be removed at the time of implantation in both rodents[189] and primates.[267] The role of MUC-1 in human endometrium is less clear, however, since it is present throughout the secretory phase in normal cycles.[268] The glycoprotein glycodelin (PP14) is a major secretory product of the glandular epithelium and seems to detect hormonally inadequate cycles.[269,270] Glycodelin may play a role in the immune response to pregnancy and has been shown to prevent egg-sperm interaction.[81] Epithelial progesterone receptors vary within the endometrium during the menstrual cycle[64] and could be used as a marker of endometrial progression. The relative levels of PR shift in cycles from women with LPD.[69] Novel cell adhesion molecules recently have been described at the time of implantation in either epithelial or stromal cells and have been suggested to play a key role in initial embryo/trophoblast interaction. These include trophinin[271] and cadherin-11.[272,273] Several of the cytokines and growth factors, including LIF,[41,102,105] Hb-EGF,[156,158] and IGF-II,[274] appear during the receptive period in humans. The classic studies by Stewart et al.[41] show that LIF is critical to implantation as the null mutant fails to undergo implantation and decidualization. Mouse embryos will adhere to cells expressing Hb-EGF,[159] suggesting multiple potential roles for this growth factor. Other marker proteins that appear critical to implantation in rodents such as the Hoxa-10 transcription factor,[42,43] calcitonin,[275] and cyclo-oygenase-2, a rate limiting enzyme in prostaglandin synthesis,[108] appear to be promising markers in the endometrium of humans as well.[276,277] Understanding the role of these gene products in endometrial-embryo interactions adds to our understanding of the mechanism of implantation, both by elucidation of function and the study of their regulation.

E. Defects in Uterine Receptivity, Infertility, and Recurrent Pregnancy Loss

The synchronous development of the endometrial and embryonic cells appears to be critical for successful implantation. Loss of this synchrony causes pregnancy loss in animal models[84] and in humans.[278] If receptivity is delayed or prevented, recurrent pregnancy loss or infertility results. Where the major insult occurs remains unclear, but may include loss of embryo viability or a failure of the timely rescue of the corpus luteum. Using specific uterine receptivity markers, scientists construct a paradigm for discussing such defects.

Luteal phase defect (LPD) is a major cause of infertility and recurrent pregnancy loss and results from an inadequate progesterone level or a diminished response to ovarian steroids.[83] LPD commonly occurs in women with unexplained infertility.[279] The use of marker proteins has been advocated for the diagnosis of LPD.[87] Women with recurrent pregnancy loss exhibit reduced levels of serum glycodelin (PP14), for example.[269] Low hCG and relaxin levels are also found in pregnancies that fail, perhaps reflecting the loss of CL function.[280] Women with recurrent pregnancy loss also display specific isoform differences that may reflect on the quality of the embryo or the embryo-uterine interaction.[30]

We[246,247,281] and others[282] have suggested that integrins could be useful to detect such alterations in endometrial development that may predispose women to infertility or pregnancy loss. The appearance of the $\alpha v \beta 3$ integrin at the time of implantation offers a useful internal marker of endometrial progression that consistently is missing in the presence of LPD and associated histologic delay.[6] In addition, the successful treatment of LPD with hormone support results in a return of the expected $\alpha v \beta 3$ expression.[247]

Evidence also exists for a second type of endometrial receptivity defect that is unrelated to endometrial histology. Such defects appear in numerous observations associated with the disorder known as endometriosis, in which the lining of the uterine cavity gains access to the peritoneal surfaces, where it attaches and grows causing pelvic pain and/or infertility. Animal[283,284] and clinical studies in donor insemination programs,[285] lower pregnancy rates in IVF cycles,[286] and beneficial effects of treatment on pregnancy rates[287] all point to an association of this disease with implantation failure. A subset of these patients also exhibit aberrant integrin expression.[246,247] We recently extended these findings to include an effect of hydrosalpinges on endometrial integrin expression.[254] Accumulating data support a detrimental effect of hydrosalpinx fluid on implantation in human reproduction.[288-292] An endometrial cavity bathed in hydrosalpingeal fluid at the time of implantation may alter the outcome of IVF or lead to infertility in women with unofficial disease. Analogous to the return of normal integrin and PR expression in women with successfully treated LPD,[69,247] salpingectomy resulted in a return of normal endometrial histology and integrin expression in most women and a high pregnancy rate in women with unilateral disease.[254] Like endometriosis, inflammatory cytokines in the peritoneal fluid or within the hydrosalpinx may alter normal endometrial function and account for this dysfunction of the endometrium.

This concept of two distinct types of uterine receptivity defects is shown in Figure 3.5. The presence of delayed histology (Type I) and occult (Type II) defects increasingly is reported using other markers, including the mucins,[87,266,293] endometrial bleeding associated factor (ebaf),[294] PP14,[270] other integrins,[282] and leukemia inhibitor factor (LIF).[105] Greater diagnostic and treatment options prompt considerable interest in establishing the existence of such defects. The study of such defects could also lead to safer or easier methods of contraception.

It is interesting to note that age of the uterus does not appear to affect implantation;[295,296] rather the age of the oocyte appears to be critical.[297] This was illustrated recently by the pregnancy and subsequent birth by a 63-year-old woman in a donor oocyte program.[298] This is not to say that age has no effect on uterine receptivity since conditions such as endometriosis, for example, may worsen with age and probably account for the increased difficulty that women experience with fertility

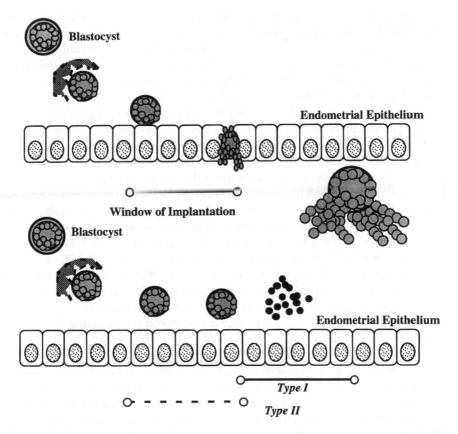

FIGURE 3.5 A proposed model of defects of uterine receptivity. The upper panel depicts the normal period of uterine receptivity corresponding to embryo attachment to the uterine lining. In the lower panel, a shift in this window of receptivity (type I defect) or an occult absence of this period of receptivity (type II defect) might result in failure of implantation. (From Lessey, B. A. et al., *Fertility and Sterility*, 63, 535, 1995. With permission.)

after delaying childbirth to their 30s. A lack of estrogen may be protective as illustrated in women who have hypothalamic amenorrhea who exhibit higher than expected cycle fecundibility compared to normal women.[299] This study also demonstrated that women with polycystic ovarian syndrome (who do not ovulate but have higher serum androgen levels) have reduced fertility compared to controls, illustrating yet another potential defect in uterine receptivity that may worsen with age.

VII. ENDOMETRIAL-EMBRYONIC DIALOGUES

Based on the information reviewed thus far, implantation materializes as an exceedingly complex and richly orchestrated series of cellular events. While much of the uterine preparation for implantation occurs without direct embryonic involvement, increasing evidence suggests that endometrium and the embryo may be targets for paracrine or juxtacrine signals that facilitate attachment and invasion. Likewise, data now exist that support a role for the endometrium in limiting placental invasion. Embryonic signals are also recognized as important to rescue the corpus luteum, but direct effects of hCG on the reproductive tract may also occur. While much remains to be learned about these signals, the information now available interprets a rich dialogue between maternal and embryonic cells.

One of the early signals for implantation in the rodent is estrogen. The presence of estrogen receptors in the early embryo has been documented,[300] and estrogen appears to be an important nidatory stimulus. Based on extensive studies with embryos transferred into delayed implantation recipients, Dey and colleagues demonstrated that the embryos' state of readiness determines the window of receptivity in this species.[39] Estrogen injection in the delayed implantation model corresponds to rapid implantation and coordinated expression of key endometrial proteins including COX-2[108] and Hb-EGF[156] which increase in response to the blastocyst.

The hatched human embryo produces hCG as cytotrophoblast differentiate into syncytiotrophoblast.[301] As outlined in Section III, hCG is critical for CL rescue and can be detected as early as post-ovulatory day 18 to 20.[26] In addition to effects on the CL, hCG also may have direct effects on the endometrium. Reshef et al. described gonadotropin receptors in the human reproductive tract as well.[302]

As mentioned earlier, ECM may play a role in embryo-endometrial signaling. Elaboration of the alternatively spliced form of fibronectin (fetal fibronectin) may form an adhesive interface between embryo and endometrium,[303] and exogenously added laminin or fetal fibronectin resulted in increased MMP-2 expression.[194] Because the early blastocyst also produces laminin,[304] MMP-2 expression by the embryo or endometrium may release proteolytic fragments of laminin that have been shown to stimulate cell migration as an early inducer of the invasive phenotype.[12] MMP production by the embryo also could release decidual or epithelial Hb-EGF[305] which itself promotes embryo development[217] and cytotrophoblast invasiveness.[306] Other factors from the endometrium may facilitate embryo quality. Embryo quality is improved when it is co-cultured with cells from the reproductive tract.[307] Factors such as LIF and others have been implicated, though embryo quality now improves through the use of defined media in IVF with excellent success rates.[308]

IL-1 derived from macrophages, endothelium, or trophoblast stimulates the epithelial and stromal cells of the endometrium to produce PGE2.[118,309] IL-1 receptor antagonist limits PGE2 production[309] and blocks implantation in the mouse.[123] This cytokine also appears to be a potentially important signal to the maternal endometrium to stimulate expression of key epithelial integrins.[310] Similar studies involving TNFα and IL-1 show bioactivity on the expression of stromal integrins, including the up regulation of αvβ3 and the down regulation of α6β1.[311] Additionally, endometrial growth factors or cytokines may alter embryonic integrins present on the blastocyst.[259] Matrilysin (MMP-7) specifically cleaves α6β4 integrin[215] suggesting a mechanism for loosening the luminal surface adhesiveness. Similar embryo-derived TNFα mechanisms could reduce epithelial integrity. Loss of adhesion was induced by TNFα and was associated with the disordered expression of cadherin/beta-catenin at the sites of cell-cell contact.[312] The precise relationship between these cytokines and implantation remain to be defined.

The cytotrophoblasts' invasive process does not go unchecked. One mechanism to prevent uncontrolled invasion is the regulated expression of endometrial TIMPs and inhibitors of plasmin. Studies involving the insulin-like growth factor binding protein 1 (IGFBP-1) have also been instructive. Jones et al. demonstrated that IGFBP-1, acting through its RGD site, interacts specifically with the $\alpha 5 \beta 1$ integrin to stimulate migration.[177] Irving and Lala also showed that TGF-β up regulates integrin expression and reduces migratory ability of the invasive trophoblast, whereas IGF-II has no effect on integrin expression, but stimulates migration. IGFBP-1, which mitigates the action of IGF molecules, might be expected to limit migration on this basis, but investigators found that it did the opposite.[313] This positive effect could be neutralized by blocking the $\alpha 5 \beta 1$ integrin. While stimulating migration, IGFBP-1 also limits invasiveness through interaction with the trophoblast $\alpha 5 \beta 1$ integrin receptor.[79]

ACKNOWLEDGMENTS

The authors would like to thank de Anne Guarino for her skillful artwork and Jendia Goodwin for her assistance with preparation of this chapter.

REFERENCES

1. Enders, A. C., Contributions of comparative studies to understanding mechanisms of implantation, in *Endocrinology of Embryo-Endometrium Interactions*, Glasser, S. R., Mulholland, J., and Psychoyos, A., Eds., Plenum Press, New York and London, 1994, 11–16.
2. Croxatto, H. B., Ortiz, M. E., Diaz, S., Hess, R., Balmaceda, J., and Croxatto, H. D., Studies on the duration of egg transport by the human oviduct. II. Ovum location at various intervals following luteinizing hormone peak, *Am. J. Obstet. Gynecol.*, 132, 629, 1978.
3. Buster, J., Bustillo, M., Rodi, I., Cohen, S., Hamilton, M., Simon, J., Thorneycroft, I., and Marshall, J., Biologic and morphologic development of donated human ova recovered by nonsurgical uterine lavage, *Am. J. Obstet. Gynecol.*, 153, 211, 1985.
4. Brenner, R. M. and West, N. B., Hormonal regulation of the reproductive tract in female mammals, *Ann. Rev. Physiol.*, 37, 273, 1975.
5. Noyes, R. W., Hertig, A. I., and Rock, J., Dating the endometrial biopsy, *Fertil. Steril.*, 1, 3, 1950.
6. Lessey, B. A., Damjanovich, L., Coutifaris, C., Castelbaum, A., Albelda, S. M., and Buck, C. A., Integrin adhesion molecules in the human endometrium. Correlation with the normal and abnormal menstrual cycle, *J. Clin. Invest.*, 90, 188, 1992.
7. Enders, A. C., Current topic: structural responses of the primate endometrium to implantation, *Placenta*, 12, 309, 1991.
8. Blankenship, T. N. and King, B. F., Developmental changes in the cell columns and trophoblastic shell of the macaque placenta: an immunohistochemical study localizing type IV collagen, laminin, fibronectin and cytokeratins, *Cell Tissue Res.*, 274, 457, 1993.

9. Aplin, J. D., Charlton, A. K., and Ayad, S., An immunohistochemical study of human endometrial extracellular matrix during the menstrual cycle and first trimester of pregnancy, *Cell Tissue Res.*, 253, 231, 1988.

10. Werb, Z., ECM and cell surface proteolysis: regulating cellular ecology, *Cell*, 91, 439, 1997.

11. Werb, Z., Tremble, P. M., Behrendtsen, O., Crowley, E., and Damsky, C. H., Signal transduction through the fibronectin receptor induces collagenase and stromelysin gene expression, *J. Cell Biol.*, 109, 877, 1989.

12. Giannelli, G., Falk-Marziller, J., Schiraldi, O., Stetler-Stevenson, W. G., and Quaranta, V., Induction of cell migration by matrix metalloproteinase-2 cleavage of laminin-5, *Science*, 277, 225, 1997.

13. Brooks, P. C., Strömblad, S., Sanders, L. C., Von Schalscha, T. L., Aimes, R. T., Stetler-Stevenson, W. G., Quigley, J. P., and Cheresh, D. A., Localization of matrix metalloproteinase MMP-2 to the surface of invasive cells by interaction with integrin $\alpha v \beta 3$, *Cell*, 85, 683, 1996.

14. Enders, A. C., Implantation (Embryology), *Encyclopedia of Human Biology*, 4, 423, 1991.

15. Kokawa, K., Shikone, T., and Nakano, R., Apoptosis in the human uterine endometrium during the menstrual cycle, *J. Clin. Endocrinol. Metab.*, 81, 4144, 1996.

16. Tabibzadeh, S., Zupi, E., Babaknia, A., Liu, R., Marconi, D., and Romanini, C., Site and menstrual cycle-dependent expression of proteins of the tumour necrosis factor (TNF) receptor family, and BCL-2 oncoprotein and phase-specific production of TNFα in human endometrium, *Hum. Reprod.*, 10, 277, 1995.

17. Kothapalli, R., Buyuksal, I., Wu, S. Q., Chegini, N., and Tabibzadeh, S., Detection of *ebaf*, a novel human gene of the transforming growth factor β superfamily—Association of gene expression with endometrial bleeding, *J. Clin. Invest.*, 99, 2342, 1997.

18. Salamonsen, L. A., Matrix metalloproteinases and endometrial remodelling, *Cell Biol. Int.*, 18, 1139, 1994.

19. Shikone, T., Yamoto, M., Kokawa, K., Yamashita, K., Nishimori, K., and Nakano, R., Apoptosis of human corpora lutea during cyclic luteal regression and early pregnancy, *J. Clin. Endocrinol. Metab.*, 81, 2376, 1996.

20. Csapo, A. I., Pulkkinen, M. O., and Wiest, W., Effects of luteectomy and progesterone replacement therapy in early pregnant patients, *Am. J. Obstet. Gyn.*, 115, 759, 1972.

21. Atkinson, L. E., Hotchkiss, J., Fritz, G. R., Surve, A. H., Neill, J. D., and Knobil, E., Circulating levels of steroids and chorionic gonadotropin during pregnancy in the rhesus monkey with special attention to the rescue of the corpus luteum in early pregnancy, *Biol. Reprod.*, 12, 335, 1975.

22. Bazer, F. W., Mediators of maternal recognition of pregnancy in mammals, *Proc. Soc. Exp. Biol. Med.*, 199, 373, 1992.

23. Bartol, F. F., Roberts, R. M., Bazer, F. W., and Thatcher, W. W., Characterization of proteins produced *in vitro* by bovine endometrial explants, *Biol. Reprod.*, 33, 745, 1985.

24. Dubois, D. H. and Bazer, F. W., Effect of porcine conceptus secretory proteins on *in vitro* secretion of prostaglandins-F2 alpha and -E2 from luminal and myometrial surfaces of endometrium from cyclic and pseudopregnant gilts, *Prostaglandins*, 41, 283, 1991.

25. Spies, H. G. and Nieswender, G. D., Levels of prolactin, LH, and FSH in the serum of intact and pelvic-neuroectomized rats, *Endocrinology*, 88, 937, 1971.

26. Bergh, P. A. and Navot, D., The impact of embryonic development and endometrial maturity on the timing of implantation, *Fertil. Steril.*, 58, 537, 1992.

27. Hertig, A. T., Rock, J., and Adams, E. C., A description of 34 human ova within the first 17 days of development, *Am. J. Anat.*, 98, 435, 1956.

28. Seshagiri, P. B. and Hearn, J. P., *In vitro* development of *in vivo* produced rhesus monkey morulae and blastocysts to hatched, attached, and post-attached blastocyst stages: morphology and early secretion of chorionic gonadotrophin, *Hum. Reprod.*, 8, 279, 1993.

29. Jameson, J. L. and Hollenberg, A. N., Regulation of chorionic gonadotropin gene expression, *Endocr. Rev.*, 14, 203, 1993.

30. O'Connor, J. F., Ellish, N., Kakuma, T., Schlatterer, J., and Kovalevskaya, G., Differential urinary gonadotropin profiles in early pregnancy and early pregnancy loss, *Prenatal Diagnos.*, 18, 1232, 1998.

31. Clark, G. F., Oehninger, S., Patankar, M. S., Koistinen, R., Dell, A., Morris, H. R., Koistinen, H., and Seppälä, M., A role for glycoconjugates in human development: the human feto-embryonic defence system hypothesis, *Hum. Reprod.*, 11, 467, 1996.

32. Psychoyos, A., Hormonal control of ovoimplantation, *Vitams Horm.*, 31, 201, 1973.

33. McLaren, A., Blastocyst activation, in *The Regulation of Mammalian Reproduction*, Segal, S. J., Crozier, R., Corfman, P. A., and Condliffe, P. G., Eds., Thomas Springfield, London, 1973, 321–334.

34. Finn, C. A. and Martin, L., The control of implantation, *J. Reprod. Fertil.*, 39, 195, 1974.

35. McLaren, A. and Michie, D., Studies on the transfer of fertilized mouse eggs to uterine foster-mothers, *J. Exp. Biol.*, 33, 394, 1954.

36. Hodgen, G. D., Surrogate embryo transfer combined with estrogen-progesterone therapy in monkeys: implantation, gestation, and delivery without ovaries, *JAMA*, 250, 2167, 1983.

37. Psychoyos, A., Uterine receptivity for nidation, *Ann. NY Acad. Sci.*, 476, 36, 1986.

38. Weitlauf, H. M., Biology of implantation, in *The Physiology of Reproduction*, Knobil, E. and Neill, J. D., Eds., Raven Press, New York, 1994, 391–440.

39. Paria, B. C., Huet-Hudson, Y. M., and Dey, S. K., Blastocyst's state of activity determines the "window" of implantation in the receptive mouse uterus, *Proc. Natl. Acad. Sci. USA*, 90, 10159, 1993.

40. Klemke, R. L. and Weitlauf, H. M., Comparison of the ontogeny of specific cell surface determinants on normal and delayed implanting mouse embryos, *J. Reprod. Fertil.*, 99, 167, 1993.

41. Stewart, C. L., Kaspar, P., Brunet, L. J., Bhatt, H., Gadi, I., Köntgen, F., and Abbondanzo, J. S., Blastocyst implantation depends on maternal expression of leukemia inhibitory factor, *Nature*, 359, 76, 1992.

42. Satokata, I., Benson, G., and Maas, R., Sexually dimorphic sterility phenotypes in Hoxa-10 deficient mice, *Nature*, 374, 460, 1995.

43. Benson, G. V., Lim, H. J., Paria, B. C., Satokata, I., Dey, S. K., and Maas, R. L., Mechanisms of reduced fertility in Hoxa-10 mutant mice: uterine homeosis and loss of maternal Hoxa-10 expression, *Development*, 122, 2687, 1996.

44. Abbondanzo, S. J., Cullinan, E. B., McIntyre, K., Labow, M. A., and Stewart, C. L., Reproduction in mice lacking a functional type 1 IL-1 receptor, *Endocrinology*, 137, 3598, 1996.

45. Hynes, R. O. and Bader, B. L., Targeted mutations in integrins and their ligands: their implications for vascular biology, *Thromb. Haemost.*, 78, 83, 1997.

46. Anderson, T. L., Olson, G. E., and Hoffman, L. H., Stage specific alterations in the apical membrane glycoprotiens of endometrial epithelial cells related to implantation in rabbits, *Biol. Reprod.*, 34, 701, 1986.

47. Tarantino, S., Verhage, H. G., and Fazleabas, A. T., Regulation of insulin-like growth factor-binding proteins in the baboon (Papio anubis) uterus during early pregnancy, *Endocrinolology*, 130, 2354, 1992.

48. Satyaswaroop, P. G., Bressler, R. S., De La Pena, M. M., and Gurpide, E., Isolation and culture of human endometrial glands, *J. Clin. Endocrinol. Metab.*, 48, 639, 1979.

49. Kliman, H. J., Nestler, J. E., Sermasi, E., Sanger, J. M., and Strauss, J. F., III, Purification, characterization, and *in vitro* differentiation of cytotrophoblasts from human term placentae, *Endocrinology*, 118, 1567, 1986.

50. Coutifaris, C., Babalola, G. O., Feinberg, R. F., Kao, L.-C., Kliman, H. J., and Strauss, J. F., III, Purified human cytotrophoblasts: surrogates for the blastocyst in *in vitro* models of implantation?, in *Advances in Assisted Reproductive Technologies*, Mashiach, S., Ed., Plenum Press, New York, 1990, 687–695.

51. Sengupta, J., Given, R. L., Carey, J. B., and Weitlauf, H. M., Primary culture of mouse endometrium on floating collagen gels: a potential *in vitro* model for implantation, *Ann. NY Acad. Sci.*, 476, 75, 1986.

52. Shiotani, M., Noda, Y., and Mori, T., Embryo-dependent induction of uterine receptivity assessed by an *in vitro* model of implantation in mice, *Biol. Reprod.*, 49, 794, 1993.

53. Thie, M., Harrach-Ruprecht, B., Sauer, H., Fuchs, P., Albers, A., and Denker, H.-W., Cell adhesion to the apical pole of epithelium: a function of cell polarity, *Eur. J. Cell Biol.*, 66, 180, 1995.

54. Classen-Linke, I., Kusche, M., Knauthe, R., and Beier, H. M., Establishment of a human endometrial cell culture system and characterization of its polarized hormone responsive epithelial cells, *Cell Tissue Res.*, 287, 171, 1997.

55. Dudley, D. J., Hatasaka, H. H., Branch, D. W., Hammond, E., and Mitchell, M. D., A human endometrial explant system: validation and potential applications, *Am. J. Obstet. Gynecol.*, 167, 1774, 1992.

56. Negishi, M., Sugimoto, Y., and Ichikawa, A., Molecular mechanisms of diverse actions of prostanoid receptors, *Biochim. Biophys. Acta*, 1259, 109, 1995.

57. Shoyab, M., Plowman, G. D., McDonald, V. L., Bradley, J. G., and Todaro, G. J., Structure and function of human amphiregulin: a member of the epidermal growth factor family, *Science*, 243, 1074, 1989.

58. Baulieu, E. E., Contragestion and other clinical applications of RU-486, an antiprogesterone at the receptor, *Science*, 245, 1351, 1989.

59. Katzenellenbogen, B. S., Dynamics of steroid hormone receptor action, *Ann. Rev. Physiol.*, 42, 17, 1980.

60. Flickinger, G. L., Elsner, C., Illington, D. V., Muechler, E. K., and Mikhail, G., Estrogen and progesterone receptors in the female genital tract of humans and monkeys, *Ann. NY Acad. Sci.*, 286, 180, 1977.

61. Sanborn, B. M., Kuo, K. S., and Held, B., Estrogen and progestogen binding site concentrations in human endometrium and cervix throughout the menstrual cycle and in tissue from women taking oral contraceptives, *J. Steroid Biochem.*, 9, 951, 1978.

62. Lessey, B. A., Wahawisan, R., and Gorell, T. A., Hormonal regulation of cytoplasmic estrogen and progesterone receptors in the beagle uterus and oviduct, *Mol. Cell Endocrinol.*, 21, 171, 1981.

63. Savouret, J. F., Chauchereau, A., Misrahi, M., Lescop, P., Mantel, A., Bailly, A., and Milgrom, E., The progesterone receptor. Biological effects of progestins and anti-progestins, *Hum. Reprod.*, 9 Suppl. 1, 7, 1994.

64. Lessey, B. A., Killam, A. P., Metzger, D. A., Haney, A. F., Greene, G. L., and McCarty, K. S., Jr., Immunohistochemical analysis of human uterine estrogen and progesterone receptors throughout the menstrual cycle, *J. Clin. Endocrinol. Metab.*, 67, 334, 1988.

65. Garcia, E., Bouchard, P., De Brux, J., Berdah, J., Frydman, R., Schaison, G., Milgrom, E., and Berrot-Applanat, M., Use of immunoctyochemistry of progesterone and estrogen receptors for endometrial dating, *J. Clin. Endocrinol. Metab.*, 67, 80, 1988.

66. Geisert, R. D., Pratt, T. N., Bazer, F. W., Mayes, J. S., and Watson, G. H., Immuno-cytochemical localization and changes in endometrial progestin receptor protein during the porcine oestrous cycle and early pregnancy, *Reprod. Fertil. Dev.*, 6, 749, 1994.

67. Mead, R. A. and Eroschenko, V. P., Changes in uterine estrogen and progesterone receptors during delayed implantation and early implantation in the spotted skunk, *Biol. Reprod.*, 53, 827, 1995.

68. Lessey, B. A., Castelbaum, A. J., Somkuti, S. G., Yuan, L., and Chwalisz, K., Clinical significance of integrin cell adhesion molecules as markers of endometrial receptivity, in *Targeting the Endometrium for Contraception*, Beier, H. and Chwalisz, K., Eds., Springer-Verlag, Berlin, 1997, 193–221.

69. Lessey, B. A., Yeh, I. T., Castelbaum, A. J., Fritz, M. A., Ilesanmi, A. O., Korzeniowski, P., Sun, J. H., and Chwalisz, K., Endometrial progesterone receptors and markers of uterine receptivity in the window of implantation, *Fertil. Steril.*, 65, 477, 1996.

70. Somkuti, S. G., Yuan, L., Fritz, M. A., and Lessey, B. A., Epidermal growth factor and sex steroids dynamically regulate a marker of endometrial receptivity in Ishikawa cells, *J. Clin. Endocrinol. Metab.*, 82, 2192, 1997.

71. Slayden, O. D., Zelinski-Wooten, M. B., Chwalisz, K., Stouffer, R. L., and Brenner, R. M., Chronic treatment of cycling rhesus monkeys with low doses of the antiprogestin ZK 137 316: morphometric assessment of the uterus and oviduct, *Hum. Reprod.*, 13, 269, 1998.

72. Joshi, S. G., Progestin-regulated proteins of the human endometrium, *Semin. Reprod. Endocrinol.*, 1, 221, 1983.

73. Bell, S. C. and Drife, J. O., Secretory proteins of the endometrium—potential markers for endometrial dysfunction, *Baillieres. Clin. Obstet. Gynaecol.*, 3, 271, 1989.

74. Fazleabas, A. T., Hild-Petito, S., and Verhage, H. G., Secretory proteins and growth factors of the baboon (Papio anubis) uterus: potential roles in pregnancy, *Cell Biol. Int.*, 18, 1145, 1994.

75. Ilesanmi, A. O., Hawkins, D. A., and Lessey, B. A., Immunohistochemical markers of uterine receptivity in the human endometrium, *Microscopy Res. Tech.*, 25, 208, 1993.

76. Rutanen, E. M., Koistinen, R., Sjoberg, J., Julkunen, M., Wahlstrom, T., Bohn, H., and Seppälä, M., Synthesis of placental protein 12 by human endometrium, *Endo-crinology*, 118, 1067, 1986.

77. Julkunen, M., Koistinen, R., Sjoberg, J., Rutanen, E. M., Wahlstrom, T., and Seppälä, M., Secretory endometrium synthesizes placental protein 14, *Endocrinology*, 118, 1782, 1986.

78. Bell, S. C., Patel, S. R., Jackson, J. A., and Waites, G. T., Major secretory protein of human decidualized endometrium in pregnancy is an insulin-like growth factor-binding protein, *J. Endocrinol.*, 118, 317, 1988.

79. Giudice, L. C., Multifaceted roles for IGFBP-1 in human endometrium during implantation and pregnancy, *Ann. NY Acad. Sci.*, 828, 146, 1997.

80. Speroff, L., The effect of aging on fertility, *Curr. Opin. Obstet. Gynecol.*, 6, 115, 1994.

81. Oehninger, S., Coddington, C. C., Hodgen, G. D., and Seppälä, M., Factors affecting fertilization: endometrial placental protein 14 reduces the capacity of human spermatozoa to bind to the human zona pellucida, *Fertil. Steril.*, 63, 377, 1995.

82. Stewart, D. R., Erikson, M. S., Erikson, M. E., Nakajima, E. T., Overstreet, J. W., Lasley, B. L., Amento, E., and Seppälä, M., The role of relaxin in glycodelin secretion, *J. Clin. Endocrinol. Metab.*, 82, 839, 1997.

83. Fritz, M. A. and Lessey, B. A., Defective luteal function, in *Estrogens and Progestogens in Clinical Practice*, Fraser, I. S., Jansen, R., Lobo, R. A., and Whitehead, M., Eds., Churchhill Livingstone, London, 437, 1998.

84. Pope, W. F., Uterine asynchrony: a cause of embryonic loss, *Biol. Reprod.*, 39, 999, 1988.

85. Horta, J. L. H., Fernandex, J. G., de Leon, B. S., and Cortes-Gallegos, V., Direct evidence of luteal phase insufficiency in women with habitual abortion, *Obstet. Gyn.*, 49, 705, 1977.

86. Joshi, S. G., Progestin-dependent human endometrial protein: a marker for monitoring human endometrial function, *Cell Mol. Biol. of the Uterus*, 1, 167, 1987.

87. Seif, M. W., Aplin, J. D., and Buckley, C. H., Luteal phase defect: the possibility of an immunohistochemical diagnosis, *Fertil. Steril.*, 51, 273, 1989.

88. Wang, H.-S., Lee, J.-D., and Soong, Y.-K., Serum levels of insulin-like growth factor I and insulin-like growth factor-binding protein-1 and -3 in women with regular menstrual cycles, *Fertil. Steril.*, 63, 1204, 1995.

89. Giudice, L. C., Growth factors and growth modulators in human uterine endometrium: their potential relevance to reproductive medicine, *Fertil. Steril.*, 61, 1, 1994.

90. Tabibzadeh, S. and Babaknia, A., The signals and molecular pathways involved in implantation, a symbiotic interaction between blastocyst and endometrium involving adhesion and tissue invasion, *Hum. Reprod.*, 10, 1579, 1995.

91. Simón, C., Mercader, A., Frances, A., Gimeno, M. J., Polan, M. L., Remohí, J., and Pellicer, A., Hormonal regulation of serum and endometrial IL-1α, IL-1β and IL-1ra: IL-1 endometrial microenvironment of the human embryo at the apposition phase under physiological and supraphysiological steroid level conditions, *J. Reprod. Immunol.*, 31, 165, 1996.

92. Clark, S. C. and Kamen, R., The human hematopoietic colony-stimulating factors, *Science*, 236, 1229, 1987.

93. Zolti, M., Ben-Rafael, Z., Meirom, R., Shemesh, M., Bider, D., Mashiach, S., and Apte, R. N., Cytokine involvement in oocyte and early embryos, *Fertil. Steril.*, 56, 265, 1991.

94. Pampfer, S., Daiter, E., Barad, D., and Pollard, J. W., Expression of the colony-stimulating factor-1 receptor (c-fms proto-oncogene product) in the human uterus and placenta, *Biol. Reprod.*, 46, 48, 1992.

95. Daiter, E., Pampfer, S., Yeung, Y. G., Barad, D., Stanley, E. R., and Pollard, J. W., Expression of colony-stimulating factor-1 in the human uterus and placenta, *J. Clin. Endocrinol. Metab.*, 74, 850, 1992.

96. Pollard, J. W., Hunt, J. S., Wkitor-Jedrzejczak, W., and Stanley, E. R., A pregnancy defect in the osteopetrotic (op/op) mouse demonstrates the requirement for CSF-1 in female fertility, *Dev. Biol.*, 148, 273, 1991.

97. Kauma, S. W., Aukerman, S. L., Eierman, D., and Turner, T., Colony-stimulating factor-1 and c-fms expression in human endometrial tissues and placenta during the menstrual cycle and early pregnancy, *J. Clin. Endocrinol. Metab.*, 73, 746, 1991.

98. Haimovici, F. and Anderson, D. J., Effects of growth factors and growth factor-extracellular matrix interactions on mouse trophoblast outgrowth *in vitro*, *Biol. Reprod.*, 49, 124, 1993.

99. Garcia-Lloret, M. I., Morrish, D. W., Wegmann, T. G., Honore, L., Turner, A. R., and Guilbert, L. J., Demonstration of functional cytokine-placental interactions: CSF-1 and GM-CSF stimulate human cytotrophoblast differentiation and peptide hormone secretion, *Exp. Cell Res.*, 214, 46, 1994.

100. Stewart, C. L., The role of leukemia inhibitory factor (LIF) and other cytokines in regulating implantation in mammals, *Ann. NY Acad. Sci.*, 734, 157, 1994.

101. Hilton, D. J. and Gough, N. M., Leukemia inhibitory factor: a biological perspective, *J. Cell Biochem.*, 46, 21, 1991.

102. Bhatt, H., Brunet, L. J., and Stewart, C. L., Uterine expression of leukemia inhibitory factor coincides with the onset of blastocyst implantation, *Proc. Natl. Acad. Sci. USA*, 88, 11408, 1991.

103. Charnock-Jones, D. S., Sharkey, A. M., Fenwick, P., and Smith, S. K., Leukemia inhibitory factor mRNA concentration peaks in human endometrium at the time of implantation and the blastocyst contains mRNA for the receptor at this time, *J. Reprod. Fertil.*, 101, 421, 1994.

104. Kojima, K., Kanzaki, H., Iwai, M., Hatayama, H., Fujimoto, M., Inoue, T., Horie, K., Nakayama, H., Fujita, J., and Mori, T., Expression of leukemia inhibitory factor in human endometrium and placenta, *Biol. Reprod.*, 50, 882, 1994.

105. Cullinan, E. B., Abbondanzo, S. J., Anderson, P. S., Pollard, J. W., Lessey, B. A., and Stewart, C. L., Leukemia inhibitory factor (LIF) and LIF receptor expression in human endometrium suggests a potential autocrine paracrine function in regulating embryo implantation, *Proc. Natl. Acad. Sci. USA*, 93, 3115, 1996.

106. Nachtigall, M. J., Kliman, H. J., Feinberg, R. F., Olive, D. L., Engin, O., and Arici, A., The effect of leukemia inhibitory factor (LIF) on trophoblast differentiation: a potential role in human implantation, *J. Clin. Endocrinol. Metab.*, 81, 801, 1996.

107. Danielsson, K. G., Swahn, M. L., and Bygdeman, M., The effect of various doses of mifepristone on endometrial leukemia inhibitory factor expression in the midluteal phase: an immunohistochemical study, *Hum. Reprod.*, 12, 1293, 1997.

108. Chakraborty, I., Das, S. K., Wang, J., and Dey, S. K., Developmental expression of the cyclo-oxygenase-1 and cyclo-oxygenase-2 genesin the peri-implantation mouse uterus and their differential regulation by the blastocyst and ovarian steroids, *J. Mol. Endocrinol.*, 16, 107, 1996.

109. Dinarello, C. A., The biology of interleukin-1, *Chem. Immunol.*, 51, 1, 1992.

110. Unanue, E. R. and Allen, P. M., The basis for the immunoregulatory role of macrophages and other accessory cells, *Science*, 236, 551, 1987.

111. Sheth, K. V., Roca, G. L., al-Sedairy, S. T., Parhar, R. S., Hamilton, C. J., and al-Abdul Jabbar, F., Prediction of successful embryo implantation by measuring interleukin-1-alpha and immunosuppressive factor(s) in preimplantation embryo culture fluid, *Fertil. Steril.*, 55, 952, 1991.

112. Frank, G. R., Brar, A. K., Jikihara, H., Cedars, M. I., and Handwerger, S., Interleukin-1β and the endometrium: an inhibitor of stromal cell differentiation and possible autoregulator of decidualization in humans, *Biol. Reprod.*, 52, 184, 1995.

113. Kauma, S., Matt, D., Strom, S., Eierman, D., and Turner, T., Interleukin-1 beta, human leukocyte antigen HLA-DR alpha, and transforming growth factor-beta expression in endometrium, placenta, and placental membranes, *Am. J. Obstet. Gynecol.*, 163, 1430, 1990.

114. Simón, C., Frances, A., Piquette, G., Hendrickson, M., Milki, A., and Polan, M. L., Interleukin-1 system in the materno-trophoblast unit in human implantation: immunohistochemical evidence for autocrine/paracrine function, *J. Clin. Endocrinol. Metab.*, 78, 847, 1994.

115. De los Santos, M. J., Mercader, A., Frances, A., Portoles, E., Remohí, J., Pellicer, A., and Simón, C., Role of endometrial factors in regulating secretion of components of the immunoreactive human embryonic interleukin-1 system during embryonic development, *Biol. Reprod.*, 54, 563, 1996.

116. Sims, J. E., March, C. J., Cosman, D., Widmer, M. B., MacDonald, H. R., McMahan, C. J., Grubin, C. E., Wignall, J. M., Jackson, J. L., Call, S. M. et al., cDNA expression cloning of the IL-1 receptor, a member of the immunoglobulin superfamily, *Science*, 241, 585, 1988.

117. Horuk, R. and McCubrey, J. A., The interleukin-1 receptor in Raji human B-lymphoma cells. Molecular characterization and evidence for receptor-mediated activation of gene expression, *Biochem. J.*, 260, 657, 1989.

118. Tabibzadeh, S., Kaffka, K. L., Satyaswaroop, P. G., and Kilian, P. L., Interleukin-1 (IL-1) regulation of human endometrial function: presence of IL-1 receptor correlates with IL-1-stimulated prostaglandin E2 production, *J. Clin. Endocrinol. Metab.*, 70, 1000, 1990.

119. Simón, C., Piquette, G. N., Frances, A., Westphal, L. M., Heinrichs, W. L., and Polan, M. L., Interleukin-1 type I receptor messenger ribonucleic acid expression in human endometrium throughout the menstrual cycle, *Fertil. Steril.*, 59, 791, 1993.

120. Simón, C., Piquette, G. N., Frances, A., El-Danasouri, I., Irwin, J. C., and Polan, M. L., The effect of interleukin-1β (IL-1β) on the regulation of IL-1 receptor type I messenger ribonucleic acid and protein levels in cultured human endometrial stromal and glandular cells, *J. Clin. Endocrinol. Metab.*, 78, 675, 1994.

121. Sahakian, V., Anners, J., Haskill, S., and Halme, J., Selective localization of interleukin-1 receptor antagonist in eutopic endometrium and endometriotic implants, *Fertil. Steril.*, 60, 276, 1993.

122. Simón, C., Frances, A., Lee, B. Y., Mercader, A., Huynh, T., Remohi, J., Polan, M. L., and Pellicer, A., Immunohistochemical localization, identification and regulation of the interleukin-1 receptor antagonist in the human endometrium, *Hum. Reprod.*, 10, 2472, 1995.

123. Simón, C., Frances, A., Piquette, G. N., El-Danasouri, I., Zurawski, G., Dang, W., and Polan, M. L., Embryonic implantation in mice is blocked by interleukin-1 receptor antagonist, *Endocrinology*, 134, 521, 1994.

124. Cole, O. F., Sullivan, M. H. F., and Elder, M. G., The "interleukin 1 receptor antagonist" is a partial agonist of prostaglandin synthesis by human decidual cells, *Prostaglandins*, 46, 493, 1993.

125. Steele, G. L., Currie, W. D., Leung, E. H., Ho Yuen, B., and Leung, P. C. K., Rapid stimulation of human chorionic gonadotropin secretion by interleukin-1β from perifused first trimester trophoblast, *J. Clin. Endocrinol. Metab.*, 75, 783, 1992.

126. Yagel, S., Lala, P. K., Powell, W. A., and Casper, R. F., Interleukin-1 stimulated human chorionic gonadotropin secretion by first trimester human trophoblast, *J. Clin. Endocrinol. Metab.*, 68, 922, 1989.

127. Van Le, L., Oh, S. T., Anners, J. A., Rinehart, C. A., and Halme, J., Interleukin-1 inhibits growth of normal human endometrial stromal cells, *Obstet. Gynecol.*, 80, 405, 1992.

128. Haimovici, F., Hill, J. A., and Anderson, D. J., The effects of soluble products of activated lymphocytes and macrophages on blastocyst implantation events *in vitro*, *Biol. Reprod.*, 44, 69, 1991.

129. Hill, J. A., Haimovici, F., and Anderson, D. J., Products of activated lymphocytes and macrophages inhibit mouse embryo development *in vitro*, *J. Immunol.*, 139, 2250, 1987.

130. Faltih, H., Duggett, D., Holtz, G., Tsang, K. Y., Lee, J. C., and Williamson, H. O., Interleukin-1: a possible role in the infertility associated with endometriosis, *Fertil. Steril.*, 47, 213, 1987.

131. Fisher, D. A. and Lakshmanan, J., Metabolism and effects of epidermal growth factor and related growth factors in mammals, *Endocr. Rev.*, 11, 418, 1990.

132. Nelson, K. G., Takahashi, T., Bossert, N. L., Walmer, D. K., and McLachlan, J. A., Epidermal growth factor replaces estrogen in the stimulation of female genital-tract growth and differentiation, *Proc. Natl. Acad. Sci. USA*, 88, 21, 1991.

133. Savage, C. R., Jr., Inagami, T., and Cohen, S., The primary structure of epidermal growth factor, *J. Biol. Chem.*, 247, 7612, 1972.

134. Watanabe, T., Shintani, A., Nakata, M., Shing, Y., Folkman, J., Igarashi, K., and Sasada, R., Recombinant human betacellulin. Molecular structure, biological activities, and receptor interaction, *J. Biol. Chem.*, 269, 9966, 1994.

135. Marquardt, H., Hunkapiller, M. W., and Todaro, G. J., Rat transforming growth factor type 1: structure and relation to epidermal growth factor, *Science*, 223, 1079, 1984.

136. Higashiyama, S., Abraham, J. A., Miller, J., Fiddes, J. C., and Klagsbrun, M., A heparin-binding growth factor secreted by macrophage-like cells that is related to epidermal growth factor, *Science*, 251, 936, 1991.

137. Beerli, R. R. and Hynes, N. E., Epidermal growth factor-related peptides activate distinct subsets of ErbB receptors and differ in their biological activities, *J. Biol. Chem.*, 271, 6071, 1996.

138. Hofmann, G. E., Scott, R. T. J., Bergh, P. A., and Deligdisch, L., Immunohistochemical localization of epidermal growth factor in human endometrium, decidua, and placenta, *J. Clin. Endocrinol. Metab.*, 73, 882, 1991.

139. Hofmann, G. E., Drews, M. R., Scott, R. T. J., Navot, D., Heller, D., and Deligdisch, L., Epidermal growth factor and its receptor in human implantation trophoblast: immunohistochemical evidence for autocrine/paracrine function, *J. Clin. Endocrinol. Metab.*, 74, 981, 1992.

140. Chegini, N., Rossi, M. J., and Masterson, B. J., Platelet-derived growth factor (PDGF), epidermal growth factor (EGF), and EGF and PDGF beta-receptors in human endometrial tissue—localization and *in vitro* action, *Endocrinology*, 130, 2373, 1992.

141. Taga, M., Sakakibara, H., Suyama, K., Ikeda, M., and Minaguchi, H., Gene expression of transforming growth factor-alpha in human endometrium during decidualization, *J. Assist. Reprod. Genet.*, 14, 218, 1997.

142. Sakakibara, H., Taga, M., Saji, M., Kida, H., and Minaguchi, H., Gene expression of epidermal growth factor in human endometrium during decidualization, *J. Clin. Endocrinol. Metab.*, 79, 223, 1994.

143. Ace, C. I. and Okulicz, W. C., Differential gene regulation by estrogen and proges-
     terone in the primate endometrium, *Mol. Cell. Endocrinol.*, 115, 95, 1995.
144. Machida, T., Taga, M., and Minaguchi, H., Effects of epidermal growth factor and
     transforming growth factor alpha on the mouse trophoblast outgrowth *in vitro, Eur.
     J. Endocrinol.*, 133, 741, 1995.
145. Wiley, L. M., Wu, J. X., Harari, I., and Adamson, E. D., Epidermal growth factor
     receptor mRNA and protein increase after the four-cell preimplantation stage in
     murine development, *Dev. Biol.*, 149, 247, 1992.
146. Maruo, T., Matsuo, H., Otani, T., and Mochizuki, M., Role of epidermal growth factor
     (EGF) and its receptor in the development of the human placenta, *Reprod. Fertil.
     Dev.*, 7, 1465, 1995.
147. Taga, M., Saji, M., Suyama, K., and Minaguchi, H., Transforming growth factor-α,
     like epidermal growth factor, stimulates cell proliferation and inhibits prolactin secre-
     tion in the human decidual cells *in vitro, J. Endocrinol. Invest.*, 19, 659, 1996.
148. Rappolee, D. A., Brenner, C. A., Schultz, R., Mark, D., and Werb, Z., Developmental
     expression of PDGF, TGF-α, and TGF-β genes in preimplantation mouse embryos,
     Science, 241, 1823, 1988.
149. Huet-Hudson, Y. M., Chakraborty, C., De, S. K., Suzuki, Y., Andrews, G. K., and
     Dey, S. K., Estrogen regulates the synthesis of epidermal growth factor in mouse
     uterine epithelial cells, *Mol. Endocrinol.*, 90, 510, 1990.
150. Paria, B. C. and Dey, S. K., Preimplantation embryo development *in vitro*: cooperative
     interactions among embryos and role of growth factors, *Proc. Natl. Acad. Sci. USA*,
     87, 4756, 1990.
151. Paria, B. C., Das, S. K., Andrews, G. K., and Dey, S. K., Expression of the epidermal
     growth factor gene is regulated in mouse blastocysts during delayed implantation,
     Proc. Natl. Acad. Sci. USA, 90, 55, 1993.
152. Das, S. K., Das, N., Wang, J., Lim, H., Schryver, B., Plowman, G. D., and Dey, S. K.,
     Expression of betacellulin and epiregulin genes in the mouse uterus temporally by
     the blastocyst solely at the site of its apposition is coincident with the "window" of
     implantation, *Dev. Biol.*, 190, 178, 1997.
153. Paria, B. C., Das, S. K., Huet-Hudson, Y. M., and Dey, S. K., Distribution of trans-
     forming growth factor alpha precursors in the mouse uterus during the periimplan-
     tation period and after steroid hormone treatments, *Biol. Reprod.*, 50, 481, 1994.
154. Das, S. K., Lim, H., Wang, J., Paria, B. C., BazDresch, M., and Dey, S. K., Inappro-
     priate expression of human transforming growth factor (TGF)-α in the uterus of
     transgenic mouse causes downregulation of TGF-β receptors and delays the
     blastocyst-attachment reaction, *J. Mol. Endocrinol.*, 18, 243, 1997.
155. Johnson, D. C. and Chatterjee, S., Embryo implantation in the rat uterus induced by
     epidermal growth factor, *J. Reprod. Fertil.*, 99, 557, 1993.
156. Das, S. K., Wang, X.-N., Paria, B. C., Damm, D., Abraham, J. A., Klagsbrun, M.,
     Andrews, G. K., and Dey, S. K., Heparin-binding EGF-like growth factor gene is
     induced in the mouse uterus temporally by the blastocyst solely at the site of its
     apposition: a possible ligand for interaction with blastocyst EGF-receptor in implan-
     tation, *Development*, 120, 1071, 1994.
157. Kim, G. Y., Besner, G. E., Steffen, C. L., Mccarthy, D. W., Downing, M. T.,
     Luquette, M. H., Abad, M. S., and Brigstock, D. R., Purification of heparin-binding
     epidermal growth factor-like growth factor from pig uterine luminal flushings, and
     its production by endometrial tissues, *Biol. Reprod.*, 52, 561, 1995.

158. Yoo, H. J., Barlow, D. H., and Mardon, H. J., Temporal and spatial regulation of expression of heparin-binding epidermal growth factor-like growth factor in the human endometrium: a possible role in blastocyst implantation, *Dev. Genet.*, 21, 102, 1997.

159. Raab, G., Kover, K., Paria, B. C., Dey, S. K., Ezzell, R. M., and Klagsbrun, M., Mouse preimplantation blastocysts adhere to cells expressing the transmembrane form of heparin-binding EGF-like growth factor, *Development*, 122, 637, 1996.

160. Habiba, M. A., Bell, S. C., and Al-Azzawi, F., Endometrial responses to hormone replacement therapy: histological features compared with those of late luteal phase endometrium, *Hum. Reprod.*, 13, 1674, 1998.

161. Zhang, Z., Funk, C., Roy, D., Glasser, S., and Mulholland, J., Heparin-binding epidermal growth factor-like growth factor is differentially regulated by progesterone and estradiol in rat uterine epithelial and stromal cells, *Endocrinology*, 134, 1089, 1994.

162. Wang, X. N., Das, S. K., Damm, D., Klagsbrun, M., Abraham, J. A., and Dey, S. K., Differential regulation of heparin-binding epidermal growth factor-like growth factor in the adult ovariectomized mouse uterus by progesterone and estrogen, *Endocrinology*, 135, 1264, 1994.

163. Zhang, Z., Funk, C., Glasser, S. R., and Mulholland, J., Progesterone regulation of heparin-binding epidermal growth factor-like growth factor gene expression during sensitization and decidualization in the rat uterus: effects of the antiprogestin, ZK 98.299, *Endocrinology*, 135, 1256, 1994.

164. Das, S. K., Chakraborty, I., Paria, B. C., Wang, X.-N., Plowman, G., and Dey, S. K., Amphiregulin is an implantation-specific and progesterone-regulated gene in the mouse uterus, *Mol. Endocrinol.*, 9, 691, 1995.

165. Clemmons, D. R. and Underwood, L. E., Clinical review 59: uses of human insulin-like growth factor-I in clinical conditions, *J. Clin. Endocrinol. Metab.*, 79, 4, 1994.

166. Giudice, L. C., Lamson, G., Rosenfeld, R. G., and Irwin, J. C., Insulin-like growth factor-II (IGF-II) and IGF binding proteins in human endometrium, *Ann. NY Acad. Sci.*, 626, 295, 1991a.

167. Giudice, L. C., Lamson, G., Rosenfeld, R. G., and Irwin, J. C., Insulin-like growth factor-II (IGF-II) and IGF binding proteins in human endometrium, *Ann. NY Acad. Sci.*, 626, 295, 1991b.

168. Zhou, J., Dsupin, B. A., Giudice, L. C., and Bondy, C. A., Insulin-like growth factor system gene expression in human endometrium during the menstrual cycle, *J. Clin. Endocrinol. Metab.*, 79, 1723, 1994.

169. Laatikainen, T. J., Tomás, E. I., and Voutilainen, R. J., The expression of insulin-like growth factor and its binding protein mRNA in the endometrium of postmenopausal patients with breast cancer receiving tamoxifen, *Cancer*, 76, 1406, 1995.

170. Hild-Petito, S., Verhage, H. G., and Fazlebas, A. T., Characterization, localization, and regulation of receptors for insulin-like growth factor I in the baboon uterus during the cycle and pregnancy, *Biol. Reprod.*, 50, 791, 1994.

171. Nonoshita, L. D., Wathen, N. C., Dsupin, B. A., Chard, T., and Giudice, L. C., Insulin-like growth factors (IGFs), IGF-binding proteins (IGFBPs), and proteolyzed IGFBP-3 in embryonic cavities in early human pregnancy: their potential relevance to maternal-embryonic and fetal interactions, *J. Clin. Endocrinol. Metab.*, 79, 1249, 1994.

172. Bell, S. C., The insulin-like growth factor binding proteins—the endometrium and decidua, *Ann. NY Acad. Sci.*, 622, 120, 1991.

173. Rosenfeld, R. G., Lamson, G., Pham, H., Oh, Y., Conover, C., De Leon, D. D., Donovan, S. M., Ocrant, I., and Giudice, L. C., Insulin-like growth factor-binding proteins, *Recent. Prog. Horm. Res.*, 46, 99, 1990.

174. Bell, S. C., Jackson, J. A., Ashmore, J., Zhu, H. H., and Tseng, L., Regulation of insulin-like growth factor-binding protein-1 synthesis and secretion by progestin and relaxin in long term culture of human endometrial stromal cells, *J. Clin. Endocrinol. Metab.*, 72, 1014, 1991.

175. Coutts, A., Murphy, L. J., and Murphy, L. C., Expression of insulin-like growth factor binding proteins by T-47D human breast cancer cells: regulation by progestins and antiestrogens, *Breast Cancer Res. Treat.*, 32, 153, 1994.

176. Irwin, J. C., de las Fuentes, L., Dsupin, B. A., and Giudice, L. C., Insulin-like growth factor regulation of human endometrial stromal cell function: coordinate effects on insulin-like growth factor binding protein-1, cell proliferation and prolactin secretion, *Regul. Pept.*, 48, 165, 1993.

177. Jones, J. I., Gockerman, A., Busby, W. H., Wright, G., and Clemmons, D. R., Insulin-like growth factor binding protein 1 stimulates cell migration and binds to the alpha 5/β1 integrin by means of its ARG-GLY-ASP sequence, *Proc. Natl. Acad. Sci. USA*, 90, 10553, 1993.

178. Damsky, C. H., Librach, C., Lim, K.-H., Fitzgerald, M. L., McMaster, M. T., Janatpour, M., Zhou, Y., Logan, S. K., and Fisher, S. J., Integrin switching regulates normal trophoblast invasion, *Development*, 120, 3657, 1994.

179. Lessey, B. A., Castelbaum, A. J., Buck, C. A., Lei, Y., Yowell, C. W., and Sun, J., Further characterization of endometrial integrins during the menstrual cycle and in pregnancy, *Fertil. Steril.*, 62, 497, 1994.

180. Ruck, P., Marzusch, K., Kaiserling, E., Horny, H.-P., Dietl, J., Geiselhart, A., Handgretinger, R., and Redman, C. W. G., Distribution of cell adhesion molecules in decidua of early human pregnancy: an immunohistochemical study, *Lab. Invest.*, 71, 94, 1994.

181. Bilalis, D. A., Klentzeris, L. D., and Fleming, S., Immunohistochemical localization of extracellular matrix proteins in luteal phase endometrium of fertile and infertile patients, *Hum. Reprod.*, 11, 2713, 1996.

182. Murphy, C. R., Swift, J. G., Mukhergee, T. M., and Rogers, A. W., Changes in the fine structure of the apical plasma membrane of endometrial epithelial cells during implantation in the rat, *J. Cell Sci.*, 55, 1, 1982.

183. Murphy, C. R. and Shaw, T. J., Plasma membrane transformation: a common response of uterine epithelial cells during the peri-implantation period, *Cell Biol. Int.*, 18, 1115, 1994.

184. Enders, A. C. and Schlafke, S., Cytological aspects of trophoblast-uterine interactions in early implantation, *Am. J. Anat.*, 125, 1, 1969.

185. Chavez, D. J. and Anderson, T. L., The glycocalyx of the mouse uterine luminal epithelium during estrus, early pregnancy, the peri-implantation period, and delayed implantation. I. Acquisition of *Ricinus communis* I binding sites during pregnancy, *Biol. Reprod.*, 32, 1135, 1985.

186. Hewitt, K., Beer, A. E., and Grinnell, F., Disappearance of anionic sites from the surface of the rat endometrial epithelium at the time of blastocyst implantation, *Biol. Reprod.*, 21, 691, 1979.

187. Murphy, C. R. and Rogers, A. W., Effects of ovarian hormones on cell membranes in the rat uterus. III. The surface carbohydrates at the apex of the lumional epithelium, *Cell Biophysics*, 3, 305, 1981.

188. Chavez, D. J., Cell surface of mouse blastocysts at the trophectoderm-uterine interface during the adhesive stage of implantation, *Am. J. Anat.*, 176, 153, 1986.

189. Carson, D. D., Rohde, L. H., and Surveyor, G., Cell surface glycoconjugates as modulators of embryo attachment to uterine epithelial cells, *Int. J. Biochem.*, 26, 1269, 1994.

190. Surveyor, G. A., Gendler, S. J., Pemberton, L., Spicer, A. P., and Carson, D. D., Differential expression of Muc-1 at the apical cell surface of mouse uterine epithelial cells, *FASEB J.*, 7, 1151a, 1993.

191. Aplin, J. D. and Hey, N. A., MUCl, endometrium and embryo implantation, *Biochem. Soc. Trans.*, 23, 826, 1995.

192. Carson, D. D., DeSouza, M. M., and Regisford, E. G. C., Mucin and proteoglycan functions in embryo implantation, *Bioessays*, 20, 577, 1998.

193. Feinberg, R. F. and Kliman, H. J., Human trophoplasts and tropho-uteronectin (TUN): a model for studying early implantation events, *Assisted Reprod. Rev.*, 3, 19, 1993.

194. Turpeenniemi-Hujanen, T., Feinberg, R. F., Kauppila, A., and Puistola, U., Extracellular matrix interactions in early human embryos: implications for normal implantation events, *Fertil. Steril.*, 64, 132, 1995.

195. Feinberg, R. F., Kliman, H. J., and Lockwood, C. J., Is oncofetal fibronectin a trophoblast glue for human implantation?, *Am. J. Pathol.*, 138, 537, 1991.

196. Armant, D. R., Kaplan, H. A., Mover, H., and Lennarz, W. J., The effect of hexapeptides on attachment and outgrowth of mouse blastocysts cultured *in vitro*: evidence for the involvement of the cell recognition tripeptide Arg-Gly-Asp, *Proc. Natl. Acad. Sci. USA.*, 83, 6751, 1986.

197. Yelian, F. D., Yang, Y., Hirata, J. D., Schultz, J. F., and Armant, D. R., Molecular interactions between fibronectin and integrins during mouse blastocyst outgrowth, *Mol. Reprod. Dev.*, 41, 435, 1995.

198. Zhang, X., Shu, M. A., Harvey, M. B., and Schultz, G. A., Regulation of urokinase plasminogen activator production in implanting mouse embryo: effect of embryo interaction with extracellular matrix, *Biol. Reprod.*, 54, 1052, 1996.

199. Bischof, P., Haenggeli, L., and Campana, A., Gelatinase and oncofetal fibronectin secretion is dependent on integrin expression on human cytotrophoblasts, *Hum. Reprod.*, 10, 734, 1995.

200. Woessner, J. F., Jr., Matrix metalloproteinases and their inhibitors in connective tissue remodeling, *FASEB J.*, 5, 2145, 1991.

201. Emonard, H. and Grimaud, J. A., Matrix metalloproteinases. A review, *Cell Mol. Biol.*, 36, 131, 1990.

202. Tabibzadeh, S., The signals and molecular pathways involved in human menstruation, a unique process of tissue destruction and remodeling, *Mol. Hum. Reprod.*, 2, 77, 1996.

203. Salamonsen, L. A. and Woolley, D. E., Matrix metalloproteinases in normal menstruation, *Hum. Reprod.*, 11 Suppl. 2, 124, 1996.

204. Nagase, H., Activation mechanisms of matrix metalloproteinases, *Biol. Chem. Hoppe Seyler*, 378, 151, 1997.

205. Coussens, L. M. and Werb, Z., Matrix metalloproteinases and the development of cancer, *Chem. Biol.*, 3, 895, 1996.

206. Gospodarowicz, D., Greenburg, G., and Birdwell, C. R., Determination of cellular shape by the extracellular matrix and its correlation with the control of cellular growth, *Cancer Res.*, 38, 4155, 1978.

207. Folkman, J. and Moscona, A., Role of cell shape in growth control, *Nature*, 273, 345, 1978.

208. Lochter, A., Galosy, S., Muschler, J., Freedman, N., Werb, Z., and Bissell, M. J., Matrix metalloproteinase stromelysin-1 triggers a cascade of molecular alterations that leads to stable epithelial-to-mesenchymal conversion and a premalignant phenotype in mammary epithelial cells, *J. Cell Biol.*, 139, 1861, 1997.

209. Welsh, A. O., Uterine cell death during implantation and early placentation, *Microsc. Res. Tech.*, 25, 223, 1993.

210. Fukai, F., Mashimo, M., Akiyama, K., Goto, T., Tanuma, S. I., and Katayama, T., Modulation of apoptotic cell death by extracellular matrix proteins and a fibronectin-derived antiadhesive peptide, *Exp. Cell Res.*, 242, 92, 1998.

211. Werb, Z., Tremble, P., and Damsky, C. H., Regulation of extracellular matrix degradation by cell-extracellular matrix interactions, *Cell Differ. Dev.*, 32, 299, 1990.

212. Sato, H., Takino, T., Okada, Y., Cao, J., Shinagawa, A., Yamamoto, E., and Seiki, M., A matrix metalloproteinase expressed on the surface of invasive tumour cells, *Nature*, 370, 61, 1994.

213. Chintala, S. K., Sawaya, R., Gokaslan, Z. L., and Rao, J. S., Modulation of matrix metalloprotease-2 and invasion in human glioma cells by α3β1 integrin, *Cancer Lett.*, 103, 201, 1996.

214. Kubota, S., Ito, H., Ishibashi, Y., and Seyama, Y., Anti-α3 integrin antibody induces the activated form of matrix metalloprotease-2 (MMP-2) with concomitant stimulation of invasion through matrigel by human rhabdomyosarcoma cells, *Int. J. Cancer*, 70, 106, 1997.

215. Von Bredow, D. C., Nagle, R. B., Bowden, G. T., and Cress, A. E., Cleavage of β4 integrin by matrilysin, *Exp. Cell Res.*, 236, 341, 1997.

216. Suzuki, N., Naruse, K., Asano, Y., Okamoto, T., Nishikimi, N., Sakurai, T., Nimura, Y., and Sokabe, M., Up regulation of integrin β3 expression by cyclic stretch in human umbilical endothelial cells, *Biochem. Biophys. Res. Commun.*, 239, 372, 1997.

217. Martin, K. L., Barlow, D. H., and Sargent, I. L., Heparin-binding epidermal growth factor significantly improves human blastocyst development and hatching in serum-free medium, *Hum. Reprod.*, 13, 1645, 1998.

218. Huppertz, B., Kertschanska, S., Demir, A. Y., Frank, H. G., and Kaufmann, P., Immunohistochemistry of matrix metalloproteinases (MMP), their substrates, and their inhibitors (TIMP) during trophoblast invasion in the human placenta, *Cell Tissue Res.*, 291, 133, 1998.

219. Shimonovitz, S., Hurwitz, A., Dushnik, M., Anteby, E., Geva-Eldar, T., and Yagel, S., Developmental regulation of the expression of 72 and 92 kd type IV collagenases in human trophoblasts: a possible mechanism for control of trophoblast invasion, *Am. J. Obstet. Gynecol.*, 171, 832, 1994.

220. Ruck, P., Marzusch, K., Horny, H. P., Dietl, J., and Kaiserling, E., The distribution of tissue inhibitor of metalloproteinases-2 (TIMP-2) in the human placenta, *Placenta*, 17, 263, 1996.

221. Marzusch, K., Ruck, P., Dietl, J. A., Horny, H. P., and Kaiserling, E., Immunohistochemical localization of tissue inhibitor of metalloproteinases-2 (TIMP-2) in first trimester human placental decidua, *Eur. J. Obstet. Gynecol. Reprod. Biol.*, 68, 105, 1996.

222. Librach, C. L., Werb, Z., Fitzgerald, M. L., Chiu, K., Corwin, N. M., Esteves, R. A., Grobelny, D., Galardy, R., Damsky, C. H., and Fisher, S. J., 92-kD type IV collagenase mediates invasion of human cytotrophoblasts, *J. Cell Biol.*, 113, 437, 1991.

223. Cross, J. C., Werb, Z., and Fisher, S. J., Implantation and the placenta: key pieces of the development puzzle, *Science*, 266, 1508, 1994.

224. Schatz, F., Papp, C., Toth-Pal, E., and Lockwood, C. J., Ovarian steroid-modulated stromelysin-1 expression in human endometrial stromal and decidual cells, *J. Clin. Endocrinol. Metab.*, 78, 1467, 1994.

225. Rodgers, W. H., Matrisian, L. M., Giudice, L. C., Dsupin, B. A., Cannon, P., Svitek, C., Gorstein, F., and Osteen, K. G., Patterns of matrix metalloproteinase expression in cycling endometrium imply differential functions and regulation by steroid hormones, *J. Clin. Invest.*, 94, 946, 1994.

226. Rawdanowicz, T. J., Hampton, A. L., Nagase, H., Woolley, D. E., and Salamonsen, L. A., Matrix metalloproteinase production by cultured human endometrial stromal cells: identification of interstitial collagenase, gelatinase-A, gelatinase-B, and stromelysin-1 and their differential regulation by interleukin-1α and tumor necrosis factor-α, *J. Clin. Endocrinol. Metab.*, 79, 530, 1994.

227. Shimonovitz, S., Hurwitz A. Barak, V., Dushnik, M., Adashi, E. Y., Anteby, E., and Yagel, S., Cytokine-mediated regulation of type IV collagenase expression and production in human trophoblast cells, *J. Clin. Endocrinol. Metab.*, 81, 3091, 1996.

228. Jeziorska, M., Nagase, H., Salamonsen, L. A., and Woolley, D. E., Immunolocalization of the matrix metalloproteinases gelatinase B and stromelysin I in human endometrium throughout the menstrual cycle, *J. Reprod. Fertil.*, 107, 43, 1996.

229. Wang, S. L., Kennedy, T. G., and Zhang, X. Q., Presence of urokinase plasminogen activator and plasminogen activator inhibitor-1 messenger ribonucleic acids in rat endometrium during decidualization *in vivo*, *Biol. Reprod.*, 55, 493, 1996.

230. Fujimoto, J., Hori, M., Ichigo, S., Hirose, R., Sakaguchi, H., and Tamaya, T., Comparative study on expression of plasminogen activator inhibitor 1 and its mRNA in endometrial cancers and normal endometria, *Tumor Biol.*, 18, 13, 1997.

231. Khamsi, F., Armstrong, D. T., and Zhang, X. Q., Expression of urokinase-type plasminogen activator in human preimplantation embryos, *Mol. Hum. Reprod.*, 2, 273, 1996.

232. Sayegh, R., Awwad, J. T., Maxwell, C., Lessey, B. A., and Isaacson, K., α₂-macroglobulin production by the human endometrium, *J. Clin. Endocrinol. Metab.*, 80, 1021, 1995.

233. Loskutoff, D. J., Sawdey, M., and Mimuro, J., Type I plasminogen activator, *Prog. Hemostasis Thromb.*, 9, 87, 1989.

234. Kruithof, E. K. O., Plasminogen activator inhibitor type 2: biochemical and biological aspects, in *Protease Inhibitors*, Takada, A., Sumama, M. M., and Collen, D., Eds., Elsevier, Amsterdam, 1990, 15–22.

235. Strickland, S., Reich, E., and Sherman, M. I., Plasminogen activator in early embryogenesis: enzyme production at the time of implantation in the mouse embryo, *Cell*, 9, 231, 1976.

236. Queenan, J. T., Kao, L. C., Arboleda, C. E., Ulloa-Aguirre, A., Gaolos, T. G., Cines, D. B., and Strauss, J. F., Regulation of urokinase-type plasminogen activator production by cultured human cytotrophoblasts, *J. Biol. Chem.*, 262, 10903, 1987.

237. Zini, J. M., Murray, S. C., Graham, C. H., Lala, P. K., Kariko, K., Barnathan, E. S., Mazar, A., Herkin, J., Cines, D. B., and McCrae, K. R., Characterization of urokinase receptor expression by human placental trophoblasts, *Blood*, 79, 2917, 1992.

238. Axelrod, H. R., Altered trophoblast functions in implantation-defective mouse embryos, *Dev. Biol.*, 108, 185, 1985.

239. Sutherland, A. E., Calarco, P. G., and Damsky, C. H., Developmental regulation of integrin expression at the time of implantation in the mouse embryo, *Development*, 119, 1175, 1993.

240. Damsky, C. H., Fitzgerald, M. L., and Fisher, S. J., Distribution patterns of extracel-
     lular matrix components and adhesion receptors are intricately modulated during first
     trimester cytotrophoblast differentiation along the invasive pathway, in vivo, J. Clin.
     Invest., 89, 210, 1992.
241. Zhou, Y., Fisher, S. J., Janatpour, M., Genbacev, O., Dejana, E., Wheelock, M., and
     Damsky, C. H., Human cytotrophoblasts adopt a vascular phenotype as they differ-
     entiate—A strategy for successful endovascular invasion?, J. Clin. Invest., 99,
     2139, 1997.
242. Zhou, Y., Damsky, C. H., and Fisher, S. J., Preeclampsia is associated with failure of
     human cytotrophoblasts to mimic a vascular adhesion phenotype—One cause of
     defective endovascular invasion in this syndrome?, J. Clin. Invest., 99, 2152, 1997.
243. Lim, K. H., Zhou, Y., Janatpour, M., McMaster, M. T., Bass, K., Chun, S. H., and
     Fisher, S. J., Human cytotrophoblast differentiation/invasion is abnormal in pre-
     eclampsia, Am. J. Pathol., 151, 1809, 1997.
244. Zhou, Y., Genbacev, O., Damsky, C. H., and Fisher, S. J., Oxygen regulates human
     cytotrophoblast differentiation and invasion: implications for endovascular invasion
     in normal pregnancy and in pre-eclampsia, J. Reprod. Immunol., 39, 197, 1998.
245. Tabibzadeh, S., Patterns of expression of integrin molecules in human endometrium
     throughout the menstrual cycle, Hum. Reprod., 7, 876, 1992.
246. Lessey, B. A., Castelbaum, A. J., Sawin, S. J., Buck, C. A., Schinnar, R., Wilkins, B.,
     and Strom, B. L., Aberrant integrin expression in the endometrium of women with
     endometriosis, J. Clin. Endocrinol. Metab., 79, 643, 1994.
247. Lessey, B. A., Castelbaum, A. J., Sawin, S. J., and Sun, J., Integrins as markers of
     uterine receptivity in women with primary unexplained infertility, Fertil. Steril., 63,
     535, 1995.
248. Meyer, W. R., Castelbaum, A. J., Harris, J. E., Levy, M., Somkuti, S., Doyle, M., and
     Lessey, B. A., Hydrosalpinges adversely affect markers of uterine receptivity, Hum.
     Reprod., 12, 1393, 1997.
249. Finn, C. A. The implantation reaction, in Biology of the Uterus, Wynn, R. M., Ed.,
     Plenum Press, New York, 1977, 245–303.
250. Clément, B., Segui-Real, B., Savagner, P., Kleinman, H. K., and Yamada, Y.,
     Hepatocyte attachment to laminin is mediated through multiple receptors, J. Cell
     Biol., 110, 185, 1990.
251. Navot, D., Scott, R. T., Droesch, K., Veeck, L. L., Liu, H. C., and Rosenwaks, Z.,
     The window of embryo transfer and the efficiency of human conception in vitro,
     Fertil. Steril., 55, 114, 1991.
252. Lessey, B. A., Ilesanmi, A. O., Sun, J., Lessey, M. A., Harris, J., and Chwalisz, K.,
     Luminal and glandular endometrial epithelium express integrins differentially
     throughout the menstrual cycle: implications for implantation, contraception, and
     infertility, Am. J. Reprod. Immunol., 35, 195, 1996.
253. Aplin, J. D., Spanswick, C., Behzad, F., Kimber, S. J., and Vicovac, L., Integrins β5,
     β3, αv are apically distributed in endometrial epithelium, Molec. Hum. Reprod., 2,
     527, 1996.
254. Meyer, W. R., Castelbaum, A. J., Somkuti, S., Sagoskin, A. W., Doyle, M., Harris,
     J. E., and Lessey, B. A., Hydrosalpinges adversely affect markers of endometrial
     receptivity, Hum. Reprod., 12, 1393, 1997.
255. Tabibzadeh, S. S. and Satyaswaroop, P. G., Progestin-mediated induction of VLA-1
     in glandular epithelium of human endometrium in vitro, 72nd Ann. Meet. Endocrine
     Soc., 700, 1990.

256. Lessey, B. A., Ilesanmi, A. O., Castelbaum, A. J., Yuan, L. W., Somkuti, S. G., Satyaswaroop, P. G., and Chwalisz, K., Characterization of the functional progesterone receptor in an endometrial adenocarcinoma cell line (Ishikawa): progesterone-induced expression of the α1 integrin, *J. Steroid Biochem. Mol. Biol.*, 59, 31, 1996.

257. Press, M. F., Udove, J. A., and Greene, G. L., Progesterone receptor distribution in the human endometrium. Analysis using monoclonal antibodies to the human progesterone receptor, *Am. J. Pathol.*, 131, 112, 1988.

258. Castelbaum, A. J., Ying, L., Somkuti, S. G., Sun, J. G., Ilesanmi, A. O., and Lessey, B. A., Characterization of integrin expression in a well differentiated endometrial adenocarcinoma cell line (Ishikawa), *J. Clin. Endocrinol. Metab.*, 82, 136, 1997.

259. Campbell, S., Swann, H. R., Seif, M. W., Kimber, S. J., and Aplin, J. D., Cell adhesion molecules on the oocyte and preimplantation human embryo, *Hum. Reprod.* 10, 1571, 1995.

260. Psychoyos, A. and Mandon, P., Etude de la surface de l'epithelium uterin au microscope electronique a balayage, *C. R. Hebd. Seances Acad. Sci. Paris*, 272, 2723, 1971.

261. Anderson, T. L., *Biomolecular Markers for the Window of Uterine Receptivity*, Adams Publishing Group, Boston, 1993, 219–224.

262. Martel, D., Frydman, R., Sarantis, L., Roche, D., and Psychoyos, A., Scanning electron microscopy of the uterine luminal epithelium as a marker of the implantation window, in *Blastocyst Implantation*, Yoshinaga, K., Ed., Adams Publishing Group, Boston, 1993, 225–230.

263. Nikas, G., Drakakis, P., Loutradis, D., Mara-Skoufari, C., Koumantakis, E., Michalas, S., and Psychoyos, A., Uterine pinopodes as markers of the "nidation window" in cycling women receiving exogenous oestradiol and progesterone, *Hum. Reprod.*, 10, 1208, 1995.

264. Edwards, R. G., Clinical approaches to increasing uterine receptivity during human implantation, *Hum. Reprod.*, 10 Suppl. 2, 60, 1995.

265. Paulson, R. J., Sauer, M. V., and Lobo, R. A., Potential enhancement of endometrial receptivity in cycles using controlled ovarian hyperstimulation with antiprogestins: a hypothesis, *Fertil. Steril.*, 67, 321, 1997.

266. Graham, R. A., Seif, M. W., Aplin, J. D., Li, T. C., Cooke, I. D., Rogers, A. W., and Dockery, P., An endometrial factor in unexplained infertility, *Br. Med. J.*, 300, 1428, 1990.

267. Hild-Petito, S., Fazleabas, A. T., Julian, J., and Carson, D. D., Mucin (Muc-1) expression is differentially regulated in uterine luminal and glandular epithelia of the baboon (*Papio anubis*), *Biol. Reprod.*, 54, 939, 1996.

268. Aplin, J. D., Seif, M. W., Graham, R. A., Hey, N. A., Behzad, F., and Campbell, S., The endometrial cell surface and implantation: expression of the polymorphic mucin MUC-1 and adhesion molecules during the endometrial cycle, *Ann. NY Acad. Sci.*, 734, 103, 1994.

269. Tulppala, M., Julkunen, M., Tiitinen, A., Stenman, U.-H., and Seppälä, M., Habitual abortion is accompanied by low serum levels of placental protein 14 in the luteal phase of the fertile cycle, *Fertil. Steril.*, 63, 792, 1995.

270. Klentzeris, L. D., Bulmer, J. N., Seppälä, M., Li, T. C., Warren, M. A., and Cooke, I. D., Placental protein 14 in cycles with normal and retarded endometrial differentiation, *Hum. Reprod.*, 9, 394, 1994.

271. Fukuda, M. N., Sato, T., Nakayama, J., Klier, G., Mikami, M., Aoki, D., and Nozawa, S., Trophinin and tastin, a novel cell adhesion molecule complex with potential involvement in embryo implantation, *Genes Dev.*, 9, 1199, 1995.

272. MacCalman, C. D., Furth, E. E., Omigbodun, A., Bronner, M., Coutifaris, C., and Strauss, J. F., III, Regulated expression of cadherin-11 in human epithelial cells: a role for cadherin-11 in trophoblast-endometrium interactions?, *Dev. Dyn.*, 206, 201, 1996.
273. Getsios, S., Chen, G. T. C., Stephenson, M. D., Leclerc, P., Blaschuk, O. W., and MacCalman, C. D., Regulated expression of cadherin-6 and cadherin-11 in the glandular epithelial and stromal cells of the human endometrium, *Dev. Dyn.*, 211, 238, 1998.
274. Giudice, L. C., Endometrial growth factors and proteins, *Semin. Reprod. Endocrinol.*, 13, 93, 1995.
275. Zhu, L. J., Bagchi, M. K., and Bagchi, I. C., Attenuation of calcitonin gene expression in pregnant rat uterus leads to a block in embryonic implantation, *Endocrinology*, 139, 330, 1998.
276. Jones, R. L., Kelly, R. W., and Critchley, H. O. D., Chemokine and cyclooxygenase-2 expression in human endometrium coincides with leukocyte accumulation, *Hum. Reprod.*, 12, 1300, 1997.
277. Taylor, H. S., Arici, A., Olive, D., and Igarashi, P., HOXA10 is expressed in response to sex steroids at the time of implantation in the human endometrium, *J. Clin. Invest.*, 101, 1379, 1998.
278. Stephenson, M. D., Frequency of factors associated with habitual abortion in 197 couples, *Fertil. Steril.*, 66, 24, 1996.
279. Blacker, C. M., Ginsburg, K. A., Leach, R. E., Randolph, J., and Moghissi, K. S., Unexplained infertility: evaluation of the luteal phase. Results of the National Center for Infertility Research at Michigan, *Fertil. Steril.*, 67, 437, 1997.
280. Stewart, D. R., Overstreet, J. W., Celniker, A. C., Hess, D. L., Cragun, J. R., Boyers, S. P., and Lasley, B. L., The relationship between hCG and relaxin secretion in normal prenancies vs peri-implantation spontaneous abortions, *Clin. Endocrinol.*, 38, 379, 1993.
281. Lessey, B. A., Castlebaum, A. J., Bellardo, L., Shell, K., Sun, J., and Somkuti, S. G., Defective endometrial receptivity: an under-appreciated cause of recurrent pregnancy loss, *Amer. Fertil. Soc. Am. Mtg.*, 526, 1995.
282. Klentzeris, L. D., Bulmer, J. N., Trejdosiewicz, L. K., Morrison, L., and Cooke, I. D., Beta-1 integrin cell adhesion molecules in the endometrium of fertile and infertile women, *Hum. Reprod.*, 8, 1223, 1993.
283. Hahn, D. W., Carraher, R. P., Foldesy, R. G., and McGuire, J. L., Experimental evidence for failure to implant as a mechanism of infertility associated with endometriosis, *Am. J. Obstet. Gynecol.*, 155, 1109, 1986.
284. Schenken, R. S., Asch, R. H., Williams, R. F., and Hodgen, G. D., Etiology of infertility in monkeys with endometriosis: luteinized unruptured follicles, luteal phase defects, pelvic adhesions, and spontaneous abortions, *Fertil. Steril.*, 41, 122, 1984.
285. Jansen, R. P., Minimal endometriosis and reduced fecundability: prospective evidence from an artificial insemination by donor program, *Fertil. Steril.*, 46, 141, 1986.
286. Arici, A., Oral, E., Bukulmez, O., Duleba, A., Olive, D. L., and Jones, E. E., The effect of endometriosis on implantation: results from the Yale University *in vitro* fertilization and embryo transfer program, *Fertil. Steril.*, 65, 603, 1996.
287. Marcoux, S., Maheux, R., Bérubé, S., Langevin, M., Graves, G., Wrixon, W., O'Keane, J., Mackay, G., Gagnon, S., Mechas, T., Fisch, P., Hamel, G., Blanchet, P., Laberge, P., Champoux, F., Dupont, P., Rioux, J. E., Richard, R., Laganière, L., Bergeron, J., Villeneuve, M., and Lacroix, M., Laparoscopic surgery in infertile, women with minimal or mild endometriosis, *N. Engl. J. Med.*, 337, 217, 1997.

288. Andersen, A. N., Yue, Z., Meng, F. J., and Petersen, K., Low implantation rate after *in vitro* fertilization in patients with hydrosalpinges diagnosed by ultrasonography, *Hum. Reprod.*, 9, 1935, 1994.

289. Kassabji, M., Sims, J. A., Butler, L., and Muasher, S. J., Reduced pregnancy outcome in patients with unilateral or bilateral hydrosalpinx after *in vitro* fertilization, *Eur. J. Obstet. Gynecol. Reprod. Biol.*, 56, 129, 1994.

290. Strandell, A., Waldenström, U., Nilsson, L., and Hamberger, L., Hydrosalpinx reduces *in vitro* fertilization/embryo transfer pregnancy rates, *Hum. Reprod.*, 9, 861, 1994.

291. Vandromme, J., Chasse, E., Lejeune, B., Van Rysselberge, M., Delvigne, A., and Leroy, F., Hydrosalpinges in *in vitro* fertilization: an unfavourable prognostic feature, *Hum. Reprod.*, 10, 576, 1995.

292. Andersen, A. N., Lindhard, A., Loft, A., Ziebe, S., and Andersen, C. Y., The infertile patient with hydrosalpinges—IVF with or without salpingectomy? *Hum. Reprod.*, 11, 2081, 1996.

293. Kliman, H. J., Feinberg, R. F., Schwartz, L. B., Feinman, M. A., Lavi, E., and Meaddough, E. L., A mucin-like glycoprotein identified by MAG (mouse ascites Golgi) antibodies: menstrual cycle-dependent localization in human endometrium, *Am. J. Pathol.*, 146, 166, 1995.

294. Tabibzadeh, S., Shea, W., Lessey, B. A., and Satyaswaroop, P. G., Aberrant expression of ebaf in endometria of patients with infertility, *Mol. Hum. Reprod.*, 4, 595, 1998.

295. Garzon, P., Navarro Ruiz, A., Garcia Estrada, J., and Gallegos, A., Steroid conjugate formed by human endometrium, *Arch. Invest. Med.*, 20, 113, 1989.

296. Legro, R. S., Wong, I. L., Paulson, R. J., Lobo, R. A., and Sauer, M. V., Recipient's age does not adversely affect pregnancy outcome after oocyte donation, *Am. J. Obstet. Gynecol.*, 172, 96, 1995.

297. Van Kooij, R. J., Dorland, M., Looman, C. W. N., te Velde, E. R., and Habbema, J. D. F., Age-dependent decrease in embryo implantation rate after *in vitro* fertilization, *Fertil. Steril.*, 66, 769, 1996.

298. Paulson, R. J., Thornton, M. H., Francis, M. M., and Salvador, H. S., Successful pregnancy in a 63-year-old woman, *Fertil. Steril.*, 68, 1154, 1997.

299. Dor, J., Itzkowic, D. J., Mashiach, S., Lunenfeld, B., and Serr, D. M., Cumulative conception rates following gonadotropin therapy, *Am. J. Obstet. Gynecol.*, 136, 102, 1980.

300. Hou, Q., Paria, B. C., Mui, C., Dey, S. K., and Gorski, J., Immunolocalization of estrogen receptor protein in the mouse blastocyst during normal and delayed implantation, *Proc. Natl. Acad. Sci. USA*, 93, 2376, 1996.

301. Kliman, H. J. and Feinberg, R. F., Differentiation of the trophoblast, in *The First Twelve Weeks of Gestation*, Barnea, E. R., Hustin, J., and Jauniaux, E., Eds., Springer-Verlag, Berlin, 1992, 3–10.

302. Reshef, E., Lei, Z. M., Rao, C. V., Pridham, D. D., Chegini, N., and Luborsky, J. L., The presence of gonadotropin receptors in nonpregnant human uterus, human placenta, fetal membranes, and decidua, *J Clin. Endocrinol. Metab.*, 70, 421, 1990.

303. Feinberg, R. F., Kliman, H. J., and Lockwood, C. J., Is oncofetal fibronectin a trophoblast glue for human implantation?, *Am. J. Pathol.*, 138, 537, 1991.

304. Shim, C., Kwon, H. B., and Kim, K., Differential expression of laminin chain-specific mRNA transcripts during mouse preimplantation embryo development, *Mol. Reprod. Dev.*, 44, 44, 1996.

305. Suzuki, M., Raab, G., Moses, M. A., Fernandez, C. A., and Klagsbrun, M., Matrix metalloproteinase-3 releases active heparin-binding EGF-like growth factor by cleavage at a specific juxtamembrane site, *J. Biol. Chem.*, 272, 31730, 1997.

306. Bass, K. E., Morrish, D., Roth, I., Bhardwaj, D., Taylor, R., Zhou, Y., and Fisher, S. J., Human cytotrophoblast invasion is up-regulated by epidermal growth factor: evidence that paracrine factors modify this process, *Dev. Biol.*, 164, 550, 1994.
307. Anderson, T. L., Sieg, S. M., and Hodgen, G. D., Membrane compostition of the endometrial epithelium: molecular markers of uterine receptivity to implantation, *Hum. Reprod.*, 513, 1988.
308. Gardner, D. K., Vella, P., Lane, M., Wagley, L., Schlenker, T., and Schoolcraft, W. B., Culture and transfer of human blastocysts increases implantation rates and reduces the need for multiple embryo transfers, *Fertil. Steril.*, 69, 84, 1998.
309. Kniss, D. A., Zimmerman, P. D., Garver, C. L., and Fertel, R. H., Interleukin-1 receptor antagonist blocks interleukin-1-induced expression of cyclooxygenase-2 in endometrium, *Am. J. Obstet. Gynecol.*, 177, 559, 1997.
310. Simón, C., Gimeno, M. J., Mercader, A., O'Conner, J. E., Remohi, J., Polan, M. L., and Pellicer, A., Embryonic regulation of integrins β3, α4, and α1 in human endometrial epithelial cells *in vitro*, *J. Clin. Endocrinol. Metab.*, 82, 2607, 1997.
311. Grosskinsky, C. M., Yowell, C. W., Sun, J. H., Parise, L. V., and Lessey, B. A., Modulation of integrin expression in endometrial stromal cells *in vitro*, *J. Clin. Endocrinol. Metab.*, 81, 2047, 1996.
312. Tabibzadeh, S., Kong, Q. F., Kapur, S., Satyaswaroop, P. G., and Aktories, K., Tumour necrosis factor-α-mediated dyscohesion of epithelial cells is associated with disordered expression of cadherin/β-catenin and disassembly of actin filaments, *Hum. Reprod.*, 10, 994, 1995.
313. Irving, J. A. and Lala, P. K., Functional role of cell surface integrins on human trophoblast cell migration: regulation by TGF-β, IGF-II, and IGFBP-1, *Exp. Cell Res.*, 217, 419, 1995.

4 Evaluation of Male Infertility

Roy A. Brandell and Peter N. Schlegel

CONTENTS

I. INTRODUCTION

Infertility is an emotionally charged problem affecting an estimated 15% of all couples. The man should be evaluated concurrently with the woman since a male factor is the primary or contributing cause in 40 to 60% of cases. In addition to detecting treatable abnormalities, evaluation of the infertile man is critical to uncover life-threatening problems associated with the symptom of infertility, as well as genetic conditions associated with male infertility that could be transmitted to offspring with assisted reproduction. New diagnostic tests and refined surgical techniques have improved treatment results and patient care. Dramatic advancements in, and widespread use of, assisted reproductive techniques such as intracytoplasmic sperm injection have created alternatives for couples who previously had little hope of reproductive success. The infertility practitioner should have a thorough understanding of the advantages and limitations of various laboratory tests as well as the indications, costs, and success rates of all treatment options. The first step in evaluation is a thorough history and physical examination with initiation of basic laboratory studies.

II. HISTORY

As with all medical problems, a complete history is the cornerstone of infertility evaluation (Table 4.1). A detailed reproductive history includes duration of the problem, previous pregnancies (together or with other partners), frequency and timing of intercourse, potency and ejaculatory function, prior methods of birth control, and the use of vaginal lubricants. Some commercially available lubricants, such as K-Y Jelly™, have been shown to inhibit sperm motility, whereas vegetable and mineral oils do not appear to have this detrimental effect. The results of all previous infertility evaluation should be obtained.

A thorough past medical history including any systemic diseases along with current or previous treatment should be noted. Diabetes, thyroid disease, and renal insufficiency are just a few of the problems that can impact fertility. It takes nearly three months for a stem cell within the testicle to proceed through two meiotic divisions, morphologically mature during spermiogenesis, and appear in the ejaculate as a mature spermatozoon. Therefore, special attention should be given to any illness occurring in this time period. High fevers or other systemic ailments can cause substantial, albeit temporary, declines in sperm quantity and quality. Also important is any history of urinary tract infection or sexually transmitted disease.

Although all surgical procedures should be listed, certain ones are more likely to affect fertility. Orchidopexy is performed in childhood for cryptorchidism (undescended testicle). Low sperm density has been reported in 30% of adults with a history of unilateral cryptorchidism and 50% with bilateral cryptorchidism.[1] Any abnormality or trauma affecting the testis on one side appears to have deleterious effects on the contralateral, "normal," testis as well. For example, torsion, testis cancer, or varicocele can all cause abnormal results on semen analysis despite an apparent unilateral abnormality.

Previous inguinal hernia repair, performed any time in life, should raise the possibility of vasal injury causing obstruction of the vas deferens or injury to the testicular blood supply resulting in testicular atrophy. Indeed, any procedure performed in the inguinal or scrotal region carries these potential complications. These include previous procedures for the evaluation or treatment of infertility such as testis biopsy and testicular or epididymal sperm extraction. Nerves of the sympathetic

---

TABLE 4.1
Infertility History Outline

  I. Sexual history
    A. Duration
    B. Previous pregnancies
      1. Present partner
      2. Previous partner
    C. Frequency and timing of coitus
    D. Sexual technique
      1. Methods of birth control
      2. Potency/ejaculation
      3. Lubricants
    E. Previous evaluation and treatment
      1. Patient
      2. Partner
  II. Medical history
    A. Systemic illnesses or infections
    B. Previous/current therapy
    C. Surgical procedures
      1. Testicular
      2. Inguinal
      3. Pelvic
      4. Retroperitoneal
      5. Prostatic or bladder
    D. Gonadotoxins
      1. Chemicals
      2. Drugs
      3. Radiation
      4. Thermal
  III. Developmental history
    A. Childhood illness
    B. Childhood surgeries
    C. Onset and progression of puberty

---

nervous system are abundant in the retroperitoneum and pelvis. Therefore, any operations undertaken in these areas, especially retroperitoneal lymph node dissection for testis cancer, can lead to abnormalities of emission and ejaculation. Procedures performed on the prostate (e.g., transurethral resection of the prostate) or bladder can cause similar problems.

A developmental history includes documentation of any procedures done during childhood, but also includes systemic illnesses. Postpubertal mumps orchitis can lead to testicular atrophy and impaired fertility. Details regarding the onset and progression of puberty should be obtained since abnormalities here may suggest an endocrinopathy.

Finally, exposure to any potential gonadotoxins should be identified. These include alcohol, tobacco, caffeine, radiation, chemotherapy (especially alkylating agents), marijuana, and anabolic steroids. Many medications such as cimetidine, sulfa drugs, nitrofurantoin, cholesterol-regulating agents, and calcium channel blockers may also affect semen quality. Elevated intrascrotal temperatures may impair spermatogenesis, and routine use of saunas or hot tubs should be discouraged. The type of undergarments used does not appear to affect sperm production significantly.

III. PHYSICAL EXAMINATION

A complete physical examination should be performed since any condition affecting overall health theoretically can cause abnormalities in sperm production. The patient's general appearance including body habitus, limb length, and degree of virilization (e.g., gynecomastia, body hair) is assessed. Head, neck, heart, lungs, abdomen, extremities, and nervous system are evaluated meticulously. Any surgical scars should be noted, especially in the inguinal regions, which may represent surgical procedures performed in infancy or childhood.

Although relatively rare, several recognized syndromes exist that should be kept in mind while completing the systemic review and exam. Kartagener's syndrome is characterized by immotile sperm, frequent respiratory infections, and situs inversus. It is caused by a defective microtubule arrangement in the axoneme of cilia and sperm tails. Kallmann's syndrome results in hypogonadotropic hypogonadism and is associated with anosmia, lack of secondary sexual characteristics, and long arms out of proportion to trunk length. It results from impaired gonadotropin releasing hormone (GnRH) secretion by the hypothalamus. Klinefelter's syndrome is a disorder resulting in azoospermia (Table 4.2), gynecomastia, and elevated serum gonadotropin levels. These patients also may display undervirilization, small, firm testes, and increased average body height. The condition is caused by meiotic nondisjunction of chromosomes during gametogenesis resulting in a 47, XXY karyotype.

TABLE 4.2
Commonly Used Terms

Term	Operational Definition
Normospermia	Sperm density greater than 20 million sperm per vol.
Azoospermia	No spermatozoa in the ejaculate
Oligospermia	Sperm density less than 20 million per ml.
Asthenospermia	Less than 50% spermatozoa with good quality movement (Grade 3 or 4)
Aspermia	No ejaculate
Pyospermia	More than 1×10^6 WBC/ml
Teratospermia	Less than 30% spermatozoa with normal morphology (WHO criteria)

Special attention should be given to the genital exam beginning with penile anatomy. Inspection of the skin may reveal any lesions indicative of sexually transmitted disease. Note the position of the urethral meatus as hypospadias may impair the patient's ability to deposit an ejaculate deep in the vagina near the cervix. The testicles are then examined for masses, tenderness, size, and consistency in both the supine and standing positions. A normal testis is over 4 cm in length with a volume greater than 16 cc. The seminiferous tubules contain the spermatogenic region of the testis and occupy 80% of its volume. A reduction in the number of tubular cells can manifest itself as testicular atrophy. Abnormally soft testicles and the presence of small, hard testes also suggest impaired spermatogenesis.

Next, attention is turned to the epididymis and spermatic cord structures. Swelling, tenderness, or scarring of the epididymis suggests current or previous infection. The epididymis also may become indurated due to obstruction. The vas deferens is usually easy to palpate through the scrotal skin. Absence of this structure usually occurs secondary to congenital absence or atresia. Some but not all of these patients will also have seminal vesicle and/or renal anomalies. Varicoceles have been reported in up to 10% of men presenting with subfertility.[2] This condition results from retrograde flow of blood into dilated, tortuous veins in the pampiniform plexus of the testis. The patient should be examined in a warm room in the standing position. The severity of a varicocele may be graded as follows: Grade I—palpable only during Valsalva maneuver, Grade II—palpable in the standing position, and Grade III—visible through the scrotal skin. Varicoceles occur primarily on the left side, but bilateral varicoceles commonly are detected with careful examination.

The exact pathophysiology of varicoceles remains poorly understood. Impaired testicular function may result from abnormally high scrotal temperature, hypoxia due to venous stasis, dilution of intratesticular substrates (testosterone), hormonal imbalances, or reflux of renal and adrenal metabolites down the spermatic vein. Data exist to both support and refute each of these possibilities.[3] Spermatogenesis in the testicle and maturation in the epididymis are highly sensitive to even minor elevations in temperature. Therefore, the effect of varicoceles on scrotal temperature has garnered the most support.

Lastly, the digital rectal examination should be performed. The size and consistency of the prostate gland is recorded. A tender or "boggy" gland indicates inflammation or infection (prostatitis). The seminal vesicles may be subtly palpable. Markedly dilated seminal vesicles are thus an important finding requiring further evaluation (discussed later in this chapter).

IV. LABORATORY STUDIES

A. SEMEN ANALYSIS

The semen analysis is not, strictly speaking, a measure of fertility. However, it does represent a critical component of the initial evaluation of the infertile man. At least three separate specimens, each with a consistent 48 to 72 hour abstinence period, collected over several months are required. Substantial fluctuations in seminal quality can occur. The entire ejaculate is collected in an appropriate container, preferably by masturbation, and transported at body temperature to the laboratory in less than 1 hour (the sooner the better). The technique of semen analysis is covered in detail elsewhere.[4]

Briefly, the physical characteristics of the specimen are assessed including color, volume, viscosity, pH, and liquefaction. Freshly ejaculated semen is a coagulum that gradually liquefies over 20 to 25 minutes. Substances in the seminal vesicles induce coagulation while proteolytic enzymes contributed by the prostate gland cause liquefaction. The seminal vesicles are responsible for most (50 to 80%) of the ejaculate volume. Seminal vesicle fluid has a slightly basic pH and contains high concentrations of fructose produced through an androgen dependent process. The seminal vesicles are the major source of fructose in the reproductive system. Patients with seminal vesicle obstruction or congenital absence typically will have a fructose-negative, low volume, low pH ejaculate that does not coagulate. Prostatic secretions are rich in zinc, prostate specific antigen, and acid phosphatases and are slightly acidic resulting in a normal seminal pH in the physiologic range.

A microscopic evaluation of the specimen quantifies three general parameters: sperm density, motility, and morphology. Studies show that average semen parameters for normal, fertile men far exceed what is necessary for conception. Therefore, it is more appropriate to discuss the "limits of adequacy" or perhaps the "low end of normal" rather than "average" values (Table 4.3). This highlights an important difference between *subfertility* and *sterility*. As semen quality declines below the limits of adequacy, the chances of pregnancy decrease statistically. The pregnancy rate does not reach zero, theoretically, until a total absence of motile sperm is demonstrated.

TABLE 4.3
Minimal Standards for
Semen Analysis

Characteristic	Standard
Volume	1.5–5 cc
Density	>20 million/cc
Motility	>50%
Forward progression	>2 (scale 1–4)
Morphology	>30% normal

Note: Plus: absence of significant agglutination, pyospermia, and hyperviscosity.

If no sperm are found on routine semen analysis, the specimen is centrifuged and the pellet resuspended in a 10 to 200 µl volume for inspection. Absence of sperm in the pellet makes a definitive diagnosis of azoospermia. If motility is low (<50%) a viability stain should be performed. Determination of the proportion of viable sperm is important since ICSI is often successful using immotile sperm so long as they are viable. Unfortunately, stained spermatozoa are destroyed by this process and cannot be used directly; the viability percentage may be used only to estimate the subsequent success of ICSI using unstained sperm.

Microscopic examination of the seminal fluid should also include identification of "round cells." These represent either immature germ cells or leukocytes. Differentiating between the two is important since abnormal levels of leukocytes (>10⁶/ml) suggest infection, which may be treatable with an appropriate antibiotic. Traditionally, a peroxidase stain was used for detecting leukocytes, but had the disadvantage of only identifying granulocytes. Immunohistochemical techniques are now available that make use of monoclonal antibodies directed against WBC surface antigens.[5] This approach allows more consistent and accurate differentiation of round cells. Pyospermia should be evaluated further with aerobic and anaerobic cultures including analysis for *Mycoplasma hominis*, *Ureaplasma urealyticum*, and *Chlamydia trachomatis*.

Finally, the semen specimen should be evaluated for sperm agglutination. This finding is not uncommon and frequently represents an artifact of specimen collection or processing. For example, when sperm are present at high concentrations, they may appear to agglutinate. Dilution of the semen specimen will allow accurate evaluation of the presence or absence of agglutination. However, persistent agglutination (especially when associated with formation of sperm "dimers") may suggest the presence of antisperm antibodies. Patients who exhibit this condition should undergo further evaluation with antisperm antibody testing.

B. Urine Analysis

Obtain a urine analysis on any patient with a history of genitourinary symptoms, prior infectious, or anatomic abnormalities. A postejaculatory specimen is preferable. Again, the presence of WBCs suggests infection and culture of urine is indicated. Microscopic examination of expressed prostatic secretions may allow localization of a subclinical infection to the prostate. The presence of sperm (>10/hpf or 20% antegrade ejaculated sperm) in the urine implies retrograde ejaculation as reviewed later. Noninfectious microscopic hematuria may suggest a benign or malignant lesion within the urinary tract from the kidneys to the tip of the urethra. Hematuria should be evaluated with renal imaging and cystourethroscopy.

C. Hormonal Studies

Normal sperm production, maturation, and transport require the presence of certain hormones in appropriate amounts. The cascade of hormonal production begins at the level of the hypothalamus with the pulsatile release of gonadotropin releasing hormone (GnRH). This stimulates the release of the gonadotropin luteinizing hormone (LH) and follicle stimulating hormone (FSH) from the pituitary. LH stimulates Leydig cells in the testicles to release testosterone. FSH acts on the Sertoli cells to quantitatively maintain spermatogenesis. Sertoli cells release inhibin and other factors that feed back to the pituitary to modulate FSH release. Testosterone is present in high concentrations in the testis and is also very important in maintaining quantitatively normal spermatogenesis. It is converted in most androgen sensitive organs into a more potent form, dihydrotestosterone, by the enzyme 5-alpha reductase.

Prolactin (PRL) is another pituitary hormone that can impact fertility. It decreases LH release and impairs libido if present in excess. Elevated prolactin levels can be idiopathic or due to macroadenomas of the pituitary. Symptoms such as severe headaches or impaired visual fields should raise clinical suspicion of a macroadenoma.

Patients with primary testicular failure may have significantly elevated gonadotropins, especially FSH , due to the absence of negative feedback. Abnormally low gonadotropin levels are secondary to hypothalamic or pituitary dysfunction. Although only 3% of male infertility cases result from a primary hormonal problem in most clinical series,[6] these blood tests are recommended for all men presenting with infertility. Radioimmunoassays for these hormones are readily available. Karyotype analysis and microdeletion analysis of the Y chromosome are indicated for men with severe oligospermia or azoospermia ($<10\times10^6$ sperm/cc) because of the frequency of genetic anomalies in men with low sperm production.

V. SPECIALIZED TESTS

After obtaining a detailed history, physical exam, and baseline laboratory studies, more specific and sophisticated laboratory evaluation may be indicated.

A. COMPUTER ASSISTED SEMEN ANALYSIS

Determinations of sperm morphology and quality of motion historically have been highly subjective. In an effort to lend objectivity to such measurements, researchers developed computer assisted semen analysis (CASA).[6] Advanced biotechnology, including time-exposure photomicrography, multiple-exposure photomicrography, and videomicrography, coupled with sophisticated computer programs, has made measurement of sperm kinematics possible. Parameters such as curvilinear velocity, straight-line velocity, and amplitude of lateral head displacement are commonly reported.[7]

CASA also may reveal the fertilizing capacity of sperm by identifying and quantitating hyperactivated sperm motility. In the area of sperm morphology, CASA can determine head length and width as well as circumference and area. Sperm density can also be measured, but superiority over conventional semen analysis has not been demonstrated. In fact, CASA is far inferior to visual evaluation of sperm concentration for severely oligozoospermic men. The program may incorrectly classify azoospermic men as having sperm in the ejaculate. CASA provides a great deal of detailed information regarding subtle parameters of sperm motility, but the value of this tool outside the research laboratory remains to be demonstrated.

B. POSTCOITAL TEST

This test evaluates the interaction between sperm from the man and the cervical mucus from the woman. Important information is obtained since sperm must travel through cervical mucus to fertilize the ova. Cervical mucus is obtained just prior to ovulation, but several hours after intercourse. The specimen is considered normal if microscopic findings show more than 10 sperm per hpf (400×) and 50% or more have progressive motility. The test is indicated in cases of hyperviscous semen, unexplained infertility, low or high volume ejaculates with good sperm density, and abnormal penile anatomy. Patients with poor quality semen analysis do not require a postcoital test since results are also invariably poor.

By comparing the results of the postcoital test with the standard semen analysis, one can localize the abnormality to the male or female partner. Alternatively, cross mucus hostility testing can be performed. Here, the wife's mucus is placed in contact with both her husband's sperm and normal donor sperm for *in vitro* comparison. The female factor can be removed entirely by analyzing the partner's sperm in bovine cervical mucus. The motility of sperm in human and bovine mucus is similar.

C. ANTISPERM ANTIBODY TESTING

A blood-testis and blood-epididymal barrier exists which prevents exposure of sperm to the immune system. When these barriers are breached, the man's immune system perceives the sperm as foreign and antisperm antibody production occurs. An association between antisperm antibodies and infertility has been apparent for many years. Although a small percentage of fertile men will exhibit antisperm antibodies in their serum, higher rates of detection of antibodies occur in infertile men, and pregnancy rates are significantly lower in couples when the man has high antibody titers.[8] Various studies show that the antibodies of greatest importance are those bound to the sperm surface. Antibodies to internal sperm antigens and those found only in serum are of questionable clinical significance.

A number of techniques help detect antisperm antibodies. The most widely used and most accurate method is the direct immunobead assay (e.g., Sperm Check™, Biorad Laboratories, Hercules, CA). Rabbit antihuman antibodies are linked with either latex microspheres or polyacrylamide beads about 1 μm in size. Washed spermatozoa are mixed with the beads which bind that portion of the sperm containing the antisperm antibodies. Binding identification requires either a phase-contrast microscope or bright field standard microscopy depending on the type of bead utilized. Indirect immunobead assays (utilizing normal donor sperm with serum) may be used to detect serum antisperm antibodies, either from the man or woman.

Another technique is the mixed agglutination reaction (SpermMar test, Ortho Diagnostic Systems, Beerse, Belgium). It is performed by mixing unwashed patient sperm with red blood cells (RBC) coated with human antibodies. If antibodies are present, agglutination of the RBCs occurs when antihuman antiserum is added. Enzyme-linked immunosorbent assays (ELISA) are also available and easy to use, but false positive results have been problematic.

Any insult to the testicle, epididymis, or spermatic cord structures can lead to antibody formation. Conditions associated with antibody formation include vasectomy, infection, reproductive tract obstruction, cancer, testis biopsy, testicular torsion, cryptorchidism, and varicoceles. Indications for antibody testing include the presence of abnormal sperm agglutination, impaired motility, an abnormal postcoital test, or unexplained infertility.

D. SPERM FUNCTION TESTS

Although sperm may be present in adequate numbers, with normal motility and morphology, there is no guarantee that the sperm are functionally competent to fertilize an ovum. Therefore, several tests of sperm function have been developed. Each has shortcomings but may be useful in certain clinical or experimental situations.

Species-specific fertilization is regulated by the zona pellucida, the acellular glycoprotein layer that surrounds the specific ovum. If this layer is removed, evaluation of sperm-oocyte interaction is possible with the sperm penetration assay (SPA). A positive (normal) SPA requires that a sperm perform several important functions: capacitation, the acrosome reaction, fusion with the oolema, and incorporation into the ooplasm.

The SPA is the most commonly performed sperm function test. Human sperm are combined with hamster oocytes *in vitro*. The total number of ova penetrated and the number of penetrations per ova are determined. Normal results vary between labs but, in general, 10% of eggs penetrated and greater than 5 penetrations per egg is desirable.

The SPA is a nonstandardized bioassay and results have been variable. This has produced controversy surrounding indications for the assay and interpretation of results. The SPA correlates with semen analysis, especially motility, in most studies and with *in vitro* fertilization (IVF) rates.[9] Patients with a positive SPA have a 95% chance of fertilizing human ova *in vitro*. This contrasts with a 50% chance in couples with a negative SPA.[10] Some studies suggest a correlation between SPA results and natural *in vivo* pregnancy as well.[11] We rarely apply the SPA in evaluation of infertile men since this test seldom provides novel information that is not available from standard semen analyses. In addition, SPA is an expensive test that rarely changes clinical management of couples with male infertility. Occasional situations when the SPA may be indicated include cases of unexplained infertility and for couples considering assisted reproduction with IVF where there are borderline indications for intracytoplasmic sperm injection (ICSI). SPA testing is unnecessary when there are clear indications to proceed with ICSI.

Another test of sperm function, less commonly performed, is the hemizona assay, which measures the ability of sperm to interact with the zona pellucida, a prerequisite to fertilization. The human zona pellucida is divided microscopically in half. Each half is then mixed with either the patient's sperm or the sperm of a fertile donor. The total number of sperm bound divided by the number of donor sperm bound to the zona pellucida produces an index. A hemizona index less than 60% correlates with decreased chance of successful IVF.[12] The need for human ova limits the usefulness of this procedure. More importantly, the hemizona assay provides limited information that will affect clinical treatment.

Sperm membrane and acrosome studies also have been developed and may be useful in some clinical and research settings. Exposing viable sperm to hypoosmotic solutions causes tail swelling which is identifiable under a light microscope. Up to 80% of sperm from normal fertile donors develop swelling, with a distinctive coiling pattern in the tail region.[13] Because the hypoosmotic swelling (HOS) test functionally evaluates sperm-membrane integrity and viability on an individual sperm without lethal toxicity, the HOS test potentially allows selection of viable sperm for ICSI. Correlation of this test with SPA and IVF has been inconsistent.[14]

Fertilization requires that sperm undergo capacitation and the acrosome reaction. Using specific stains with light microscopy or transmission electron microscopy we may differentiate those sperm that undergo the acrosome reaction and those that do not.[15,16] This information could be used to identify the subgroup of patients whose infertility is secondary to abnormalities in the acrosome reaction. Many of these men, typically treated with ICSI, already may have been identified as candidates for ICSI based on severe morphologic abnormalities.

VI. RADIOLOGIC STUDIES

Radiographic evaluation serves as a valuable adjunct in determining the etiology of a patient's infertility. Scrotal ultrasonography is one of the most commonly performed studies. As discussed earlier, varicoceles are the most common correctable abnormalities in men presenting for infertility evaluation. Using ultrasonography, the diameter of dilated veins in the pampiniform plexus can be measured and retrograde flow confirmed using color Doppler flow imaging. This technology is so sensitive that "subclinical varicoceles" can be diagnosed. Subclinical varicoceles are too small to be detected on physical exam. The need for diagnosing and treating these lesions is controversial. In general, if the scrotal venous diameter is greater than 2.7 mm, then these veins can be detected on physical examination.

Scrotal ultrasound identifies other pathology as well. The testicular parenchyma can be visualized and size accurately assessed. Masses such as tumors, hydroceles, and spermatoceles can be evaluated. Color flow analysis also has been used to rule out testicular torsion in patients presenting with acute scrotal pain. Abdominal ultrasonography is indicated for evaluation of the inferior vena cava and retroperitoneum for men with large varicoceles that do not collapse in the supine position. Men with vasal anomalies also require renal evaluation. Unilateral congenital absence of the vas deferens is associated with agenesis of the ipsilateral kidney in up to 90% of cases, whereas men with congenital bilateral absence have a 10 to 15% prevalence of unilateral renal anomalies.

Transrectal ultrasound (TRUS) has gained widespread use in urology, mainly in evaluating men for prostate cancer. However, this technology also can easily image the seminal vesicles and ejaculatory ducts. The presence of dilated seminal vesicles or ejaculatory ducts suggests obstructed ejaculatory ducts. Absence or atresia of the seminal vesicles is found in patients with a nonpalpable scrotal vas deferens and can be used as a confirmatory test of physical findings. When the scrotal vas is not present, a retroperitoneal vas rarely can be detected on TRUS.

Identifying sites of obstruction in the vas deferens often requires vasography. A vasogram should only be performed at the time of planned reconstruction, not concurrent with a diagnostic testis biopsy. A Foley catheter is placed into the bladder and gentle traction used to occlude the bladder neck. The vas is cannulated through a hemi-vasotomy and injected with contrast medium while plain radiographs of the pelvis are obtained. The finding of contrast in the urethra rules out obstruction. The catheter prevents the bladder from filling with contrast than can obscure the distal ejaculatory ducts. Never attempt retrograde injection of contrast toward the testicle. This may result in epididymal rupture and injury to the testicle.

VII. TESTICULAR BIOPSY

A testicular biopsy is indicated for the evaluation of azoospermic patients to differentiate ductal obstruction from abnormal spermatogenesis. It can be accomplished under general or local anesthesia through a small "window" scrotal incision. Needle biopsy has been performed, but a percutaneous needle biopsy provides so few tubules for analysis that the clinical usefulness of this approach remains debatable. Bilateral biopsy is indicated whenever two testes are present. Testicular biopsy is not indicated in cases of oligospermia since the results will rarely alter therapy.

Microscopic evaluation of biopsy specimens initially should be quantified by evaluating the average number of elongating spermatids per round seminiferous tubule. If more than 15 to 20 mature spermatids per tubule are present in an azoospermic patient, then a diagnosis of obstruction can be made.

Seminiferous tubules frequently appear in a mosaic of different spermatogenic patterns in a single testis. These tubules generally fall into the following categories:

A. NORMAL

Seminiferous tubules are separated by a thin interstitium containing acidophilic Leydig cells, macrophages, blood vessels, lymphatics, and connective tissue. Sertoli cells and spermatogonia line the basement membrane of the tubules. Germ cells are visible in all stages of spermatogenesis. Normal findings are typically found in azoospermic men with ductal obstruction.

B. HYPOSPERMATOGENESIS

In this condition, seminiferous tubules contain a reduced number of all germinal elements. The germinal epithelium may be disorganized in places with immature germ cells in the lumen. The interstitium and Leydig cells are normal. Diffuse hypospermatogenesis may manifest clinically with oligospermia or azoospermia.

C. MATURATION ARREST

These testes display normal spermatogenesis proceeding up to a specific stage of development, but no further. The arrest may be early (primary or secondary spermatocyte) or late (spermatid). Mixed patterns occur occasionally, and some cases of late maturation arrest may be difficult to differentiate from normal spermatogenesis. A touch prep or wet prep of testicular tissue may help to evaluate complete spermatogenesis during the testis biopsies. Most patients with maturation arrest have nonobstructive azoospermia.

D. SERTOLI CELL ONLY SYNDROME

Also known as germinal aplasia, this condition appears histologically as a complete absence of germ cells. Seminiferous tubule diameter is reduced and the interstitium may be minimally altered or demonstrate Leydig cell hyperplasia. The Sertoli cells are identified easily by their basal location in the seminiferous tubules and by the single prominent nucleolus in the nucleus of each cell. Typically, these patients have bilateral atrophic, soft testicles and elevated levels of FSH.

E. Sclerosis

Seminiferous tubules and the surrounding interstitium are sclerotic and hyalinization may be apparent. Germ cells are absent and Leydig cells may be present in hypertrophic nodules. On physical exam, these testes usually feel small and firm. Patients with Klinefelter's syndrome may exhibit these symptoms.

Testicular biopsy findings rarely are pathognomonic and do not, by themselves, provide a clinical diagnosis. Oftentimes, biopsy simply confirms what is already suspected clinically.

VIII. ETIOLOGY AND TREATMENT

Men presenting for infertility evaluation generally will fall into one of four groups based upon their semen analysis results: (1) all parameters normal, (2) azoospermia, (3) abnormalities in all semen parameters, or (4) isolated problems restricted to one parameter. Categorizing patients in this manner helps to organize subsequent work-up and treatment.

A. Normal

If all semen parameters appear normal, a thorough evaluation of the female partner should be completed. If her evaluation proves normal, or if identified problems are treated adequately but pregnancy still does not result, then a post-coital test and antisperm antibody evaluation should be performed, followed by more sophisticated testing of sperm function, if appropriate. This subfertile condition is referred to as unexplained (or idiopathic) infertility. A sperm penetration assay occasionally helps to direct further evaluation and treatment (e.g., to proceed directly to ICSI rather than IUI or IVF if no penetrations are seen).

B. Azoospermia

If an initial semen analysis shows a complete absence of sperm, the diagnosis should be confirmed by centrifuging the specimen and examining the pellet. It is not uncommon to find a few sperm, in which case, complete obstruction has been ruled out. Hormonal evaluation is indicated in all patients with azoospermia including individuals with an obvious cause such as previous vasectomy or congenital absence of the vas deferens.

Serum FSH reflects the completeness of spermatogenesis in the seminiferous tubules. In general, FSH appears to reflect the number of germ cells present in the testes.[17] So, a man with normal spermatogenesis in a solitary testis will have an elevated FSH. However, a man with nonobstructive azoospermia and maturation arrest in both testes typically will have a normal serum FSH level, but may have no sperm present within the testes. In addition, a man with diffuse Sertoli cell only pattern but isolated pockets of spermatogenesis typically will have an elevated FSH but have an excellent chance of sperm retrieval with testicular sperm extraction (TESE). Conversely, with maturation arrest (despite a frequently normal FSH), no mature sperm appear despite intensive efforts at TESE. If the FSH level is more than two to three times normal values, the patient has some degree of testicular failure and the chance of finding obstruction is very low. Testicular biopsy may be performed for confirmation to evaluate the prognosis for sperm retrieval and to rule out intratubular germ cell neoplasia (testicular carcinoma *in situ*). Potential causes of nonobstructive azoospermia include acquired (e.g., mumps orchids), genetic (e.g., Klinefelter's), or idiopathic. Patients with a Sertoli cell only pattern on testis biopsy have an elevated FSH in 90% of cases. Luteinizing hormone (LH) and testosterone (T) typically are normal. Men with primary testicular failure may achieve fertility depending on the ability of physicians to extract sperm of adequate quality and maturity from the testis. Intracytoplasmic sperm injection (ICSI) has made fertility possible for many men who just a few years ago would have been labeled as sterile.

A low FSH and LH combined with a reduced serum testosterone level is indicative of hypogonadotrophic hypogonadism. The condition may be congenital (e.g., Kallman's syndrome), acquired (e.g., pituitary tumor), or idiopathic. Such conditions require imaging of the pituitary with magnetic resonance imaging (MRI) along with further hormonal testing. Prolactin (PRL) levels also should be obtained. Evaluation of adrenocorticotropic hormone (ACTH), thyroid stimulating hormone (TSH), and growth hormone (GH) is rarely indicated for the infertile male. In the presence of acquired or congenital hypogonadotrophic hypogonadism, some patients will have panhypopituitarism while others might show significant elevations in an isolated hormone such as PRL. High circulating PRL levels cause decreased gonadotropin release and may have direct detrimental effects on the testes as well. Tumors usually are managed medically with oral bromocriptine or cabergoline. Resistant or symptomatic macroadenomas may require surgical management or radiation. Idiopathic elevations in PRL usually respond to bromocriptine administration. Deficiencies in GnRH or gonadotropins (LH and FSH) are managed with hormone replacement (partially purified or recombinant LH or FSH).

If FSH, LH, and T levels are normal, retrograde ejaculation or obstruction should be considered as a cause for the azoospermia. Retrograde ejaculation usually has an obvious cause such as diabetes or prior retroperitoneal surgery (e.g., retroperitoneal lymph node dissection for testis tumor). The prostate and bladder neck are densely populated with α-adrenergic receptors. Failure of the bladder neck to close during emission results in retrograde flow of semen into the bladder instead of down the urethra. This abnormality is diagnosed upon finding sperm in the urine on post-ejaculatory urinalysis (greater than 10 sperm per HPF). Treatment begins with sympathomimetic agents that help to close the bladder neck prior to emission and ejaculation. If unsuccessful, sperm may be retrieved from a post-ejaculatory urine specimen by centrifugation and used for insemination (e.g., IUI). However, urine is very toxic to sperm. Therefore, the post-ejaculatory urine should be centrifuged promptly to minimize contact of sperm with urine. Alternatively, the patient may be catheterized immediately before ejaculation, the bladder filled with sperm-wash buffer (e.g., HEPES-buffered human tubal fluid) and the post-ejaculatory urine used to extract spermatozoa for IUI.

If no sperm appear in the post-ejaculatory urine, evaluation of the ejaculatory ducts and seminal vesicles should be done. The absence of fructose in a low volume (<1 cc), acidic (pH<7) ejaculate and appearance of swollen seminal vesicles on transrectal ultrasound (TRUS) indicate ejaculatory duct obstruction. Prior to treatment, confirmation of the presence of vasa in the scrotum (on physical exam) and retroperitoneum (by TRUS) is mandatory. Ejaculatory duct obstruction may be treated endoscopically using transurethral resection of the ejaculatory ducts (TUR-ED), whereas congenital absence of the vas deferens requires sperm retrieval with assisted reproduction.

Azoospermic patients with normal FSH, palpable vasa, and no evidence of ejaculatory duct obstruction should undergo testis biopsy. If quantitatively limited spermatogenesis is found (less than 10 to 15 mature spermatids per tubule), TESE-ICSI, adoption, and donor insemination are management options. If biopsy results are normal, then exploration for obstruction, beginning with sampling of intravasal fluid and vasography, is indicated. Points of focal obstruction often can be repaired with the microsurgical techniques of vasoepididymostomy or vasovasostomy. If no sperm appear in the vasal fluid and the testis biopsy is normal, then a diagnosis of epididymal obstruction is warranted. Epididymal blockage frequently can be bypassed by microsurgical vasoepididymostomy. These procedures are straightforward, but technically demanding. Meticulous attention to detail is essential. Another therapeutic option, especially if the obstruction is beyond repair, is retrieval of spermatozoa through microsurgical epididymal sperm aspiration (MESA) for subsequent IVF and ICSI.[18] This approach is a primary treatment option for patients with congenital absence of the vas. To avoid subsequent sperm retrieval procedures if the microsurgical reconstruction is unsuccessful, sperm retrieval should be considered during the reconstructive procedure.

Occasionally, aspermia can result from failure of seminal emission (anejaculation). For these men, semen does not enter the urethra or bladder following climax despite an absence of ejaculatory duct obstruction. This results from complete functional failure of the entire ejaculatory mechanism. Some cases are idiopathic, but most are secondary to nervous system damage (e.g., following spinal cord injury or retroperitoneal surgery). Psychotherapeutic intervention can help in idiopathic/psychogenic cases, and sympathomimetic agents should be tried, but penile vibratory stimulation or electroejaculation is usually required to effect emission.

Genetic abnormalities are commonly present in men with azoospermia.[19] Men with congenital bilateral absence of the vas deferens (CBAVD) usually carry cystic fibrosis (CF) gene mutations, and testing of the female partner is mandatory before proceeding to sperm retrieval with assisted reproduction. CBAVD also corresponds to a 10 to 15% rate of renal anomalies. Men with idiopathic epididymal obstruction frequently carry CF gene mutations. If the female partner is a carrier as well, then the chance of having an affected child with CF approaches 50%.

Of men with nonobstructive azoospermia, 15 to 27% will show definable genetic abnormalities using screens for Y chromosome microdeletions and standard karyotype analyses. Common defects include deletions of the AZFb or AZFc (DAZ) region of the Y chromosome. For men who have AZFc deletions, sperm commonly are found in the ejaculate or with TESE. However, men with AZFb deletions appear far less likely to have sperm, even with extensive TESE procedures.[20] Karyotype abnormalities include Klinefelter's syndrome, other sex chromosome anomalies (e.g., XYY), and autosomal translocations. If a genetic anomaly is detected, genetic counseling is mandatory before proceeding to treatment with assisted reproduction. In some cases, preimplantation genetic diagnosis can be used to analyze each embryo during IVF to avoid transfer of genetically abnormal embryos. This process minimizes the risks of transmitting genetic anomalies.

C. DIFFUSE SEMEN ABNORMALITIES

Many patients present abnormalities involving all semen parameters: density, motility, and morphology. Repeated specimens are needed since transient stresses like high fever can cause a temporary decline in overall semen quality. For men with impaired semen quality, an appropriate search for correctable etiologies is necessary. This includes hormonal abnormalities, varicoceles, anti-sperm antibodies, heat/environmental factors, infections, mechanical/sexual dysfunction, certain prescription medications, or toxins that can affect sperm quality.

Scrotal varicoceles commonly cause diffuse bulk parameter defects.[21] They are diagnosed by physical exam and often confirmed with scrotal ultrasound. Varicoceles can be corrected surgically using a variety of techniques. The dilated veins are either ligated or occluded. Improved semen parameters occur in approximately 70% of patients but pregnancy rates average only 40 to 50%.[22] Not all varicoceles cause infertility and require treatment. However, if a man has a clinically detectable varicocele, semen abnormalities, and subfertility, then treatment may increase the chances of conception if the female partner is normal.

Sometimes diffuse semen analysis defects occur in the absence of an identifiable etiology. This is termed idiopathic subfertility. Empiric therapy with antiestrogens such as clomiphene citrate, either alone or in combination with supplemental gonadotropins, reveals inconsistent results. These patients often require assisted reproductive techniques (IUI or IVF/ICSI). Intrauterine insemination is best reserved for men with greater than 10 million motile sperm per ejaculate; however, IUI with ovarian stimulation often may be attempted even with only 5,000,000 motile sperm per ejaculate prior to proceeding with more invasive forms of assisted reproduction such as IVF.

D. SINGLE PARAMETER ABNORMALITIES

Low sperm motility with impaired forward progression (asthenospermia) is the most common isolated semen parameter abnormality. This problem is often due to anti-sperm antibodies and evidence of agglutination may be present. The microscopic finding of two sperm joined head to head or tail to tail (dimers) is almost pathognomonic for the presence of antibodies. The diagnosis ultimately is made using the previously described direct immunobead assays. Treatment with immunosupressive steroids has been reported, but results have been inconsistent, and this approach remains controversial because of the risk of aseptic necrosis associated with steroid administration.[23] Semen processing followed by IUI or IVF-ICSI is the most commonly pursued therapeutic option.

Poor motility also may result from genital tract infection. The presence of leukocytes in the semen along with positive urine culture results indicate a genital tract infection. Manage any suggestion of infection with antibiotics prior to embarking on a more involved and expensive work-up or treatment course. The choice of antibiotics also may affect sperm production, as some agents including nitrofurantoin and sulfa drugs appear to be toxic to the testis or sperm themselves. The quinolones (e.g., ciprofloxacin) and tetracyclines (e.g., doxycycline) generally are considered to be safe and effective for most pathogens in the genitourinary tract.

Partial ejaculatory duct obstruction or severe hypoandrogenic states also cause isolated parameter abnormalities (e.g., low semen volume) on rare occasions. These problems are diagnosed and treated as discussed previously. Nonspecific epididymal dysfunction or partial obstruction may occur as well and diagnosis is difficult. Isolated problems with sperm density can be managed with semen processing and IUI or other assisted reproductive techniques once treatable conditions have been ruled out. Accumulating poor quality ejaculates by freezing samples over time may be limited by the low freeze-thaw survival rate observed for sperm with poor motility.

Patients with low volume ejaculates (less than 1 cc) should be evaluated for ejaculatory duct obstruction or malformation of the vas/seminal vesicles. High volume ejaculates result in sperm dilution with an indeterminate effect on fertility. High semen volumes should be treated only if the postcoital test is abnormal. Mechanical concentration by centrifugation or use of a split ejaculate can be performed and are relatively straightforward tools. Hyperviscosity as an isolated problem also should be treated only if the postcoital test is poor. Oral treatment with vitamin C (250 mg/day), mucolytics (guanefisen), or sperm processing followed by IUI are treatment options. The treatable and/or correctable etiologies of male infertility are summarized in Table 4.4.

TABLE 4.4
Correctable and/or Treatable Causes of Male Infertility

Etiology	Treatment
Varicocele	Microsurgical varicocele ligation
Obstruction	Microsurgical reconstruction
Immunologic	Systemic steroid administration
Ejaculatory dysfunction	Sympathomometic agents
Endocrinologic	Medical/surgical treatment as indicated by diagnosis
Infection	Appropriate antibiotics

IX. CONCLUSIONS

The number of couples who seek medical attention for subfertility appears to rise each year. Men and women marry at a later age and often delay parenthood until after career development. As divorce rates rise, second and third marriages become commonplace, and many couples find themselves in a race against the woman's "biological clock." Traditionally, infertility evaluation occurred only after 12 months of attempted conception. Today, investigation may begin earlier as many couples have a limited time window for conception due to advanced female age. Evidence exists that the longer a couple remains subfertile, the less likely they are to conceive.[24]

Public awareness about fertility issues is also rising. Because of the large number of couples involved and the highly emotional nature of these problems, media attention has been intense. Recent reports have generated concern about a progressive, global decrease in sperm quality.[25] Although these studies had design flaws and may have drawn inappropriate conclusions, they did point out the possible detrimental effects of environmental toxins on reproductive function, an area that clearly deserves further investigation.[26]

The development of new diagnostic tests and treatment alternatives brings hope to many couples. There is still much we do not know, however, especially in the area of impaired spermatogenesis. Perhaps the most dramatic breakthrough in recent years has been the advent and success of ICSI. Couples formerly labeled sterile and encouraged to adopt or undergo donor insemination are now capable of bearing their own biologic offspring. An unfortunate consequence has been the tendency to bypass thorough evaluation and specific, effective treatment of the male by proceeding directly to assisted reproductive techniques. This practice is not only costly, but potentially dangerous. It may subject the woman to unnecessary hormonal manipulation and procedural intervention. Multiple gestations are common and carry their own costs and risks. It should also be remembered that impaired sperm production may be a symptom of a more complex and significant illness in the man such as a testis tumor or hormonal abnormality that requires appropriate investigation and therapy. Finally, optimal pregnancy and delivery rates may occur when a male factor is identified and properly treated.[27,28]

REFERENCES

1. Kogan, S. J., Cryptorchidism, in *Clinical Pediatric Urology*, Kelalis, P. P., King, L. R., and Belman, A. B., Eds., W. B. Saunders, Philadelphia, 1985, 876.
2. Cockett, A. T. K., Takihara, H., and Cosentino, M. J., The varicocele, *Fertil. Steril.*, 41, 5, 1984.
3. Turek, P. J. and Lipshultz, L. I., The varicocele controversies. I. Etiology and pathophysiology, *AUA Update Series*, Vol. XIV, Lesson 13, 1995.
4. World Health Organization. WHO laboratory manual for the examination of human semen and sperm-cervical mucus interaction, 4th ed., Cambridge University Press, 1999.
5. Homyk, M., Anderson, D. J., and Wolff, H., Differential diagnosis of immature germ cells in semen utilizing monoclonal antibodies MHS-10, *Fertil. Steril.*, 53, 323, 1990.

6. Baker, H. W. G., Burger, H. G., and de Kretser, D. M., Relative incidence of etiologic disorders in male infertility, in *Male Reproductive Dysfunction. Diagnosis and Management of Hypogonadism, Infertility, and Impotence*, Santen, R. J. and Swerdloff, R. S., Eds., Marcel Dekker, New York, 1986.

7. Mortimer, D., Aitken, R. J., Mortimer, S. T., and Pacey, A. A., Workshop report: clinical CASA—the quest for consensus, *Reprod. Fertil. Dev.*, 7, 951–9, 1995.

8. Rumke, P., Van Amstel, N., Messa, E. M., and Rezemar, P. D., Prognosis of fertility in men with sperm agglutins in the serum, *Fertil. Steril.*, 24, 35, 1973.

9. Swanson, R. J., Mayer, J. F., Jones, K. H., Lanzendorf, S. E., and McDowell, J., Hamster ova/human sperm penetration: correlation with count, motility, and morphology for *in vitro* fertilization, *Arch. Androl.*, 10, 69, 1983.

10. Smith, R. G., Johnson, A., Lamb, D. J., and Lipshultz, L. I., Functional tests of spermatozoa: sperm penetration assay, *Urol. Clin. North Am.*, 14, 451, 1987.

11. Corson, S. L., Batzer, F. R., Marmar, J., and Maislin, G., The human sperm-hamster egg penetration assay: prognostic value, *Fertil. Steril.*, 49, 328, 1988.

12. Burkman, L. J., Coddington, C. C., Fraken, D. R., Kruger, T. F., Rosenwaks, Z., and Hodgen, G. D., The hemizona assay (HZA): development of a diagnostic test for the binding of human spermatozoa to the human hemizona pellucida to predict fertilization potential, *Fertil. Steril.*, 49, 688, 1988.

13. Jeyendran, R. S., Van der Van, H. H., Perez-Pelaez, M., Crabo, B. G., and Zaneveld, L. J. D., Development of an assay to assess the functional integrity of the human sperm membrane and its relationship to other semen characteristics, *J. Reprod. Fertil.*, 70, 219, 1984.

14. Chan, S. Y. W., Fox, E. J., Chan, M. M. C., Tsoi, W., Wang, C., Tang, L. C. H., Tang, J. W. K., and Ho, P., The relationship between the human sperm hypoosmotic swelling assay, routine semen analysis and the human sperm zona-free hamster ovum penetration assay, *Fertil. Steril.*, 44, 668, 1985.

15. Talbot, P. and Chacon, R. S., A triple stain technique for evaluating normal acrosome reactions of human sperm, *J. Exp. Zool.*, 215, 201, 1981.

16. Cross, N. L., Morales, P., Overstreet, J. W., and Hanson, F. W., Two simple methods for detecting acrosome-reacted human sperm, *Gamete Res.*, 15, 213, 1986.

17. Kim, E. D., Gilbaugh, J. H., Patel, V. R., Turek, P. J., and Lipshultz, L. I., Testis biopsies frequently demonstrate sperm in men with azoospermia and significantly elevated follicle stimulating hormone levels, *J. Urol.*, 157, 144, 1997.

18. Schlegel, P. N., Palermo, G. D., Alikani, M., Adler, A., Reing, A. M., Cohen, J., and Rosenwaks, Z., Micropuncture retrieval of epididymal sperm with *in vitro* fertilization: importance of *in vitro* micromanipulation techniques, *Urology*, 46, 236, 1995.

19. Mak, V. and Jarvi, K. A., The genetics of male infertility, *J. Urol.*, 156, 1245, 1996.

20. Brandell, R. A., Mielnik, A., Liotta, D., Ye, Z., Veeck, L. L., Palermo, G. D., and Schlegel, P. N., AZFb deletions predict the absence of sperm with testicular sperm extraction: preliminary report of a prognostic genetic test, *Hum. Reprod.*, 13, 2812–2815, 1998.

21. Dubin, L. and Amelar, R. D., 986 cases of varicocelectomy: a 12 year study, *Urology*, 10, 446, 1977.

22. Brown, J. S., Varicocelectomy in the subfertile male: a 10 year experience in 295 cases, *Fertil. Steril.*, 27, 1046, 1976.

23. Hendry, W. F., Hughes, L., Scammell, G., Prior, J. P., and Hargreave, T. B., Comparison of prednisolone and placebo on subfertile men with antisperm antibodies to spermatozoa, *Lancet*, 335, 85, 1990.

24. Lamb, D. J., Prognosis for the infertile couple, *Fertil. Steril.*, 23, 320, 1972.

25. Auger, J., Kunstmann, J. M., and Czyglik, F., Decline in semen quality among fertile men in Paris during the past 20 years, *N. Engl. J. Med.*, 332, 281, 1995.
26. Lipshultz, L. I., Fisch, H., Lamb, D. J., Meacham, R. B., and Neiderberger, C. S., Is semen quality declining?, *Contemporary Urol.*, 8, 50, 1996.
27. Pavlovich, C. P. and Schlegel, P. N., Fertility options after vasectomy: a cost-effectiveness analysis, *Fertil. Steril.*, 67, 133, 1997.
28. Schlegel, P. N., Is assisted reproduction the optimal treatment for varicocele-associated male infertility? A cost-effectiveness analysis, *Urology*, 49, 83, 1997.

5 Female Infertility

Pasquale Patrizio, M. Esposito,
S. Kulshrestha, and O. Khorram

CONTENTS

I. INTRODUCTION

Infertility affects approximately 10 to 15% of couples in the U.S. and is defined as the inability at reproductive age for a couple to achieve a pregnancy after one year of unprotected intercourse.

Overall, about 50% of infertile couples experience inability to conceive secondary to a female factor, about 35% to a male factor, and the remaining 15% fall in the group of unexplained infertility. Specifically, female factor infertility conditions include tubal factor (20 to 30% of the cases); hypothalamic pituitary ovarian dysfunction (25 to 30%), which includes anovulatory infertility, and primary and secondary amenorrhea; endometriosis (25 to 30% of infertile women); uterine anomalies (5%); and finally, recurrent pregnancy losses and autoimmunity. This chapter will discuss the different etiologies of female infertility and the approaches to diagnosis and treatment. In the last section, some of the common therapies offered in infertility, such as ovulation induction for both intrauterine insemination and *in vitro* fertilization, will be presented.

II. ENDOCRINOLOGY OF FEMALE INFERTILITY

Amenorrhea is defined as the absence of menarche by the age of 16 regardless of the presence of normal growth and appearance of secondary sexual characteristics (primary amenorrhea) or the absence of menses for the duration of 3 or more cycle intervals, or 6 months, in women with prior menses (secondary amenorrhea). Amenorrhea is physiologic in prepubertal girls, during pregnancy, during lactation, and after menopause.

The production of a menstrual flow requires an intact and functional axis between the central nervous system (hypothalamus, i.e., release of GnRH), pituitary (release of FSH, LH), ovary (folliculogenesis and steroidogenesis), and uterus (endometrial development, decidual changes, menstrual shedding). The entire system is regulated by a complex set of hormonal signals, autocrine and paracrine release of peptide and steroid factors, and interaction with target cell receptors. Any dysfunction along the system may result in amenorrhea.

A. PRIMARY AMENORRHEA

Patients with primary amenorrhea may be hypergonadotropic secondary to ovarian failure or hypogonadotropic as a result of hypothalamic-pituitary dysfunction. They also may be eugonadal, but have primary amenorrhea secondary to an obstruction or developmental defect in the Mullerian system.

1. Genetic Abnormalities

Genetic abnormalities are the most common cause of primary amenorrhea occurring in about 30% of patients with this symptom.[1] Gonadal failure mostly results from a partial or complete X chromosome deletion. In Turner's syndrome (45 XO), symptoms include hypergonadotrophic hypogonadism, a short stature, "shield-like chest," webbed neck, and coarctation of the aorta. Patients usually deplete their follicular reserve long before puberty. Approximately 3% of patients, however, have sufficient ova to experience a short period of normal gonadal activity. Approximately 12% of patients with XO/XX mosaicism have a brief period of ovarian function.[2]

Some patients with hypergonadotrophic primary amenorrhea have a normal XX karyotype. Etiologies of their ovarian failure include microdeletions of the X chromosome, autoimmune disease, and galactosemia.

Other genetic disorders are characterized by low levels of FSH and LH (hypogonadotrophic hypogonadism). Deletions of the Kallmann gene (KALIG-1) on Xp appear in some subjects with X-linked forms of Kallman's syndrome. This gene seems to encode a cell adhesion protein that facilitates the migration of the GnRH neurons from the medial olfactory placode to the hypothalamus. Patients with Kallman's syndrome present with congenital hypogonadotrophic hypogonadism associated with anosmia or hyposmia. They have undetectable levels of LH and FSH. Ovarian follicles never mature past the primordial stage unless stimulated via exogenous gonadotropin. These patients respond well to pulsatile GnRH treatment and exogenous gonadotropins in the establishment of menses and fertility.

2. Anatomic Abnormalities

Any abnormality of the outflow tract (vagina, cervix, uterus) may block menstrual flow despite normal gonadotropin levels and folliculogenesis. Rokitansky–Mayer–Kuster–Hauser syndrome is the most common anatomic genital abnormality associated with primary amenorrhea. These patients have an absence or hypoplasia of the vagina. The uterus may be normal, but may not be connected to the introitus or may have only a rudimentary horn. Ovarian function is normal. The inheritance pattern is sporadic and multifactorial.

Complete androgen insensitivity or testicular feminization is a disorder characterized by a missing uterus, missing fallopian tubes, and the presence of only the lower one third of the vagina. It is responsible for about 10% of all cases of primary amenorrhea. The condition is a maternal X-linked recessive disorder and affects the androgen intracellular receptor. The patient has a female phenotype, but a male karyotype and testes. On physical exam, the patient has scanty or absent pubic/axillary hair, a shortened vagina, and an absent uterus and cervix. Laboratory findings include an elevated LH, mildly elevated testosterone, and a high estradiol.

Other disorders of differentiation of the Mullerian system lead to distal genital tract obstruction. Instances where patients have functional but obstructed genital tracts include transverse vaginal septum and imperforate hymen. Surgical intervention usually renders these patients sexually functional and restores menses.

B. Secondary Amenorrhea

Some of the causes of secondary amenorrhea are listed below. They may include disorders of the hypothalamic-pituitary axis, ovarian dysfunction, peripheral effects, and anatomic causes. Secondary amenorrhea may or may not be associated with chronic anovulation.

1. Hypothalamic-Pituitary Disorders

Hypothalamic-pituitary axis dysfunction is the most common cause of amenorrhea in the adult female population and is responsible for about 15% of cases.[2] As the hypothalamic-pituitary axis is the major regulator of folliculogenesis and the menstrual cycle, any central abnormalities directly within or influencing the production of GnRH, FSH, and LH will lead to menstrual dysfunction. Effects at the level of the hypothalamus with a resulting alteration in the secretion of GnRH occur in eating disorders such as anorexia nervosa and bulimia, seen with changes in diet and exercise and in systemic illnesses and stress. Damage to the hypothalamus or pituitary leads to an alteration or loss of adequate FSH/LH production and subsequent decreases in estrogen production from the ovary.

a. Hypothalamic chronic anovulation

This type of hypothalamic dysfunction is characterized by a low to normal gonadotropin level and a relative hypoestrogenism. Factors that may induce this state include stress, increased exercise levels, a precipitous decrease in body weight, or the development of an inappropriate ratio of lean body mass to fat.

Initially the patient has normal gonadotropin levels with an appropriate ratio of LH:FSH and will respond to a progestin challenge with withdrawal bleeding. However, when this state increases (as in anorexia nervosa or strenuous athletic exercise), a decrease in the LH and FSH levels, an inversion of the LH:FSH ratio, and a failure to respond to a progestin challenge occur.

In response to starvation, endogenous levels of neuropeptide Y increase.[3] This release inhibits gonadotropin secretion presumably through the inhibition of the GnRH pulse generator. Decreasing body fat has been postulated to stimulate the peripheral conversion of estradiol to its inactive catecholestrogen form. This could interfere with the feedback estrogen exerts at the pituitary level.

As many as 66% of runners are anovulatory or have short luteal phases. Acute exercise has been associated with a decreased FSH and LH. However, prolactin, growth hormone, testosterone, ACTH, adrenal steroids, and endorphins are all increased.[2]

Excess endogenous opioids, dopamine, melatonin, or a combination of these contribute to low GnRH secretion in some women with hypothalamic dysfunction. Patients with hypothalamic amenorrhea also have been found to have an increased circulating cortisol level.[4] Primate research shows that corticotropin-releasing hormone inhibits gonadotropin secretion.[5] A similar mechanism may exist in humans.

Low gonadotropin levels can result from head trauma, space occupying lesions of the CNS, infiltrative diseases, granulomatous diseases (syphilis and TB), and medications (minor tranquilizers, MAO inhibitors, and drugs that alter serotonin metabolism). In some patients, the hypothalamic-pituitary suppression of oral contraceptives persists for several months after their discontinuation. This should not last for more than six months as the incidence of amenorrhea after six months is 0.8% which is equivalent to that of non-OCP users.[6]

With the exception of clomiphene citrate, ovulation induction with GnRH, FSH/LH, or purified FSH works well in establishing fertility. Intravenous pulsatile administration of GnRH is associated with a near universal restoration of ovulation and an increased rate of unifollicular cycles.[7] These patients are hypoestrogenic and should be given hormone replacement therapy to prevent osteoporosis and to relieve the symptoms of hot flushes, decreased libido, and vaginal dryness.

Due to the central-acting nature of clomiphene citrate, this drug typically is ineffective. Normally, the drug activates the neuroendocrine secretion of GnRH. The GnRH (and therefore FSH and LH) frequency does increase. However, in anovulatory women, this pulse frequency is not increased.[8,9]

b. Hyperprolactinemia

The most common cause of pituitary dysfunction is hyperprolactinemia. It occurs in about 15% of patients with amenorrhea. Numerous physiologic, pharmacologic, and pathologic causes of prolactin elevation exist. Prolactin is produced by the lactotrophs in the anterior pituitary and its secretion is regulated by dopamine. Thyrotropin-releasing hormone, GnRH, and beta-endorphin stimulate prolactin release. Researchers speculate that hyperprolactinemia may inhibit GnRH secretion and may affect dopamine, which then influences GnRH pulses. Many also think that hyperprolactinemia acts directly on the ovary thereby affecting ovulation.

The four main causes of hyperprolactinemia are pituitary hyperplasia (which may be the result of dopamine dysfunction), prolactinomas (micro <10 mm, macro >10 mm), hypothyroidism, and drug intake (tranquilizers, antidepressants, steroids, OCPs, antihypertensives, H2 receptor antagonists). Additional less common causes include CNS trauma, tumors and infection, cavernous sinus thrombosis, temporal arteritis, chest trauma, surgery, or burn, herpes zoster, breast manipulation, and renal failure.

Prolactin is secreted in a sleep related circadian rhythm. Serum levels rise after sleep onset and peak between 3 and 5 a.m. When checking levels, blood should be obtained between 9 and 12 p.m. Stimuli such as nipple stimulation, sexual intercourse, increased meal protein and fat content all stimulate secretion and should be avoided.

The symptoms of hyperprolactinemia are galactorrhea and menstrual irregularity. Galactorrhea is a nonpuerperal watery or milky breast secretion that does not contain pus or blood. Microscopically, fat globules can be seen. If the patient is symptomatic and the prolactin is less than 40 ng/ml, levels should be monitored yearly. If the prolactin level is between 40 and 100 (and the TSH is normal) a coned-down view of the sella is recommended to evaluate possible microadenomas. If the prolactin level is greater than 100 or if the patient has headaches or visual field defects an MRI or CT is recommended.

Treatment options for patients with prolactinomas include surgery and medical management. Transsphenoidal resection provides complete resolution in 40% of patients with macroadenoma and 80% of patients with microadenomas.[10] Bromocriptine is a dopamine agonist and mimics dopamine inhibition of pituitary prolactin secretion. Macroadenomas will regress with bromocriptine therapy. In some cases, the resolution is prompt (days) and in other cases it may take more than six months. Therapy must continue indefinitely. Bromocriptine is highly effective in patients with hyperprolactinemia but no detectable tumor. In 22 clinical trials, 80% of such patients had menses restored with an average treatment time of 5.7 weeks.[11] Today, newer ergoline derivatives on the market have dopaminergic activity. These include the medications Pergolide™, Cabergoline™, Quinagolide™, Lysuride™, and

Terguride™. Most patients with hyperprolactinemia are hypoestrogenic and should also receive hormone replacement.

c. Sheehan's syndrome

Sheehan's syndrome results from acute necrosis of the pituitary gland due to post-partum hemorrhage and shock. The symptoms of hypopituitarism usually appear early in the postpartum period, especially failure of lactation and loss of pubic and axillary hair. In Sheehan's syndrome a general pan-hypopituitarism occurs, and this condition may be life threatening as a result of the adrenal insufficiency and loss of corticosteroid and mineralocorticoid production.

2. Ovarian Dysfunction

a. Polycystic ovarian disease (PCO or PCOS)

PCO is a heterogeneous disease that has a variable presentation but is typically characterized by anovulation and hyperandrogenism. It affects about 5% of repro-ductive age women and is the most common cause of hyperandrogenic anovulatory infertility with oligomenorrhea. Its prevalence has been estimated to be as high as 73% in women with anovulatory infertility. The patient with PCO has menstrual irregularity caused by oligoovulation or anovulation. The patient may have signs of hyperandrogenism, obesity, and infertility secondary to anovulation. PCO is char-acterized biochemically by an increased LH/FSH ratio (> 2.5:1) and increased circulating levels of androgens (testosterone and androstenedione). Additionally, insulin resistance is a common feature of women who have PCO.

Theories regarding the pathogenesis of the disease include (1) a primary hypo-thalamic etiology leading to abnormal LH secretion, (2) peripheral hyperinsulinism, (3) a central androgen effect, (4) subnormal induction of cytochrome P450 aro-matase, and (5) alterations in the paracrine/autocrine system in the ovary.[2,12,13] Recently, Urbanek et al. tested a carefully chosen collection of 37 candidate genes for linkage and association with PCO. These included genes involved in steroid hormone metabolism and action, gonadotropin action, obesity and energy regulation, and insulin action. They found the strongest evidence of linkage with follistatin, an activin-binding protein.[14]

The increase in circulating LH seen in PCO is secondary to a marked increase in LH pulse amplitude and a modest increase in LH pulse frequency. The increase in LH amplitude is secondary to excess GnRH secretion or an excessively sensitive pituitary response to LH. The increase in LH frequency is secondary to an increase in the GnRH pulse frequency and may involve hypothalamic opioid and catechola-mine systems. The chronic androgen overproduction may result from chronic expo-sure of the ovary to excess LH, increased sensitivity of the ovary to LH, or other growth factors (IGF-1 or somatomedin C) that act in concert with LH to stimulate ovarian androgen production.

The pathogenesis of the insulin resistance seen in PCO has been studied. Insulin receptor gene analysis reveals no mutations and equal expression of both gene alleles in affected patients.[15] Dunaif et al. reported increased insulin receptor beta-subunit serine phosphorylation.[16] This leads to decreased beta-subunit tyrosine kinase activity, thereby impeding intracellular phosphorylation in patients with PCO. It is presumed that the major lesion in insulin action is a post-binding effect in the insulin receptor and/or in postreceptor signal transduction.

Clomiphene citrate is the first line agent used for ovulation induction in the infertile woman with PCO. Additionally, insulin-sensitizing agents such as metformin and Troglitazone™ increase ovulation success and restore menstrual cyclicity.[17] Hirsutism is controlled with the oral contraceptive pill and if severe, spironolactone may be used. Weight loss corresponds to a decreased free testosterone, fasting insulin levels, and an increased rate of ovulation.[18]

b. Premature ovarian failure

Premature ovarian failure (POF) is defined as the cessation of menses before age 35. It may be due to genetic (galactosemia, X chromosome abnormalities), autoimmune, chemical (alkylating agents), radiation, or idiopathic causes. Additionally, damage to follicles as a result of infection, decreased blood supply, or surgical removal may lead to insufficient estrogen production, which is required for endometrial growth and menses. In POF, findings include a repeatedly elevated FSH (usually greater than 40) with amenorrhea or oligoovulation.

One of the more attractive hypotheses regarding the cause of premature ovarian failure is an autoimmune one. The polyglandular syndromes associated with ovarian failure include hypoparathyroidism, adrenal insufficiency, and thyroiditis. The antithyroid antibody is the most common antibody seen in patients with POF.[19] Some patients with myasthenia gravis and systemic lupus erythematosus and accompanying POF exhibited a substance in their sera which inhibited *in vitro* binding of FSH to its receptor and an FSH receptor auto-antibody.[2] Another study showed that 69% of karyotypically normal patients with myasthenia gravis, pernicious anemia, idiopathic thrombocytopenic purpura, rheumatoid arthritis, vitiligo, and hemolytic anemia had sera positive for oocyte or ovarian antibodies.[20] It is recommended that in patients with premature ovarian failure a CBC, glucose, electrolytes, calcium, morning cortisol, ANA, RF, TSH, and thyroid antibodies be checked.

Premature ovarian failure occurs more frequently with a partial deletion of an X chromosome, such cases being sometimes familial. Two genes appear to be related to premature ovarian failure. They include the POF1 gene, which is localized to the Xq21.3-q27 region,[21] and the POF2 gene localized to Xq13.3-q21.2.[22]

Galactosemia may also lead to premature ovarian failure. Women with galactosemia have inactive gonadotropin molecules secondary to an abnormal carbohydrate component. There may also be a direct effect of galactose on germ cell migration from the yolk sac to the genital ridge resulting in a smaller reserve of oogonia.

In general, the ovaries resist infection. However, it is thought that approximately 10% of women who have mumps develop a diffuse oophoritis. This may cause premature ovarian failure in a small percentage as a result of the tissue destruction.

Older women are more susceptible than younger women to the effects of irradiation. The detrimental effect may manifest only years later. Radiation effects depend on the patient age and the dose.[23,24] At a dose of 60 rads to the ovary, no effects occur. At 150 rads, patients over 40 experience some risk. Between 250 to

800 rads, 60 to 70% of patients between age 15 and 40 will be sterilized, and over 800 rads, 100% are permanently sterilized.[10]

Alkylating agents are highly toxic to the gonads. As with radiation, older women are more susceptible. Other chemotherapeutic agents also have potential for ovarian damage, but have been less well studied.

The most successful modality in treating infertility in this population is oocyte donation and IVF. Lydic et al. showed that patients with this treatment regimen had the same pregnancy rate as women who had oocyte donation for other reasons.[25]

3. Peripheral Sources

Ovulation and normal menstrual cyclicity may be affected by the release of hormones in the periphery which have either direct effects on the intra-ovarian environment or on the feedback mechanisms involving the hypothalamus and pituitary. These include disorders of androgen excess of adrenal and/or ovarian origin (neoplasm, polycystic ovarian disease, congenital adrenal hyperplasia), disorders of estrogen excess (neoplasms, liver or renal disease, obesity), Cushing's disease, and acromegaly.

a. Hypothyroidism

Hypothyroidism can lead to menstrual dysfunction. The patient's symptoms may include fatigue, easy weight gain, dry skin, lethargy, and constipation. The TSH will be elevated but the T4 may be normal. Additionally, hypothyroidism may lead to hyperprolactinemia and galactorrhea. Hypothyroidism seems to correspond to a decline in the hypothalamic content of dopamine, which influences GnRH secretion. Treatment involves thyroid hormone replacement.

b. Congenital adrenal hyperplasia

Congenital adrenal hyperplasia is a unique group of genetic disorders involving mutations in the enzymes of adrenal steroidogenesis. Symptoms can appear identical to hyperandrogenic chronic anovulation (PCO). Five enzymes are required to convert cholesterol to cortisol. Genetic disorders in three of these enzymes (21-hydroxylase, 11-OHylase, and 3β-hydroxy-steroid-dehydrogease-isomerase) can lead to overproduction of adrenal androgens and hyperandrogenic chronic anovulation.

The defect in the 21-hydroxylase gene, which lies on chromosome 6, is the most common and is seen in 2 to 4% of hyperandrogenic women.[26] As a result of this defect, production of 17-alpha-hydroxy-progesterone, androstenedione, DHEA, DHEAS, and testosterone increases.

If the mutation is near complete, adrenal androgen production increases *in utero* and females are born with the classic form of CAH. Symptoms include clitoromegaly, labioscrotal fusion, and an abnormal course of the urethra. With a modest decrease in 21-OHylase activity, the phenotype may be nonclassical and present as late-onset adrenal hyperplasia. Such patients will present with the symptoms of chronic anovulation, hirsutism, and menstrual irregularities and may appear to have PCO. The distinction is important because patients with CAH need replacement treatment with both hydrocortisone and 9-fluorohydrocortisone.

4. Anatomic Causes

Any acquired genital tract obstruction may lead to secondary amenorrhea. If severe enough, these may include entities such as cervical stenosis, intrauterine adhesions, and tumor. Intrauterine adhesions may develop from PID and Asherman's syndrome (post-curettage or endometritis). Intrauterine adhesions or synechiae can obliterate the endometrial cavity and produce secondary amenorrhea as described later in the chapter.

C. CLINICAL APPROACH TO THE PATIENT WITH AMENORRHEA

The evaluation of the patient with amenorrhea involves the acquisition of a good history and physical. In the history, the patient should be asked about the onset and duration of the amenorrhea, dietary and exercise habits, stress, medications, family history of amenorrhea or genetic anomalies, infection, and previous surgery. Review of systems should involve asking about galactorrhea, headaches, menopausal symptoms such as hot flushes, energy level, weight fluctuations, and patterns of hair growth and acne.

On physical examination, a complete internal and external genital exam should be performed. An imperforate hymen, vaginal septum, and vaginal/uterine aplasia will be obvious. A breast exam should evaluate for the presence of galactorrhea. A thyroid exam should be performed. The patient should be evaluated for evidence of estrogenization and hyperandrogenism. Symptoms of hyperandrogenism include acne, hirsutism, and if severe, deepening of the voice, balding, clitoromegaly, and altered lean body:fat distribution.

Initial laboratory evaluation should involve testing hCG, LH, FSH, prolactin, and TSH. The most common cause of secondary amenorrhea is pregnancy. In a normal adult female, the serum FSH is 5 to 30 IU/L with the ovulatory midcycle peak about twice as high as the basal level. The serum LH is between 5 to 20 IU/L with the ovulatory midcycle peak about three times the basal level. In a hypogonadotropic state, as in hypothalamic and pituitary dysfunction, both the FSH and LH are less than 5 IU/L. In a hypergonadotropic state as in premature ovarian failure, the FSH is greater than 30 IU/L and the LH is greater than 40 IU/L.[10] If the patient has an elevated prolactin, then further evaluation in the form of imaging should be performed as described in the section on hyperprolactinemia above. If the patient's TSH is elevated, a complete thyroid profile should be obtained and the patient should be given thyroid replacement if she is indeed hypothyroid. An FSH greater than 40 suggests ovarian failure. If this occurs in a younger woman and there is concern for premature ovarian failure, further testing should be conducted. This may include obtaining markers of autoimmune disease such as a sedimentation rate, thyroid antibodies, ANA, CBC, RF, and a karyotype.

If the patient shows evidence of hirsutism, then free and total testosterone, DHEAS, and 17-hydroxy-progesterone should be checked. However, because not all hyperandrogenic women are hirsute, some authors also recommend routine testing of testosterone, DHEAS, and 17-alpha-hydroxy-progesterone. Conversely, circulating androgen levels sometimes occur normally in hirsute women because of an alteration in the metabolic clearance of androgens and in SHBG, and because of varying activity of 5-alpha-reductase. In PCO, patients will usually have an LH greater than 20 mIU/ml and an LH:FSH ratio greater than 2.5. They also may have a slightly increased testosterone, and perhaps DHEAS.

Free and total testosterone measurements indicate the severity of disease. In normal women, the range is between 30 and 75 ng/ml. If testosterone is greater than 200 ng/ml, one suspects the presence of a tumor. Likewise, a DHEAS level greater than 700 μg suggests an adrenal tumor. 17-alpha-hydroxy-progesterone is a distinguishing screen between nonclassical late-onset adrenal hyperplasia and heterozygous 21-hydroxylase deficiency. If the level is greater than 4 ng/ml, the diagnosis may be nonclassical CAH. If the level is greater than 10 ng/ml the patient may have 21-hydroxylase deficiency.

III. TUBAL FACTOR INFERTILITY

Infertility affects approximately 10 to 15% of couples in the United States and is defined as the inability of a reproductive aged couple to achieve a pregnancy after one year of unprotected intercourse. Of this group, 30% experience inability to conceive secondary to a tubal factor, and of those with tubal disease, about 15% suffer from proximal tubal obstruction.[27] Tubal disease may result from a variety of disorders; however, the most common is that stemming from an infectious etiology, most notably pelvic inflammatory disease, which has increased in incidence in the U.S., along with other sexually transmitted diseases. Other conditions resulting in tubal disease and infertility include endometriosis, previous peritonitis, prior tubal surgery, a history of ectopic pregnancy, or congenital malformations. In the case of distal tubal obstruction leading to development of a hydrosalpinx, the prognosis for achieving pregnancy is poor.[28,29]

Tubal pathology may result from any insult causing injury to the internal tube, external tube, or both. Adhesion formation may cause mechanical disruption of normal anatomic relationships and may result from any inflammatory process stemming from infection, foreign body reaction, endometriosis, or ischemia and hemorrhage from a surgical procedure on or near the tube.[30] Infection, however, is the most common inciting event, and researchers note that *Chlamydia trachomatis*, which has in recent years surpassed gonococcal infection in incidence, has become the most common sexually transmitted disease in the U.S.[31] In the infertile population, both serologic and bacterial cultures reveal that up to 90% of females screened have been exposed. In women younger than 25, 60% of cases of pelvic inflammatory disease are the result of sexually transmitted diseases. Other infectious microorganisms known to cause salpingitis are *Neisseria gonorrhoeae*, *Mycoplasma hominis*, *Ureaplasma urealyticum*, *Mycobacterium tuberculosis*, and endogenous anaerobes. Damage to the endosalpinx may include intraluminal adhesions, flattening of the rugal folds, and disruption of the cilia, all leading to deranged transport mechanisms. Hydrosalpinges, arising from closure of the distal tubal ostia leading to significant ampullary dilation and deciliation,[32] carries a poor prognosis. This corresponds to alteration in the tubal fluid pH and electrolyte content, along with dysfunctional contractile function of the myosalpinx.[33]

Proximal tubal disease also may result from those conditions affecting the distal tube, namely endometriosis, infection, traumatic occlusion, and salpingitis isthmica nodosa (SIN), a condition unique to the proximal tube. Salpingitis isthmica nodosa is a diverticular disease of the tube, where the endosalpinx everts into the tubal muscularis, often leading to blockage.[30] Investigators do not know whether the inciting event leading to SIN is infectious, autoimmune, or congenital in nature; however, based on HSG studies, SIN is thought to be a progressive disease.[34] In a study by Musich and Behrman,[35] SIN appeared in up to 70% of patients with proximal tubal obstruction. In approximately 7% of patients with proximal tubal obstruction, endometriosis is diagnosed from the surgical specimen at the time of proximal tubal anastomosis.[36] Interestingly, medical therapy of the endometriosis appears to resolve the proximal obstruction and therefore should be attempted prior to surgery. However, as in distal tubal obstruction, infection is the most common cause of proximal tubal obstruction.[30]

A. Diagnosis of Tubal Disease

A number of diagnostic modalities accurately assess tubal disease. The most commonly used modality is the hysterosalpingogram. This test involves instilling contrast medium into the uterus (either water or oil soluble) under fluoroscopy and directly visualizing the uterine cavity contour, tubal patency, mucosal integrity (manifest by the normal rugal folds), and the presence of salpingitis isthmica nodosa (SIN). It has been demonstrated that the use of oil soluble contrast media may increase post-HSG fertility rates perhaps by dislodging mucous plugs or debris from the tube.[37] The HSG is performed after menses, but prior to ovulation so that disruption of a pregnancy will not occur. A hysterosalpingogram should not be done if any suspicion of a latent infection exists, for fear of reactivation. Although the test is extremely useful, it has some drawbacks. In some women, the test produces a moderate to severe amount of cramping. Pre-procedural use of a nonsteroidal anti-inflammatory drug will alleviate the cramping. There is also a 0.3 to 3.1% incidence of inflammatory reactions,[38] and a high rate of false positive occlusions of the proximal tube, which may result from mere spasm. This problem may be overcome with selective cannulation of the ostia of the blocked tube under fluoroscopic guidance prior to dye instillation.[39] Other diagnostic modalities include salpingoscopy, which is the placement of a flexible fiberoptic scope into the tubal lumen that will allow direct visualization and assessment of mucosal integrity.[40] Laparoscopy allows the clinician to evaluate the external tube for the presence of peritubal adhesions, fimbrial stenosis, and ampullary dilatation. Severity of the damage to the tubes and pelvis, most commonly resulting from infection, may be graded, according to the degree of dilatation in centimeters (> 4 cm is a very poor prognosis). Treatment prognosis depends on many factors, some of which include mucosal integrity of the tube, density of periovarian or peritubal adhesions, and whether disease is unilateral or bilateral.[41]

B. Treatment of Tubal Disease

Until the advent of *in vitro* fertilization (IVF), tubal surgery was the mainstay of therapy. Years ago, before the use of laparoscopy, tubal surgery was done by laparotomy. Today, operative laparoscopy largely has replaced open surgery. The main advantages over laparotomy are decreased hospital stay or outpatient treatment, lower total cost of the procedure, and faster recovery.[42] Not all diseased tubes, however, are amenable to surgical repair, and the clinician must choose his or her surgical candidates wisely and methodically.

During any pelvic reconstructive surgery on the tubes, one must apply microsurgical techniques meticulously, as these have helped to nearly double the pregnancy rates following surgery.[31] Gentle handling of tissues, achieving adequate hemostasis, minimizing tissue trauma and inflammation, and adhering to general microsurgical principles will increase the chances for a successful outcome. The surgeon's armamentarium includes several procedures: salpingolysis and ovariolysis, fimbrioplasty, salpingostomy, reversal of tubal steriliztion, and repair of proximal tubal occlusion.

Salpingolysis and ovariolysis are procedures that involve lysing peritubal or periovarian adhesions. Adhesions may be lysed via laparotomy or laparoscopy, using sharp scissor dissection, blunt dissection, laser, or electrocautery.[42] With the removal of adhesions, the surgeon hopes to restore the normal pelvic architecture, thereby increasing the resulting pregnancy rates. A study by Tulandi et al.,[43] demonstrated that the pregnancy rate in patients who had undergone salpingo-ovariolysis was three times higher than in those who were not treated. Gomel demonstrated an intrauterine pregnancy rate of 62% and an ectopic pregnancy rate of 5.4% in 92 patients followed for a period of 9 months or more.[44] It must be remembered that any surgical procedure, even one that is done meticulously to remove adhesions, may result in the formation of new ones. Luciano et al.[45] demonstrated in rabbits that de novo adhesion formation was less following laparoscopy than laparotomy. It has also been shown that patients who have very thick, vascular, and more extensive adhesions do less well with surgery,[46] and in these patients, or those who have failed to conceive 1 year following surgery, IVF is a more suitable option.[42]

Surgery success also depends on coexisting disease of the endosalpinx. Fimbrioplasty involves lysis of fimbrial adhesions, so as to enable the fimbria to capture the oocyte from the ovary at the time of ovulation. Salpingo-ovariolysis and fimbrioplasty produce similar pregnancy rates.[42] Neosalpingostomy involves making a cruciate or stellate incision into the agglutinated tubal fimbria and placing sutures so as to evert the edges of the newly created ostium to maintain patency. This procedure also may be accomplished with the laser. Transuterine instillation of blue dye at the end of the procedure is used to confirm tubal patency. As with any procedure, the results are variable, and depend significantly on the extent of tubal damage. Studies show that term pregnancy rates after this procedure are usually below 30%, with 5 to 15% of these being ectopic pregnancies.[47]

The presence of a hydrosalpinx, as stated previously, is often associated with a poor surgical prognosis. According to the criteria set forth by Boer-Meisel et al.[48] researchers examined five parameters to determine which cases of hydrosalpinx would be amenable to surgery and which ones would not: (1) extent of adhesions,

(2) the nature of the adhesions, (3) the diameter of the hydrosalpinx, (4) the macroscopic condition of the endosalpinx, and (5) tubal wall thickness. The two most important prognostic factors were the amount of adhesions present and condition of the endosalpinx. Patients fell into three groups based on their prognoses for success with surgery, and it was found that in the poor prognosis group, the probability of success in achieving an intrauterine pregnancy was only 3% vs. 77% in the good prognosis category and 21% in the intermediate prognosis group. A study by Schlaff et al. of 95 women undergoing surgery (terminal neosalpingostomy) for distal tubal disease demonstrated that in those with severe disease the intrauterine pregnancy rate was 12% compared with 70% for those with mild disease.[49]

Approximately 1% of women undergoing tubal sterilization procedures in the U.S. will desire reversal in the future. Pregnancy rates resulting from microsurgical tubal anastomosis range from 50 to 90%, attesting to the fact that patients who undergo surgery on less damaged tubes tend to have superior outcomes. The final success rate depends largely on the post-operative length of tube after anastomosis, with a length of greater than 4 cm associated with optimal results. Also, sterilization procedures that cause the least damage to the tubes result in the best outcome.

Lately, many have considered prophylactic salpingectomy or proximal tubal occlusion for patients with hydrosalpinx prior to undergoing IVF, as evidence exists of intermittent drainage of the hydrosalpinx fluid into the uterine cavity at around the time of embryo transfer.[30] Recent investigations report that pregnancy, implantation, and live birth rates are approximately one half of what they are in patients without hydrosalpinges.[50] Researchers speculate that the fluid from a hydrosalpinx contains microorganisms, cytokines, debris, and possibly other toxic agents that may damage the embryo and endometrium.[51] Aboulghar et al. observed that ultrasound monitoring of follicular development during an ovulation induction cycle was thwarted in the presence of hydrosalpinges.[52] Shelton et al. performed a prospective study that showed that removal of hydrosalpinges in patients who had multiple repeated IVF failures resulted in a better pregnancy outcome.[53] The patients served as their own control, and pre-salpingectomy, the ongoing pregnancy rate per transfer was 0%, with a 25% rate post-salpingectomy. Several retrospective studies in the literature support surgical treatment of hydrosalpinx prior to an IVF cycle.[54,55]

Proximal tubal occlusion may be corrected surgically with tubocornual anastomosis. Pregnancy rates have ranged from 50%[31] to 71%.[56] Successful cannulation of proximally occluded tubes also may be achieved using epidural catheters, ureteral catheters, balloon angiographic catheters, guide wires, and more recently, coaxial systems, under fluoroscopic, hysteroscopic, or ultrasound guidance.[27]

In summary, tubal disease is one of the leading causes of female infertility encountered in practice. Although it may result from a number of conditions, the primary cause is infectious, mostly related to sexually transmitted diseases, which are not only preventable, but curable. The treatment of tubal disease depends, in part, on where in the tube the obstruction occurs. A thorough diagnostic evaluation can lead to appropriate treatment. The whole infertility evaluation should be completed in these patients for the purpose of ruling out other confounding diagnoses that may contribute to the problem. After this, the patient may be channeled to the appropriate treatment for her situation, namely surgery or IVF.

IV. ENDOMETRIOSIS

Endometriosis is a condition frequently encountered by gynecologists and is thought to affect approximately 5 to 10% of premenopausal women, with most cases diagnosed between the ages of 25 and 30.[57] The disease prevalence may be up to 30% in the female infertile population.[58] For a woman with an affected first degree relative, the risk appears to increase approximately 10-fold over the baseline population. The symptoms of this disease vary from absent to severe, not necessarily correlating with the amount of disease present at diagnostic laparoscopy.

The etiology of this condition remains a mystery. One of the favored theories is that proposed by Sampson of "retrograde menstruation."[59] This theory proposes that endometriosis results from endometrial implants that lodge ectopically in the pelvic and abdominal cavities as a result of menstrual fluid refluxing through the fallopian tubes. Evidence for this theory comes from laparoscopies performed during the perimenstrual period which demonstrated that approximately 90% of patients had bloody peritoneal fluid.[60] The theory of retrograde menstruation is supported further by the association of an increased incidence of endometriosis in adolescent females with Mullerian anomalies leading to outflow tract obstruction. A second theory is that of coelomic metaplasia which asserts that peritoneal mesothelial cells undergo metaplastic transformation, under the influence of an unspecified stimulus, to endometrial cells.[61] No firm scientific evidence supports this theory. A third hypothesis proposes that estrogenic stimulation of remnant Mullerian cell rests induces these cells to differentiate into functional glands and stroma, which may explain the few cases of endometriosis seen in male patients treated with estrogens.[62] Evidence also demonstrates that patients with previous gynecologic surgery may have direct transplantation of endometrial cells iatrogenically following the surgery,[63] as may be evidenced by implants in the scars. One study suggests that dysfunctional immune recognition, endometrium specific, may contribute to the pathogenesis.[64]

We know that women with endometriosis have larger amounts of macrophages in the peritoneal fluid, which may contribute to the phagocytosis of sperm or altering of sperm function. A study by Wang et al. observed a statistically significant increase in the volume of peritoneal fluid in patients with endometriosis, speculated to be secondary to either increased secretion or decreased reabsorption of fluid from ectopic implants.[65] Ovulation also may be impaired secondary to the large amounts of free radicals, prostaglandins, and toxic metabolites elaborated by macrophages. Scientists speculate that antibodies to implants cross react with normal endometrium and ovarian tissue, also leading to aberrant implantation or abnormal ovulatory mechanisms.[66]

Visualization of the implants by thorough inspection of the peritoneum at the time of diagnostic laparoscopy is the most effective way to diagnose endometriosis in conjunction with multiple peritoneal biopsies. The appearance of implants varies widely, and therefore, the ability to diagnose endometriosis visually may require physician experience. Biopsies of normal appearing peritoneum in infertility patients reveal endometriosis in approximately 6% of patients, underscoring the importance of the biopsy and pathologic diagnosis.[67] Endometriotic implants typically appear like red-blue nodules or brown and powder burnt appearing. Atypical lesions, however, are much more difficult to recognize. These lesions appear clear and vesicular, white opacified, or as glandular excrescences. Sometimes, retraction and scarring of the peritoneum may be all that is seen at the time of surgery. The presence of endometrial glands and stroma is needed to make a true histologic diagnosis

The most common symptoms of endometriosis include dysmenorrhea (pain with menses), dyspareunia (painful intercourse), premenstrual spotting, chronic pelvic pain, and bowel or bladder symptoms (many patients have involvement of the bowel or bladder with disease). The most common signs of endometriosis include the presence of friable perineal implants, a laterally deviated cervix, a fixed and retroverted uterus, uterosacral nodularity, adnexal masses, and excessive pain to palpation on pelvic exam. Interestingly, the extent of disease does not always correlate with the severity of symptoms, as patients with very minimal disease often have the most pain, while infertility patients may have extensive disease and be completely pain free, with only infertility as the chief complaint.

The dysmenorrhea is a result of increased uterine contractions resulting from elevated levels of prostaglandins in the menstrual fluid. Both prostaglandin and histamine levels are elevated in these patients.[68] Pain also results from leaking implants leading to peritoneal irritation. The pain may precede the onset of flow and is accentuated when flow begins. Another common complaint encountered in the sexually active woman is that of dyspareunia. It is important to inquire specifically about this symptom, since many patients are reluctant or embarrassed to discuss this with the physician. The dyspareunia commonly accompanies deep thrust penetration and is worse premenstrually.

Premenstrual spotting is not an uncommon symptom, and has been reported to occur in as many as 35% of patients with endometriosis.[69] It usually occurs several days prior to flow. Investigators believe that the fallopian tubes "pick up" menstrual material released by ectopic endometrial implants and deliver it to the cervix, or alternatively, that premature shedding of the endometrium occurs secondary to elevated levels of prostaglandins.

Lateral deviation of the cervix may appear on speculum exam, secondary to scarring and retraction of the ipsilateral uterosacral ligament from endometriotic implant involvement. Palpation of the uterus often reveals it to be in a fixed and retroverted position, while the uterosacral ligaments are nodular and tender. Palpation of the adnexae may identify adnexal masses, most commonly secondary to endometriomas (endometriotic cysts). Endometriotic nodules, painful to palpation, may also be palpable in the rectovaginal septum.

Endometriosis is not exclusive to the pelvis. It may occur in rare locations. Outside of the reproductive organs, the GI tract is the most common site of endometriosis.[70] Patients with bowel involvement may experience abdominal distention, rectal bleeding, and bowel function disturbances. Endometriosis also may affect the urinary tract, including the bladder, kidney, and ureters, although less commonly than the GI tract. Patients may experience urgency, frequency, and dysuria. With renal involvement, hematuria and flank pain may be present. Interestingly, patients with lung and thorax involvement can experience hemoptysis and chest pain with menses.

Endometriosis treatment is challenging, and factors such as age of the patient, severity of symptoms, and desire for future reproduction must factor into the equation.[66] Before treating, one must establish the extent of disease, and this is best accomplished with the use of laparoscopy. Keep in mind that patients with a chief complaint of infertility should undergo a full diagnostic evaluation in order to rule out other confounding factors.[57] Treatment options include medical, surgical, or expectant management. Although expectant management is not often considered a treatment, several studies show that patients with stage I or II endometriosis have conception rates of 55 to 75% with expectant management alone.[71] One should therefore wait a period of 5 to 12 months before initiating treatment in these patients. This is certainly not the case for the patients with stage III or IV disease who are better served by surgical treatment.[72]

Medical therapy essentially is hormonal. Various hormonal regimens appear to suppress endometrium, thereby suppressing ectopically located implants as well. These therapies include progestins, oral contraceptives, GnRH agonists, and anti-progestational agents.[73] A commonly used, nonhormonal treatment for the pain of endometriosis is nonsteroidal anti-inflammatory drugs, which help to offset the elevated levels of prostaglandins in the menstrual and peritoneal fluids. These drugs, although relatively benign, may induce gastrointestinal side effects, due to binding of both cyclooxygenase-1 and cyclooxygenase-2 enzymes involved in prostaglandin production. This problem may be partially or completely offset with the advent of the new, specific cyclooxygenase-2 inhibitors.

Progestins promote atrophy and decidualization of endometriotic implants and are good therapy for the pain associated with endometriosis.[66] The most commonly utilized progestin is medroxyprogesterone acetate in a dose of 30 mg/day for six months. In most cases, menstruation is suppressed, but breakthrough bleeding remains a significant problem. Side effects include nausea, depression, weight gain, fluid retention, and breakthrough bleeding; however, these are reversible. Similarly, oral contraceptive pills lead to decidualization and atrophy of implants[59,68] and, given continuously, curtail retrograde menstruation through the induction of an amenor-rheic state. The degree of dysmenorrhea reduces drastically when given for a period of at least 6 to 12 months. Breakthrough bleeding is also commonly encountered with this therapy.

Danazol is a synthetic derivative of testosterone and has been used for the treatment of endometriosis since the 1970s. The medication functions as an ago-nist/antagonist of the progesterone receptor and an agonist of the glucocorticoid and androgen receptors.[66] Up to 90% of patients with mild to moderate disease gain pain relief after 6 months of therapy;[74] however, symptoms recur after therapy ceases. The androgenic properties of this medication may lead to adverse side effects including weight gain, acne, hot flushes, vaginitis, muscle cramps, altered libido, hirsutism, and increased atherogenic index, precluding its use in patients at risk for cardiovascular disease.[75] The usual dose is 800 mg/day in divided doses, although some practitioners begin therapy with a dose of 400 mg/day and titrate upward if needed. Gestrinone is an antiprogestational derivative of 19-Nortestosterone™ and acts as an agonist at the androgen receptor level and an agonist/antagonist at the progesterone receptor. It also induces atrophy of implants and appears to be effective in relieving pain.

Gonadotropin releasing hormone agonists are one of the more commonly used therapies for patients with endometriosis. These medications suppress ovarian function, leading to a pseudo-menopausal state, which causes atrophy of implants secondary to the low circulating estrogen levels. These medications are effective in pain relief,[76,77] but may be associated with menopausal side effects including hot flushes, vaginal dryness, irregular vaginal bleeding, decreased libido, depression, insomnia, irritability, fatigue, and headache. Concern arises about leaving patients on this therapy for more than six months, as it has been associated with bone demineralization, leading to osteoporosis. Evidence supports the use of estrogen plus progestins or progestins alone to reduce the incidence of adverse side effects from this therapy, specifically those resulting from hypoestrogenism.[78]

Surgical therapy consists of conservative versus definitive treatment. For a reproductive age woman who is interested in maintaining future reproductive ability, conservative therapy is the best option. This usually involves laparoscopy and the use of laser, electrocautery, or excision of endometriotic implants and cysts (endometriomas), thereby restoring normal anatomic relationships.

Maintenance of microsurgical technique and delicate handling of tissues seems to best prevent or decrease postoperative adhesion formation. Studies demonstrate that 37 to 100% of patients have a complete resolution of pain, and 18 to 80% report a reduction of symptoms 6 months postoperatively.[79–82] Definitive surgery is the treatment of choice for patients who have not been helped by more conservative approaches and usually includes total abdominal hysterectomy and bilateral salpingo-oophorectomy.[57] This surgery, including the removal of all visible disease, alleviates pain in approximately 90% of patients.

Aside from pain, many patients with endometriosis present with a chief complaint of infertility, either primary or secondary. Some of these patients have no somatic symptoms, and the diagnosis of endometriosis comes as a surprise at the time of diagnostic laparoscopy. Patients with stage I and II endometriosis show decreased monthly fecundity rates, though a direct cause and effect relationship has not been demonstrated.[83] Medical therapy is not very effective for the treatment of infertility, but five controlled studies compared laparoscopy with expectant management with respect to pregnancy outcome.[84–88] The patients who had surgery had significantly higher conception rates. The mechanisms by which endometriosis interferes with infertility are largely unknown, however several hypotheses have been proposed. Because patients with endometriosis have a larger number of macrophages and other inflammatory mediators in the peritoneal fluid, researchers think that tubal motility may be altered as well as the process of fertilization, or perhaps patients with endometriosis have abnormal endometrium, subsequently leading to abnormal implantation.[89] Some also postulate that patients with endometriosis may develop abnormal oocytes with further development of defective embryos.

Superovulation and intrauterine insemination have been used for the treatment of infertility. Physicians most commonly prescribe clomiphene citrate and gonadotropins. By stimulating the ovaries with the above medications, more than one dominant follicle will be recruited to dominance, and thus the patient will ovulate more than one oocyte, thereby increasing the chances for pregnancy. In a study of patients undergoing therapy with clomiphene citrate and IUI, cycle fecundity was

10% in those treated vs. 3% in the control group.[90] Results from two studies of patients treated with gonadotropins and IUI demonstrated that in women with endometriosis fertility improved with therapy, even when age, stage of disease, and time since surgery were taken into account.[91,92]

In vitro fertilization is one of the assisted reproductive technologies that has helped patients with endometriosis. However, the data on the use of IVF for patients with endometriosis are confusing and conflicting, as some results suggest that patients with endometriosis do less well with IVF than those without,[93–95] while other studies suggest that pregnancy rates are about equal to those in women with other diagnoses.[96,97]

V. UTERINE INFERTILITY

A. UTERINE MYOMAS

The incidence of infertility attributable to uterine causes, whether structural or endometrial, appears to be approximately 5 to 10%.[98] Structural uterine abnormalities include uterine leiomyomas (also know as fibroids), intrauterine synechiae (also known as Asherman's syndrome), and the structural abnormalities secondary to defects in embryogenesis, specifically those affecting Mullerian structures. Endometritis, or infection of the endomerium, has been linked to reproductive failure and recurrent abortion, and may result from a multitude of organisms such as gonococcus, *Chlamydia trachomatis*, and *Ureaplasma urealyticum*. A less commonly encountered condition in the U.S. is pelvic tuberculosis, which may lead to extensive intrauterine synechiae and pelvic involvement.

Uterine myomas are the most common solid pelvic tumors encountered in women, with approximately 20 to 50% of women over the age of 30 affected and with the incidence increasing with age.[99,100] Myomas may occur in all areas of the uterus, including cervix, and may even extend into the supporting uterine structures, such as the broad ligament. The three most common locations are submucosal (impinging into the uterine cavity), intramural (residing in the myometrial layer), and subserosal (projecting off of the exterior surface of the uterus). The pathophysiology is unclear, but it is thought that fibroids are unicellular in origin. Many uterine myomas are asymptomatic and are diagnosed incidentally on ultrasound exam. However, myomas, especially of the submucosal variety, correspond to preterm delivery, postpartum hemorrhage, puerperal sepsis, abnormal fetal presentation, and increased risk of spontaneous abortion.[101–103] Researchers suspect that myomas interfere with normal uterine contractility and gamete transport and may alter endometrial blood flow, leading to atrophy or ulceration and decreased implantation rates.[104–107] Aside from pertubations in reproductive function, myomas, depending on size and location, also may lead to abnormal bleeding patterns causing anemia, pain, or bowel and bladder disturbances.

Many diagnostic modalities help diagnose myomas. Usually, the first step is the routine pelvic and abdominal exam. Palpation of the abdomen may reveal a mass, and depending on size and location of the myomas, the uterus may feel enlarged and irregular in contour on pelvic exam, often prompting further investigation with an ultrasound examination of the pelvis. One cannot guarantee that the mass is uterine in nature, as ovarian neoplasms and myomas may be indistinguishable both on pelvic and ultrasound exam. Ultrasound will detect intramural and subserosal myomas; however, submucosal myomas are not detected reliably on routine ultrasound exam. If one suspects that a patient has a submucosal myoma, a sonohysterography, hysteroscopy, or hysterosalpingogram may be performed.

A sonohysterography is a simple procedure that involves instilling normal saline into the uterine cavity, through a special catheter system, while performing a transvaginal ultrasound. The fluid appears very dark, or echolucent, and outlines the lighter (echogenic) submusocal myoma impinging into the cavity. Hysteroscopy is the insertion of a fiberoptic scope with a light source into the uterus. A uterine distention media, such as carbon dioxide gas or one of several liquids used for this purpose, allows the gynecologist to visualize the cavity directly. If any abnormalities appear (such as fibroids or polyps), they can be removed surgically through electrocautery or laser resection. Hysterosalpingogram involves instillation of a water or oil soluble contrast media into the uterine cavity, under pressure. This will outline any filling defects in the uterine cavity, while also confirming tubal patency. Intramural and subserosal myomas appear at the time of diagnostic laparoscopy or laparotomy.

Treatment of uterine myomas may be either medical or surgical. The medical methods are hormonal and are aimed at inducing a hypoestrogenic state. It is known that myomas are estrogen responsive tumors that tend to proliferate during the reproductive years, especially during pregnancy, and regress after the menopause.[98] Research shows that high dose progestins, primarily medroxyprogesterone acetate, have the ability to induce fibrosis and degeneration.[108] RU-486, an antiprogestin, also causes degeneration and shrinkage of myomas.[109] Gonadotropin releasing hormone agonists are used to create a pseudo-menopausal state with resulting hypoestrogenism. This class of medications may be used preoperatively to shrink myomas, making the surgical procedure less difficult.[110,111] Blood loss during the procedure also will be reduced after preoperative use of a GnRH agonist. For patients who are anemic, preoperative GnRH agonist will suppress menstruation and vaginal bleeding and, in combination with supplemental iron therapy, will allow patients to rebuild their blood stores in preparation for surgery. Treatment usually proceeds for at least 3 months. However, second to the serious side effect of bone demineralization leading to osteoporosis, therapy is not usually continued for longer than 6 months. Therefore, medical therapy helps temporarily, but surgical therapy is the definitive way of treating myomas.

Surgical treatment of myomas may include laparotomy, or open abdominal surgery, or laparoscopy, where a fiberoptic scope with a light source is placed into the abdomen through a small incision at the umbilicus. Depending on the complexity of the procedure, anywhere from one to three small incisions will be made in the lower abdomen for accessory instruments.

Atlee was the first to describe myomectomy in the literature.[112] Semm and Mettler were the first to describe laparoscopic myomectomy.[113] Since that time, many have published reports on the safe use of laparoscopy for myomectomy.[114–117] Of course, as with any other operative laparoscopic procedure, the success of the surgery depends on the skill of the surgeon. During a myomectomy, the myometrial defects created from fibroid removal must be carefully sutured and repaired, or else the risk of scar rupture during labor and/or delivery increases. This is more difficult using the laparoscopy versus the laparotomy approach and is one of the major disadvantages of laparoscopic myomectomy, especially if the surgeon is not adept at suturing through the laparoscope. However, subserosal myomas, especially those on a stalk, respond well to laparoscopic resection. A recent retrospective analysis of 143 myomectomies by Darai et al.[118] attempted to determine the limits and complications of laparoscopic myomectomy and the fertility and pregnancy outcomes. They concluded that laparoscopic myomectomy may be used for patients with fewer than 4 myomas, all less than 7 cm in diameter. They also showed a 38.8% pregnancy rate in those patients undergoing the laparoscopic approach for a history of unexplained infertility, which parallels the results of 16.7 to 66.7% published in other studies of laparotomy[100,119] and 33% following laparoscopic myomectomy.[120]

Although uterine myomas are known to disrupt various aspects of reproduction, their direct role in causing infertility is less well known. Buttram and Reiter, in 1981, investigated whether myomas cause infertility by analyzing fertility performance after myomectomy in women with otherwise unexplained infertility.[121] They found that 54% of patients became pregnant after abdominal myomectomy. Fertility results improved after submucous myoma resection via hysteroscopy[122,123] and after laparoscopic myomectomy.[118,120] A study by Eldar-Geva et al.[124] examined whether subserosal, intramural, or submucosal myomas impacted pregnancy rates and live birth rates. Their retrospective comparative study demonstrated that subserosal myomas did not affect pregnancy or implantation rates. However, in those patients with intramural or submucosal myomas, even if the cavity was undisturbed, the pregnancy and implantation rates diminished significantly. They therefore concluded that patients should consider therapy for intramural or submucosal myomas if planning for one of the assisted reproductive technologies. On the other hand, a retrospective controlled study by Ramzy et al.[125] concluded that patients with uterine myomas, less than 7 cm, not impinging into the uterine cavity, may not need myomectomy, as implantation and miscarriage rates were not affected in the IVF and ICSI cycles that they studied.

In summary, uterine myomas are a common problem and the decision of when and how to treat a symptomatic patient may not always be clear cut. In the case of submucous myomas, the data seem to support surgical removal in patients who are attempting pregnancy; however, the case for intramural myomas causing no cavity distortion is less clear.

B. ASHERMAN'S SYNDROME

Intrauterine adhesions, also known as synechiae, are one of the more common structural abnormalities of the uterus. Joseph Asherman was the first to describe "Amenorrhoea Traumatica" in 1948,[126] and since that time, Asherman's syndrome, or intrauterine adhesions, has been recognized as a challenging entity to diagnose and treat. Any type of insult to the endometrium, specifically the basalis layer, may result in the development of intrauterine adhesions. Asherman's syndrome often is diagnosed after such procedures as puerperal dilation and curettage for retained placental fragments, or curettage for voluntary interruption of pregnancy or evacuation of an incomplete abortion.[127]

Presentation of a patient with Asherman's syndrome is characteristic in many instances. Typically, a woman who has had a uterine curettage or intrauterine infection presents with the onset of secondary amenorrhea or oligomenorrhea. Not all women will have amenorrhea, and some, in fact, will have cyclic, painless menses, although this is far less common. The degree of uterine bleeding usually corresponds to the amount of intrauterine scarring. Patients with these adhesions usually are ovulatory and will often complain of menstrual symptoms including moderate to severe, cyclic, abdominal discomfort.

Intrauterine adhesions also have been implicated in causing infertility, recurrent abortion, or fetal death *in utero*, and if pregnancy does occur, they may increase the incidence of premature labor or abnormal placentation, such as placenta previa or accreta.[128] Decreased uterine blood flow, smaller cavity size, and myometrial fibrosis have been proposed as the underlying causes of the above complications.[129,130] Researchers also postulate that hypoestrogenism, such as occurs in a postpartum lactating woman, may predispose to the development of intrauterine adhesions. In fact, in a study by Westendorp et al.,[131] lactating women had significantly increased risk of developing this condition, although the number of patients was small. Their results also suggested a decreased incidence of hypoestrogenism in oral contraceptive users, with a relative risk of 0.55, although this finding was not statistically significant.[131]

A hysterosalpingogram is the most common method of diagnosis of Asherman's syndrome, with the pattern of contrast media distribution demonstrating one or multiple filling defects in the uterine cavity of various shapes and sizes.[132] Sometimes, no filling of the cavity occurs, suggesting complete obstruction by adhesions. Additional information from the hysterosalpingogram confirms tubal patency. Hysterosalpingography is an excellent procedure if the physician suspects intrauterine adhesions. If the results of the test are normal, then further testing, for instance diagnostic hysteroscopy, need not be performed.[135] Schlaff et al. wondered if transvaginal ultrasonography of the endometrium could reliably predict surgical outcome in a group of seven patients with amenorrhea and Asherman's syndrome.[127] The results of their study indicated that a uniform endometrial stripe thickness of ≥6 cm on preoperative ultrasound exam predicted good success with hysteroscopic repair, with resumption of menses and recreation of a near normal or normal cavity. In the patients with a preoperative stripe thickness of ≤2 cm, amenorrhea persisted after surgical repair, likely representing an obliterated cavity. Although the sample size was small, the results suggest that patients with thin endometrial stripes on ultrasound will have a poor prognosis after surgical repair.

Hysteroscopy may confirm the presence of intrauterine adhesions and also may be used to treat the adhesions once diagnosed. This is not always a simple and straightforward task. When the uterine cavity is completely obliterated by adhesions, the surgeon cannot find the correct plane of dissection when trying to lyse the adhesions.[133] In attempts to correct the deformity surgically, if in the wrong plane of dissection, the physician may injure the myometrium, thereby complicating the surgery with excess bleeding and perhaps even perforation of the uterus.[134] Many surgeons advocate the simultaneous use of laparoscopy so that the uterus may be visualized directly during the hysteroscopic procedure with the hope of avoiding uterine perforation. Hysteroscopic lysis of intrauterine adhesions may be performed with scissor dissection, electrocautery, or laser, and the dissection proceeds in a caudad to cephalad direction. In some patients, actual hysterotomy (surgical opening of the uterus) may be necessary to gain access to the fundus of the uterus if the cervix and lower uterine segment are badly involved with disease.[135]

Many surgeons advocate the use of postoperative conjugated estrogens for 60 days, with medroxyprogesterone acetate added during the last five days of therapy,[136] as high dose sequential therapy promotes re-eptihelialization of the endometrium denuded from surgery. Some other adjuvants used to promote healing are an inflated Foley catheter balloon in the cavity for approximately one week[137] or a loop IUD for 2 months, to help prevent apposition of raw endometrial surfaces.[138] One also should obtain a postoperative HSG to confirm patency of the cavity, as some patients will require more than one procedure. Pregnancy rates after surgical treatment have been shown to range from 60 to 75%;[139,140] however, even higher rates of 93% have been demonstrated in patients with only minimal disease compared to 57.4% in those with severe disease. When the majority of the cavity is obliterated, the prognosis is dismal, and surrogacy motherhood should be considered.

C. DES EXPOSURE

Structural abnormalities of the uterus may also result from *in utero* exposure to diethylstilbestrol (DES). DES is a synthetic nonsteroidal estrogen that was given between the years of 1940 and 1971 to women in the U.S. with a history of recurrent miscarriage.[141] Smith, in 1948, reported that DES decreased the incidence of early pregnancy loss, preterm delivery, intrauterine fetal demise, and pregnancy-induced hypertension in those with a poor obstetric history.[142] This was later disproven by a prospective, randomized, double-blind, placebo-controlled study of 1646 patients by Dieckmann et al. in 1953.[143] Approximately 2 million women in the U.S. have been exposed to DES. In a study of 267 patients, HSG abnormalities typical of DES exposure occurred in 69% of exposed women.[144] DES binds to estradiol receptors during fetal development and adversely affects development of Mullerian structures.[98] Some of the more common anomalies encountered in patients who have been exposed *in utero* include T-shaped uterine cavity, a small uterine cavity with irregular borders, dilation of the lower uterine segment, and tubal changes including sacculations, pinpoint ostia, and fimbrial abnormalities.[145] Other abnormalities may involve the vaginal mucosa (vaginal adenosis) and cervix (collars, cockscombs, septae, and hoods).[144,146,147]

Women who have been exposed to DES *in utero* have an increased risk for conceiving an ectopic pregnancy, more than two times as likely according to several case-control studies.[148] The cause is largely uncertain; however, it is thought to result from structural abnormalities of the tube, which is a Mullerian structure and subject to the influence of this synthetic estrogen. Uterine anomalies, most commonly hypoplasia, may contribute to incompetent cervix, preterm labor, and recurrent first and second trimester abortion.[148] *In utero* exposure to DES has been shown to increase a woman's risk of developing clear cell adenocarcinoma of the vagina.[149]

Data on the prevalence of infertility in this population of women are conflicting. In a study by Senekjian et al.,[150] the incidence of primary and secondary infertility was higher in the exposed group. Kaufman et al.[151] showed that of women with uterine anomalies, constriction bands and a T-shaped cavity predisposed to a higher incidence of infertility

Treatment of DES exposed women with infertility may include IVF. A study by Karande et al.[152] demonstrated that DES exposed women, as compared to their counterparts with tubal factor infertility, had similar numbers of oocytes retrieved and fertilized, and similar resulting pregnancy rates. The pregnancy outcome was worse for the DES exposed group, however. Of all the assisted reproductive technologies, IVF is the one most strongly recommended, as these patients are already at higher risk for ectopic pregnancy.[147] For the DES exposed patients with a history of spontaneous abortion, cervical cerclage may be considered; however, the evidence for prophylactic cerclage is conflicting.

VI. RECURRENT PREGNANCY LOSS (RPL)

Recurrent pregnancy loss (RPL) is a common clinical condition that affects 0.5 to 1% of pregnant women. The miscarriage rate for clinically recognized pregnancies approximates 15 to 20%.[153] What constitutes recurrent pregnancy loss or habitual abortion fuels debate and varies in the literature, but classically it is defined as three or more spontaneous abortions (SAB). Investigators sometimes make a distinction between primary and secondary RPL. Primary RPL refers to women who have never delivered a liveborn infant, whereas women with secondary RPL have at least one liveborn child. Data from a number of studies indicate that after one spontaneous abortion the couple has a small increase in the 15% baseline risk for having another miscarriage, and after two miscarriages this risk increases to 25% (range, 17 to 35%). After three SABs the risk for having a fourth is 33% (range, 25 to 49%).[154] Disagreement exists as to when to begin an evaluation of couples with RPL. Some investigators advocate starting a work-up after two miscarriages although the common recommendation is to begin an evaluation after three losses.

A. ETIOLOGY

An etiology for RPL can be ascertained in approximately half of the cases. These include chromosomal (3.5%), anatomic (16%), endocrine (20%), infectious (0.5%), and immunologic causes (20%).[155] In the remaining cases the cause remains unexplained, although some postulate that immunologic factors cause these unexplained cases of RPL.

B. ENDOCRINOLOGIC

The most common endocrine cause of RPL is luteal phase defect which is defined as inadequate production of progesterone by the corpus luteum. Researchers have solidly established that successful implantation and maintenance of early pregnancy require progesterone. The diagnosis is made by an endometrial biopsy, which is considered to be out of phase when the histologic dating lags behind the menstrual dating by three days or more. A midluteal progesterone level also indicates this diagnosis, although significant controversy exists as to what constitutes a normal level. A widely accepted treatment for this condition has been to use supplemental progesterone in the luteal phase, although a meta analysis of randomized controlled trials found that progesterone therapy was ineffective.[156] Other endocrine causes of RPL may be maternal hyper and hypothyroidism. The mechanism by which these disorders lead to RPL is unknown. Diabetes mellitus also has been associated with RPL. Recent evidence suggests this is a problem when the disease is not well-controlled. Disorders of androgen secretion may occur in women with RPL, particularly in polycystic ovary syndrome where hypersecretion of LH occurs. Researchers postulate that this may result from premature ovulation of an oocyte that is unfertilizable, or the fertilized embryo is prone to early loss.[157]

C. GENETIC ABNORMALITIES

Genetic abnormalities may account for 3.5 to 6% of cases of RPL.[155–158] This is the only uncontested cause of RPL that occurs as a result of structural chromosome aberrations in one or both partners.[159] Abnormalities also can result from recurrent aneuploidy in the conceptus which in part may be related to the age of the mother. Balanced translocations account for the largest proportion of such abnormalities, affecting 2 to 3% of couples. The more common types of translocations are reciprocal and simple, followed by Robertsonian translocation (fusion of acrocenteric chromosomes). When either parent is a carrier of such translocations the conceptus may have normal chromosomes, be a balanced carrier, or have abnormal chromosomes. The overall risk of miscarriage in couples with reciprocal or simple translocations is approximately 25 to 50%, and the overall risk of an offspring carrying an unbalanced translocation is approximately 10%. Although routine cytogenetic testing of abortus specimens is not indicated at this time, analysis of parental karyotypes is a part of the work-up of RPL.

D. INFECTIONS

To date no infectious agent has been proven to be a cause of RPL. However, associations have been found between infectious agents and RPL. Women with RPL appear to have higher rate of endometrial colonization with *Ureaplasma urealyticum* suggesting an association.[160] Other organisms such as *Toxoplasma gondii* and viruses such as rubella, herpes simplex virus, cytomegalovirus, measles virus, and Coxsackie virus have been linked to abortion, but none has clearly been shown to cause RPL.

E. UTERINE ABNORMALITIES

Uterine anomalies account for 10 to 15% of cases of RPL. The most common malformations associated with RPL include bicornuate, septate, and didelphic uterus. Exposure to diethylstilbestrol (DES), submucosal leiomyomata, and endometrial polyps also correspond to RPL. These defects lead to pregnancy loss possibly secondary to inadequate space or poor vascularization of the endometrium and can be diagnosed by hysterosalpingography, ultrasonography, and hysteroscopy. Cervical incompetence, which is defined as painless dilation of the cervix during the second trimester leading to rupture of membranes and fetal expulsion, can cause RPL. This condition results from previous cervical trauma, congenital defects, or *in utero* DES exposure. Placement of a cervical cerclage helps prevent future losses. For uterine anomalies, corrective surgery, particularly hysteroscopic resection of a septum, produces favorable pregnancy outcome.

F. IMMUNOLOGICAL FACTORS

Immunologic causes of RPL include autoimmune and alloimmune factors. Autoimmunity refers to induction of an immune response to self antigens and results in failure of self tolerance. Antiphospholipid antibodies are antibodies that bind to negatively charged phospholipids and have been associated with RPL, arterial and venous thrombosis, autoimmune thrombocytopenia, and autoimmune hemolytic anemia. Women who have these antibodies also have pregnancy complications such as preeclampsia, intrauterine growth retardation, abnormal fetal heart tracings, and preterm delivery. The two antibodies of proven clinical relevance are lupus anticoagulant and anticardiolipin. In one study the rate of pregnancy loss in women with lupus anticoagulant was reported to be more than 90%.[161] The incidence of antiphospholipid antibodies in women with RPL varies depending on the study, and figures of 3 to 48% have been reported.[162] The mechanism(s) by which antiphospholipid antibodies (APA) cause RPL is unknown. Proposed mechanisms include inhibition of prostacyclin production, leading to vasoconstriction and thrombosis,[163] interference with protein C activation,[164] or inhibition of syncytial trophoblast formation.[165] Antinuclear antibodies (ANA) have been measured by some in women with RPL. Most authors consider a titer of 1:40 as significant. Although earlier studies showed an association between ANA and RPL, more recent prospective studies failed to show a difference in ANA titers between women with habitual abortion and controls. Therefore, testing for ANA is no longer recommended.[166] Antithyroid antibodies also appear to be associated with increased risk of RPL. Women with these antibodies did not have clinically overt thyroid disease, thus suggesting that thyroid autoantibodies may be an independent marker for increased risk for miscarriage.[167] Whether thyroid antibodies cause RPL currently is unknown. Their presence simply may reflect a nonspecific activation of the immune system.

Allogeneic factors may be a cause of otherwise unexplained RPL. An earlier proposed mechanism was that parental HLA heterozygosity was necessary for successful reproduction. Multiple studies now refute this concept, and testing of couples for HLA sharing is no longer recommended. Another proposed alloimmune mechanism includes deficient blocking antibodies in women with RPL. Blocking antibodies are thought to be antiidiotype antibodies that mask fetal trophoblast antigens or cover maternal lymphocyte receptors thereby preventing a maternal immune response against the conceptus. The lack of reliable methods for measuring these antibodies presents problems. Furthermore, these blocking antibodies lack predictive value for determining the outcome of future pregnancies.[168]

One other alloimmune factor important in RPL is a change in the resident immune cells of the endometrium. Natural killer (NK) cells, which are large granular lymphocytes, have been detected in decidua in early pregnancy. NK cells can kill human trophoblast cells after stimulation with interleukin-2. Women with RPL were reported to have higher NK cell activity than controls, and immunotherapy lowered this activity.[169–170] More recent studies failed to confirm these findings.[171] The possibility exists that alteration in the resident immune cells also results in altered cytokine secretion, some of which may be embryotoxic. Hill et al. provided evidence for this concept by showing that antigen-activated lymphocytes obtained from women with RPL produced embryotoxic factors.[172] Interferon gamma was identified as one of these embryotoxic cytokines produced by lymphocytes of these women.

G. TESTING AND THERAPY

The standard and currently accepted evaluation of RPL includes parental peripheral blood karyotype analysis, hysterosalpingogram or hysteroscopy or both for evaluation of the endometrial cavity. Endocrine testing includes thyroid function tests, serum prolactin, fasting glucose, and luteal phase endometrial biopsy. Immunologic testing for RPL comprises measurement of anticardiolipin antibodies and lupus anticoagulant (activated partial thromboplastin time or Russell's Viper Venom). Some investigators suggest measurement of additional APA. However, a recent study reported no utility of this additional assessment.[173] Infectious assessment includes cervical cultures for mycoplasma and chlamydia.

When chromosomal abnormality occurs in one or both partners no corrective measures are possible, and genetic counseling is warranted before another pregnancy attempt. In cases of Robertsonian translocation, donor oocytes or sperm are indicated since this abnormality always results in an aneuploidic conception. Uterine abnormalities generally are treated by hysteroscopic techniques. Certain congenital anomalies such as bicornuate uterus with a prior poor pregnancy outcome respond to laparatomy and reconstructive procedures to unify the two uterine cavities. Various techniques of cerclage correct cervical incompetence. Luteal phase deficiency is treated by either ovulation induction with clomiphene citrate or menotropins or exogenous luteal phase progesterone supplementation. When thyroid dysfunction is found, Synthroid helps cases of hypothyroidism, especially when this may be the cause of ovulatory dysfunction. Women who have hyperprolactinemia should receive dopaminergic agonists such as bromocriptine. When cervical cultures reveal the presence of mycoplasma, treatment with doxycycline is effective in eliminating the organism. Women treated with antibiotics for mycoplasma experienced a significant reduction in pregnancy loss compared with nontreated women.[174]

The treatment of immune mediated RPL remains the most controversial, particularly alloimmune mediated loss. The most widely accepted therapy for women with antiphospholipid antibodies combines low dose aspirin with heparin, although other treatments such as prednisone in combination with heparin have also been tried, but produced more serious side effects, such as aseptic hip necrosis. Low dose aspirin alone is not as effective as aspirin with heparin,[175] and aspirin alone carries an increased risk of abruptio placentae.

Immunotherapies proposed for the treatment of alloimmune RPL include intravenous immunoglobulin (IVIG) and leukocyte therapy. The rationale for leukocyte immunization was that it elicited potentially beneficial blocking antibodies in the mother. Few randomized prospective studies have examined the efficacy of leukocyte therapy, and most of the studies showing a benefit are anecdotal. Another problem with the clinical trials has been the lack of uniformity, with use of different doses, route, and frequency of administration, and the patient population selected for treatment. An analysis of the world wide data on leukocyte immunization for treatment of RPL showed a small treatment effect, with immunotherapy helping 8 to 10% of affected couples. However, investigators lack the proper diagnostic tests that would identify this small subset of patients who may benefit from this treatment.[176]

The rationale for the use of IVIG in RPL is based on its efficacy in treatment of other autoimmune-related conditions. These preparations may contain both idiotype and antiidiotype antibodies against trophoblast antigens, and may be beneficial to women with RPL who do not produce sufficient antiidiotype antibodies. Again a paucity of properly designed studies test this treatment. A German multicenter prospective randomized placebo-controlled trial failed to show a beneficial effect,[177] whereas an American study showed a beneficial effect in reducing the incidence of intrauterine fetal death.[178] Presently, both leukocyte therapy and IVIG remain unproven and costly treatments for alloimmune RPL.

H. AUTOIMMUNITY AND INFERTILITY

Several studies show an increased incidence of antiphospholipid antibodies in patients undergoing IVF, and this has been linked to implantation failure.[179–181] The proposed mechanism(s) is that phospholipids function as adhesion molecules during the formation of syncytiotrophoblast, and antibodies attaching to surface phospholipids may cause direct cellular injury.[172] Based on these observations, some investigators propose treating all antiphospholipid antibody positive women with heparin and aspirin and report higher pregnancy rates for women treated with this combination.[179] In a more recent study,[182] although women undergoing IVF had APA more frequently than controls, treatment with heparin and aspirin did not improve their implantation or pregnancy rates. Until more studies address this issue, routine testing and treatment of patients undergoing IVF for APA is not warranted.

VII. UNEXPLAINED INFERTILITY

In 10 to 15% of infertile couples, the standard tests for infertility yield normal results. In these couples the monthly fecundity is 1.5 to 3%, in contrast to 25% in normal couples, and approximately 60% of these couples with less than 3 years of infertility will become pregnant within 3 years.[183,184] Attempts to identify potential causes of infertility in these women persist.

Although the diagnostic tests presently available are not sensitive enough to identify all the causes of infertility, attempts have been made to elucidate subtle problems in these couples. The endometrium features prominently in these studies. Luteal phase endometrium from women suffering from primary unexplained infertility showed a deficiency of $\alpha_4\beta_1$ (VLA-4) integrin expression by epithelial cells, and this can lead to failure of the blastocyst to attach via fibronectin to its endometrial counter receptor at implantation.[185] Alterations in the resident population of endometrial lymphocytes also occur in women with unexplained infertility, with increased numbers of CD4-positive T-cells, decreased numbers of CD8-positive cells, and decreased numbers of CD56-positive granulated lymphocytes.[186]

Another proposed cause of unexplained infertility is subtle ovulatory dysfunction which can not be diagnosed by a luteal phase endometrial biopsy or luteal progesterone levels. In a group of women who met these stringent criteria, mean progesterone levels measured in the serum every other day from the onset of menstruation until the first day of the next menstrual period were found to be lower than the control population. Also, the ratio of integrated estradiol to progesterone was significantly greater in women with unexplained infertility. The magnitude of the LH surge, rate of follicular growth, and maximum follicular diameter did not differ in these women.[187]

Immunologic factors also may influence unexplained infertility, and as discussed earlier, some affected women may have APA. Subtle fertilization problems, which cannot be identified by available diagnostic tests, could be another cause of unexplained infertility. Schatten et al. described the steps at which fertilization may fail at a cellular and molecular level. Some of these defects stem from intrinsic problems with the cytoskeletal elements of the oocyte or the sperm's ability to organize microtubule assembly.[188,189] Current tests, such as the hamster sperm penetration assay, which is designed to test the sperm's fertilizing capacity, have poor predictive value and have been abandoned by most centers.[190] Diagnostic tests are being developed to identify subtle defects in fertilization, many of which stem from cytoskeletal abnormalities.[191]

Regardless of the underlying cause of infertility in these couples, the recommended first line treatment has been superovulation and intrauterine insemination. Recently, a large randomized controlled trial demonstrated this treatment's efficacy. In this trial, in 932 couples in which the woman had no identifiable infertility factor and the man had motile sperm, superovulation with intrauterine insemination was twice as likely to result in pregnancy as superovulation or intrauterine insemination alone.[192] Earlier studies also showed that superovulation and intrauterine insemination increased cycle fecundity from 3 to 15% in these couples.[193] IVF would be the next treatment modality offered to these couples if superovulation fails.

VIII. THERAPY FOR FEMALE INFERTILITY

A. AGENTS FOR OVULATION INDUCTION

The agents commonly used for ovulation induction are clomiphene citrate, gonadotropins in the form of human menopausal gonadotropins (hMG) and follicle stimulating hormones (FSH), both extracted from urine of postmenopausal women, and recently recombinant FSH (r-FSH). The different ways to plan ovulation induction depend on the pathology that is being treated. The most common indications for ovulation induction are listed in Table 5.1.

**TABLE 5.1
Indications for
Ovulation Induction**

Hypothalamic amenorrhea
Chronic anovulation
Endometriosis
Unexplained infertility
Tubal factor
Mild male factor

---

1. Clomiphene Citrate

Clomiphene citrate consists of two isomers: the en clomiphene isomer, which is more biologically active, and the zu clomiphene isomer, which is less active. Its mechanism of action is the selective blockage of estrogen receptors, and for this reason it is also called an antiestrogen in the hypothalamus and pituitary. As a consequence, estrogen cannot exert a negative feedback and GnRH, FSH, and LH secretion increases. Thus, folliculogenesis is stimulated. The starting dose is usually 50 mg a day, 1 tablet a day for 5 days, and it may be given from days 3 to 7 of the menstrual cycle. If ovulation does not occur with the dosage of 50 mg, the subsequent cycle dose can be increased to 100 mg or even to 150 mg. If ovulation does not take place with 150 mg, further increases rarely help the condition, and at this point a more aggressive approach, such as using injectable gonadotropins, is warranted. To monitor ovulation, the patient can measure the basal body temperature, or the physician can order a midluteal phase progesterone level, usually 7 days after the last tablet of clomiphene. Follicular development can also be monitored with ultrasound, beginning the monitoring from day 11 or 12 of the menstrual cycle. Ovulation rates with clomiphene are about 70% after four cycles, and pregnancy rates when the primary indication is anovulation are about 20% per cycle or a cumulative pregnancy rate of 50 to 60% after a total of four cycles. If no pregnancy occurs after a total of four well-timed cycles, in spite of clearly documented ovulation, no benefit remains in continuing the same treatment. The risks of clomiphene citrate therapy include multiple pregnancy at a rate of about 10 to 15% per cycle. The drug also can cause nausea and occasionally bloating. Patients rarely reported headache. It is also not advisable to use ovulation predictor kits based on the presence of urinary LH content with use of clomiphene citrate because not only FSH but also LH is released from the pituitary which can create a false positive reading on the test kit. No increase in birth defects has been reported.

2. Urinary and Recombinant Gonadotropins

Gonadotropins are urinary products and are subdivided into human menopausal gonadotropins (hMG) and follicle stimulating hormones (FSH). An additional type, extra purified urinary gonadotropins, contain minimal amounts of other urinary contaminants allowing the subcutaneous route of administration. The new class of gonadotropins comprises a recombinant FSH and recombinant LH. Gonadotropins are derived from the urine of postmenopausal women and the final purified preparation contains a 1:1 ratio of FSH and LH. Although used extensively, these preparations contain other urinary contaminants that do not allow subcutaneous administration and therefore require an intramuscular injection. High purification of the urinary extracted gonadotropins was introduced into clinical practice in 1993, and since 1997 in the U.S., patients could benefit from the availability of recombinant FSH. In clinical practice, the use of gonadotropins for ovulation induction requires careful monitoring of the patient's response to these agents. This includes serial ultrasound exams and blood tests to evaluate the rise in estradiol. Commonly used protocols involve the administration of two ampules of 75 units a day, starting from day 2 of the cycle, of any of the urinary or recombinant products. After the first 3 days of therapy, the patient's response dictates dose adjustment. The goal is to achieve a mono- or bifollicular development. However, this is not easy to obtain, especially in patients diagnosed with chronic anovulation due to polycystic ovarian disease. In the latter, the ideal protocol is yet to be described, but it is common practice to begin stimulation either with a single ampule of gonadotropins (75 IU) for prolonged periods of time or to begin with two ampules (150 IU) a day for the first 2 or 3 days of the cycle and then use the so-called step down protocol where only one ampule a day is continued until a leading follicle is detected on ultrasound. Patients with polycystic ovaries represent a challenging population to treat, since the risk for multiple ovulation, and thus multiple pregnancies, and for ovarian hyperstimulation syndrome is very high. During ovulation induction with gonadotropins, when a leading follicle of 18 to 20 mm in mean diameter appears on ultrasound, an intramuscular injection of human chorionic gonadotropin (hCG), at the dosage of 10,000 units, is given to trigger ovulation. This allows the release 24 to 36 hours later of an oocyte. If the couple is scheduled for a cycle of intrauterine insemination, this will be performed 36 hours after hCG, although in some cases it is common practice to carry out two inseminations 24 and 48 hours after hCG. For couples planning timed intercourse, they are instructed to have intercourse the night of hCG administration and again the following day.

B. OVULATION INDUCTION AND ASSISTED REPRODUCTION

In cases of tubal factor infertility, or after having failed a total of four to six well-timed intrauterine inseminations with ovulation induction, the couple is advised to undergo a cycle of assisted reproduction consisting of *in vitro* fertilization or, if the etiology of infertility is male factor, intracytoplasmic sperm injection (ICSI). In addition to the gonadotropins administered during ovulation, an agent to suppress the endogenous release of FSH and LH is also added to the protocol. This agent is known as GnRH analog, and the most frequently used is leuprolide acetate (Lupron™). According to the type of female factor infertility being treated, the ovarian stimulation protocols can be divided into two groups: (1) long or luteal phase protocol; and (2) short or follicular phase protocol.

The long protocol incorporates GnRH analogs beginning on day 21 of the previous menstrual cycle in order to obtain suppression by the time the patient will have her menses. On day 2 of the next menstrual cycle, after establishing hormonal suppression by measuring estradiol (usually < 30 pg/ml), the physician adds gonadotropins to the protocol. The dosage varies according to the patient's age, weight, etiology of infertility, and previous response to gonadotropins. The GnRH analog continues until the day of hCG administration when about 50% or more of the follicles recruited are above 17 to 18 mm in mean diameter.

The short protocol is also called flare up protocol. It is usually reserved for patients who are known to have poor response, for older patients (defined as patients older than 40 years old), or for patients with borderline elevated FSH (every laboratory should have its own standard reference values). Short or flare up protocol involves the administration of GnRH analog on day 1 of the menstrual cycle, followed from day 2 on with gonadotropins. The potential benefit of this protocol in this specific group of patients is the massive release of FSH and LH stored in the pituitary creating the so-called flare up effect during the first three days of administration of the analog. hCG is administered when the leading follicles are above 18 mm in diameter. During both of these protocols, the dosage of gonadotropins can be adjusted according to the ovarian response and the level of estradiol.

Lately, recombinant gonadotropins (r-FSH) have been introduced in the U.S. market in an attempt to replace the old urinary product. The first human pregnancy with the product was reported in 1992;[194] it was approved for use in Europe in 1995 and then in the U.S. in 1997. The specific bioactivity of r-FSH is the highest with more than 10,000 IU of FSH per mg of protein. Furthermore, the product has a purity greater than 99% with complete absence of LH activity. Recombinant FSH requires fewer days of stimulation (shorter by one day than other urinary gonadotropins). Also, the dosage of gonadotropins is lower compared to intramuscular products and a slightly higher number of eggs are collected. However, no differences in pregnancy rates and no differences in implantation rates appear. The main advantages of r-FSH products are high purity and specificity, no batch-to-batch variability, no risk of shortage in supply, and patients' acceptance of the subcutaneous administration. About 34 to 38 hours after administration of hCG, transvaginal oocyte aspiration under ultrasound guidance is performed. Intravenous sedation is usually accomplished by using Propoxyfol™ and/or Versed™. After routine *in vitro* fertilization or ICSI procedures, embryo transfers are scheduled for either day 3 from egg collection or day 5 at the blastocyst stage.

Generally, the luteal phase is supported with daily administration of progesterone via intramuscular injections (50 mg/day) or via vaginal gel applicators or vaginal suppositories.

Replacement of more than one embryo, usually three per cycle, corresponds to high (20 to 25%) multiple pregnancy rates. To reduce this risk, limit the number of embryos transferred to two. By transferring one or two blastocyst stage embryo(s), the number of high order pregnancies (triplet or more) should become a rare event. While there are no doubts that women with more than ten follicles or more than three embryos at the eight-cell stage on day 3 of culture have high pregnancy rates with blastocyst transfer,[195,196] it is still unclear whether blastocyst transfer is indicated for women with poorer prognoses.

REFERENCES

1. Rosen, D. L., Kaplan, B., and Lobo, R. A., Menstrual function and hirsutism in patients with gonadal dysgenesis, *Obstet. Gynecol.*, 17, 677, 1988.
2. Santoro, N. F. and Tortoriello, D. V., Amenorrhea: etiologies and therapies, in *Int. Frontiers in Reproductive Endocrinology*, Serono Symposia USA Inc., 1999, 307–330.
3. Levine, J. E., Chappell, P., Besecke, L. M., Bauer-Dantoin, A. C., Wolfe, A. M., Porkka-Heiskanen, J. et al., Amplitude and frequency modulation of pulsatile luteinizing hormone-releasing hormone release, *Cell Mol. Neurobiol.*, 15, 117–39, 1995.
4. Suh, B. Y., Liu, J. H., Quigley, M. E., Laughlin, G. A., and Yen, S. S., Hypercortisolism in patients with hypothalamic amenorrhea, *J. Clin. Endocrinol. Metab.*, 66, 733–9, 1988.
5. Olster, C. H. and Ferin, M., Corticotrophin-releasing hormone inhibits gonadotropin secretion in the ovariectomized rhesus monkey, *J. Clin. Endocrinol. Metab.*, 65, 262–7, 1987.
6. Fries, H., Nillus, S. J., and Petterson, F., Epidemiology of secondary amenorrhea: a retrospective evaluation of etiology with special regard to psychogenic factors and weight loss, *Am. J. Obstet. Gynecol.*, 118, 473, 1974.
7. Santoro, N., Wierman, M. E., Filicor, M., Waldstreicher, J., and Crowley, W. F., Intravenous administration of pulsatile gonadotropin-releasing hormone in hypothalamic amenorrhea: effects of dosage, *J. Clin. Endocrinol. Metab.*, 62, 109–116, 1986.
8. Kerin, J. F., Liu, J. H., Phillipou, G., and Yen, S. S. C., Evidence for a hypothalamic site of action of clomiphene citrate in women, *J. Clin. Endocrinol. Metab.*, 61, 265, 1985
9. Kettel, L. M., Roseff, S. J., Berga, S. L., Mortola, J. F., and Yen, S. S. C., Hypothalamic-pituitary-ovarian response to clomiphene citrate in women with polycystic ovarian syndrome, *Fertil. Steril.*, 59, 532, 1993.
10. Speroff, L., Glass, R. H., and Kase, N. G., Amenorrhea, in *Clinical Gynecologic Endocrinology and Infertility*, 5th ed., Williams & Wilkins, Baltimore, MD, 1994.
11. Cuellar, F. G., Bromocriptine mesylate (Parlodel) in the management of amenorrhea/galactorrhea associated with hyperprolactinemia, *Obstet. Gynecol.*, 278, 1980.
12. DeZiegler, D., Steungold, K., Cedars, M., Lu, J. H. K., Meldrum, D. R., Judd, H. L. et al., Recovery of hormone secretion after chronic gonadotropin-releasing hormone agonist administration in women with polycystic ovarian disease, *J. Clin. Endocrinol. Metab.*, 68, 1111–7, 1989.
13. Adashi, E. Y., Hsueh, A. J. W., and Yen, S. S. C., Insulin enhancement of luteinizing hormone and follicle-stimulating hormone release by cultured pituitary cells, *Endocrinology*, 108, 1441–9, 1981.

14. Urbanek, M., Legro, R. S., Driscoll, D., Azziz, R., Ehrman, D. A., Norman, R. J., Strauss, J. F., Spielman, R. S., and Dunaif, A., Thirty-seven candidate genes for polycystic ovary syndrome: strongest evidence for linkage is with follistatin, *Proc. Natl. Acad. Sci.*, 96, 8573–8578, 1999.

15. Sorbara, L. R., Tang, A. Z., Cama, A., Xia, J., Schenker, E., Kohanski, R. A. et al., Absence of insulin receptor gene mutations in three insulin-resistant women with the polycystic ovary syndrome, *Metabolism*, 43, 1568–74, 1994.

16. Dunaif, A., Xia, J., Book, C. B., Schenker, E., and Tang, Z., Excessive insulin receptor serine phosphorylation in cultured fibroblasts and in skeletal muscle (A potential mechanism for insulin resistance in the polycystic ovary syndrome), *J. Clin. Invest.*, 8, 801–10, 1995.

17. Nestler, J. E., Jakubowicz, D. J., Evans, W. S., and Pasquali, R., Effects of metformin on spontaneous and clomiphene-induced ovulation in the polycystic ovary syndrome, *N. Engl. J. Med.*, 338, 1876–80, 1998.

18. Guzick, D. S., Wing, R., Smith, D., Berg, S. L., and Winters, S. J., Endocrine consequences of weight loss in obese, hyperandrogenic anovulatory women, *Fertil. Steril.*, 61, 598–604, 1994.

19. Belvisi, L., Bombelli, F., Sironi, L., and Doldi, N., Organ-specific autoimmunity in patients with premature ovarian failure, *J. Endocrinol. Invest.*, 16, 889–92, 1993.

20. Luborsky, J. L., Visintin, I., Boyers, S., Asari, T., Caldwell, B., and DeCherney, A., Ovarian antibodies detected by immobilized antigen immunoassay in patients with premature ovarian failure, *J. Clin. Endocrinol. Metab.*, 70, 69–75, 1990.

21. Kraus, C. M., Turskoy, R. N., Atkins, L., McLaughlin, C., Brown, L. G., and Page, D. C., Familial premature ovarian failure due to an interstitial deletion of the long arm of the X chromosome, *N. Engl. J. Med.*, 16, 125–31, 1987.

22. Powell, C. M., Taggart, R. T., Drumheller, T. C., Wangsa, D., Qian, C., Nelson, L. M. et al., Molecular and cytogenetic studies of an X autosome translocation in a patient with premature ovarian failure and review of the literature, *Am. J. Med. Genet.*, 52, 19–26, 1994.

23. Gradishan, W. J. and Schilsky, R. L., Ovarian function following radiation and chemotherapy, *Seminars Oncol.*, 16, 425, 1989.

24. Wallace, W. H., Shalet, S. M., Crowne, E. C., Morris-Jones, P. H., and Gattamanen, H. R., Ovarian failure following abdominal irradiation in childhood: natural history and prognosis, *Clin. Oncol.*, 1, 75, 1989.

25. Lydic, M. L., Liu, J. H., Rebar, R. W., Thomas, M. A., and Cedars, M. I., Success of donor oocyte *in vitro* fertilization-embryo transfer in recipients with and without premature ovarian failure, *Fertil. Steril.*, 65, 98–102, 1996.

26. Chantilis, S. J. and Bradshaw, K. D., Clinical and molecular aspects of steroidogenic enzyme deficiencies, *Infertil. Reprod. Clin. N. Am.*, 5, 81–104, 1994.

27. Flood, J. T. and Grow, D. R., Transcervical tubal cannulation: a review, *Obstet. Gynecol. Surv.*, 48, 768–776, 1993.

28. Marana, R., Rizzi, M., Muzii, L., Catalano, G. F., Caruana, P., and Mancuso, S., Correlation between the American Fertility Society classifications of adnexal adhesions and distal tubal occlusion, salpingoscopy, and reproductive outcome in tubal surgery, *Fertil. Steril.*, 64, 924–929, 1995.

29. Bahamondes, L., Bueno, J. G. R., Hardy, E., Vera, S., Pimental, E., and Ramos, M., Identification of main risk factors for tubal infertility, *Fertil. Steril.*, 61, 478–482, 1984.

30. Sauer, M V., Tubal infertility: the role of reconstructive surgery, in *Mishell's Textbook of Infertility, Contraception, and Reproductive Endocrinology*, 4th ed., Lobo, R. A., Mishell, D. R., Jr., Paulson, R. J., and Shoupe, D., Eds., Blackwell Science, Inc., Malden, MA, 1997, 604–622.

31. Gomel, V. and Yarali, H., Infertility surgery: microsurgery, *Curr. Opin. Obstet. Gynecol.*, 4, 390, 1992.

32. Donnez, J., Casanas-Roux, F., Ferin, J., and Thomas, K., Fimbrial ciliated cells percentage and epithelial height during and after salpingitis, *Eur. J. Obstet. Gynecol. Reprod. Biol.*, 17, 293, 1984.

33. David, A., Garcia, C. R., and Czernobilisky, B., Human hydrosalpinx: histologic study and chemical composition of fluid, *Am. J. Obstet. Gynecol.*, 105, 400, 1969.

34. McComb, P. F. and Rowe, T. C., Salpingitis isthmica nodosa: evidence it is a progressive disease, *Fertil. Steril.*, 51, 542, 1989.

35. Musich, J. R. and Behrman, S. J., Surgical management of tubal obstruction at the uterotubal junction, *Fertil. Steril.*, 40, 423, 1983.

36. Donnez, J. and Casanas-Roux, F., Histology: a prognostic factor in proximal tubal occlusion, *Eur. J. Obstet. Gynecol. Reprod. Biol.*, 29, 33, 1988.

37. Schwabe, M. G., Shapiro, S. S., and Haning, R. V., Hysterosalpingography with oil contrast medium enhances fertility in patients with infertility of unknown etiology, *Fertil. Steril.*, 40, 604, 1983.

38. Stumpf, P. G. and March, C. M., Febrile morbidity following hysterosalpingography: identification of risk factors and recommendations for prophylaxis, *Fertil. Steril.*, 33, 487, 1980.

39. Novy, M., Thurmond, A. S., Patton, P. et al., Diagnosis of cornual obstruction by transcervical fallopian tube cannulation, *Fertil. Steril.*, 50, 434, 1988.

40. Kerin, J. F., Daykhosvsky, L., Segalowitz, J., Surrey, E., Anderson, R., Stein, A., Wade, M., and Grundfest, W., Falloposcopy: a microendoscopic technique for visual exploration of the human fallopian tube from the uterotubal ostium to the fimbria using a transvaginal approach, *Fertil. Steril.*, 54, 390–400, 1990.

41. Hull, M. G. R. and Cahill, D. J., *Female Infertility*, Endocrinology and Metabolism Clinics of North America, 27, 851–876, 1998.

42. Benadiva, C. A., Kligman, I., Davis, O., and Rosenwaks, Z., *In vitro* fertilization versus tubal surgery: is pelvic reconstructive surgery obsolete?, *Fertil. Steril.*, 64, 1051–1061, 1995.

43. Tulandi, T., Collins, J. A., Burrows, E., Jarrell, J. F., McInnes, R. A., Wrixon, W. et al., Treatment-dependent and treatment-independent pregnancy among women with periadnexal adhesions, *Am. J. Obstet. Gynecol.*, 162, 354–357, 1990.

44. Gomel, V., Salpingo-ovariolysis by laparoscopy in infertility, *Fertil. Steril.*, 40, 607–611, 1983.

45. Luciano, A. A., Maier, D. B., Koch, E. I., Nulsen, J. C., and Whitman, G. F., A comparative study of postoperative adhesions following laser surgery by laparoscopy versus laparotomy in the rabbit model, *Obstet. Gynecol.*, 74, 220–224, 1989.

46. Hulka, J. F., Adnexal adhesions: a prognostic staging and classification system based on a five-year survey of fertility surgery results at Chapel Hill, North Carolina, *Am. J. Obstet. Gynecol.*, 144, 141–148, 1982.

47. Bateman, B. G., Nunley, J. W. C., and Kichin, J. D., Surgical management of distal tubal obstruction: are we making progress?, *Fertil. Steril.*, 48, 523, 1987.

48. Boer-Meisel, M. E., te Velde, E. R., Habbema, J. D. F., and Kardaun, J. W. P. F., Predicting the pregnancy outcome in patients treated for hydrosalpinx: a prospective study, *Fertil. Steril.*, 45, 23–29, 1986.

49. Schlaff, W. D., Hassiakos, D. K., Damewood, M. D., and Rock, J. A., Neosalpingostomy for distal tubal obstruction: prognostic factors and impact of surgical technique, *Fertil. Steril.*, 54, 984–990, 1990.

50. Anderson, A. N., Yue, Z., Meng, F. J., and Petersen, K., Low implantation rate after *in vitro* fertilization in patients with hydrosalpinges diagnosed by ultrasonography, *Hum. Reprod.*, 9, 1935, 1994.

51. Nackley, A. C. and Muasher, S. J., The significance of hydrosalpinx in *in vitro* fertilization, *Fertil. Steril.*, 69, 373–384, 1998.

52. Aboulghar, M., Mansour, R., Serour, G., Sattar, M., Awad, M., and Amin, Y., Transvaginal ultrasonic needle guides aspiration of pelvic inflammatory cystic masses before ovulation induction for *in vitro* fertilization, *Fertil. Steril.*, 53, 311–314, 1990.

53. Shelton, K. E., Butler, L., Toner, J. P., Oehninger, S., and Muasher, S. J., Salpingectomy improves the pregnancy rate in *in vitro* fertilization with hydrosalpinx, *Hum. Reprod.*, 11, 523–525, 1996.

54. Vandromme, J., Chasse, E., Lejeune, B., Van Rysselberge, M., Delvigne A., and Leroy, F., Hydrosalpinges in *in vitro* fertilization: an unfavorable prognostic feature, *Hum. Reprod.*, 10, 576–579, 1995.

55. Kassabji, M., Sims, J., Butler, L., and Muasher, S., Reduced pregnancy rates with unilateral or bilateral hydrosalpinx after *in vitro* fertilization, *Eur. J. Obstet. Gynecol. Reprod. Biol.*, 56, 129–132, 1994.

56. Meldrum, D. R., Microsurgical tubal reanastomosis: the role of splints, *Obstet. Gynecol.*, 57, 613–619, 1981.

57. Lu, P. Y. and Ory, S. J., Endometriosis: current management, *Mayo Clin. Proc.*, 70, 453–463, 1995.

58. Barbieri, R. L., Endometriosis 1990. Current treatment approaches, *Drugs*, 39, 502–510, 1990.

59. Sampson, J. A., Perforating hemorrhagic (chocolate) cysts of the ovary: their importance and especially their relation to pelvic adenomas of endometrial type (adenomyoma of the uterus, rectovaginal septum, sigmoid, etc.), *Arch. Surg.*, 3, 245, 1921.

60. Halme, J., Hammond, M. G., Hulka, J. F., Raj, S. G., and Talbert, L. M., Retrograde menstruation in healthy women and in patients with endometriosis, *Obstet. Gynecol.*, 64, 151–154, 1984.

61. Ridley, J. H., A review of facts and fancies, *Obstet. Gynecol. Surv.*, 23, 1–35, 1968.

62. Schrodt, G. R., Alcorn, M. O., and Ibanez, J., Endometriosis of the male urinary system: a case report, *J. Urol.*, 124, 722–723, 1980.

63. Chatterjee, S. K., Scar endometriosis: a clinicopathologic study of 17 cases, *Obstet. Gynecol.*, 56, 81–84, 1980.

64. Vigano, P., Vercellini, P., Di Blasio, A. M., Colombo, A., Candiani, G. B., and Vignali, M., Deficient antiendometrium lymphocyte-mediated cytotoxicity in patients with endometriosis, *Fertil. Steril.*, 56, 894–899, 1991.

65. Wang, Y., Sharma, R. K., Falcone, T., Goldberg, J., and Agarwal, A., Importance of reactive oxygen species in the peritoneal fluid of women with endometriosis or idiopathic infertility, *Fertil. Steril.*, 68, 826–830, 1997.

66. Hurst, B. S. and Rock, J. A., Endometriosis: pathophysiology, diagnosis, and treatment, *Obstet. Gynecol. Surv.*, 44, 297–304, 1989.

67. Tureck, R. W., Endometriosis, *Hospital Physician Obstetrics and Gynecology Board Review Manual*, Turne White Communications, Inc., Wayne, PA, 3(3), 1–5, 1997.

68. Rock, J. A., Dubin, N. H., Ghotgaonkar, R. B. et al., Cul-de-sac fluid in women with endometriosis: fluid volume and prostanoid concentration during the proliferative phase of the cycle-days 8 to 12, *Fertil. Steril.*, 37, 747–750, 1982.

69. Wentz, A. C., Premenstrual spotting: its association with endometriosis but not luteal phase inadequacy, *Fertil. Steril.*, 33, 605–607, 1980.
70. Rock, J. A. and Markham, S. M., Extrapelvic endometriosis, in *Endometriosis*, Wilson, E. A., Ed., Alan R. Liss, New York, 1987, 185.
71. Hull, M. E., Moghissi, K. S., Magyar, D. F., and Hayes, M. F., Comparison of different treatment modalities of endometriosis in infertile women, *Fertil. Steril.*, 47, 40–44, 1987.
72. Olive, D. L. and Lee, K. L., Analysis of sequential treatment protocols for endometriosis-associated infertility, *Am. J. Obstet. Gynecol.*, 154, 613–619, 1986.
73. Reiter, R. C., Management of endometriosis, in *Drug Therapy in Obstetrics and Gynecology*, Rayburn, W. F. and Zuspan, F. P., Eds., Mosby Year Book, St. Louis, MO, 1992, 384–399.
74. Bayer, S. R., Seibel, M. M., Saffan, D. S., Berger, M. J., and Taymor, M. L., Efficacy of danazol treatment for minimal endometriosis in infertile women: a prospective, randomized study, *J. Reprod. Med.*, 33, 179–183, 1988.
75. Buttram, V. C., Jr., Belue, J. B., and Reiter, R. C., Interim report of a study of danazol for the treatment of endometriosis, *Fertil. Steril.*, 37, 478–483, 1982.
76. Kauppila, A., Changing concepts of medical treatment of endometriosis, *Acta Obstet. Gynecol. Scand.*, 72, 324–336, 1993.
77. Rock, J. A., Truglia, J. A., and Caplan, R. J., Zoladex Endometriosis Study Group. Zoladex (goserelin acetate implant) in the treatment of endometriosis: a randomized comparison with danazol, *Obstet. Gynecol.*, 82, 198, 1993.
78. Barbieri, R. L. and Gordon, A.-M. C., Hormonal therapy of endometriosis: the estradiol target, *Fertil. Steril.*, 56, 820–822, 1991.
79. Porpora, M. G. and Gomel, V., The role of laparoscopy in the management of pelvic pain in women of reproductive age, *Fertil. Steril.*, 68, 765–779, 1997.
80. Daniell, J. F., Kurtz, B. R., and Gurley, L. D., Laser laparoscopic management of large endometriomas, *Fertil. Steril.*, 55, 692–695, 1991.
81. Fayez, J. A. and Vogel, M. F., Comparison of different treatment methods of endometriomas by laparoscopy, *Obstet. Gynecol.*, 78, 660–665, 1991.
82. Sutton, C. J. G., Ewen, S. P., Whitelaw, N., and Haines, P., Prospective, randomized, double-blind, controlled trial of laser laparoscopy in the treatment of pelvic pain associated with minimal, mild, and moderate endometriosis, *Fertil. Steril.*, 62, 696–700, 1994.
83. Candiani, G. B., Vercellini, P., Fedele, L., Colombo, A., and Candiani, M., Mild endometriosis and infertility: a critical review of epidemiologic data, diagnostic pitfalls, and classification limits, *Obstet. Gynecol. Surv.*, 46, 374, 1991.
84. Marcoux, S., Maheux, R., and Berube, S., Laparoscopic surgery in infertile women with minimal or mild endometriosis. Canadian Collaborative Group on Endometriosis, *N. Engl. J. Med.*, 337(4), 217–222, 1997.
85. Tulandi, T. and Mouchawar, M., Treatment-dependent and treatment-independent pregnancy in women with minimal and mild endometriosis, *Fertil. Steril.*, 56, 790–791, 1991.
86. Fayez, J. A., Collazo, L. M., Vernon, C. et al., Comparison of different modalities of treatment for minimal and mild endometriosis, *Am. J. Obstet. Gynecol.*, 159, 927–932, 1988.
87. Nowroozi, K., Chase, J. S., Check, J. H. et al., The importance of laparoscopic coagulation of mild endometriosis in infertile women, *Int. J. Fertil.*, 32, 442–444, 1987.

88. Adamson, G. D., Lu, J., and Subak, L. L., Laparoscopic CO_2 laser vaporization of endometriosis compared with traditional treatments, *Fertil. Steril.*, 50, 704–710, 1988.
89. Smith, S. K., Endometriosis and infertility: pathogenesis and work-up, in *Female Infertility Therapy Current Practice*, Shoham, Z., Howles, C. M., and Jacobs, H. S., Eds., Martin Dunitz Ltd., London, United Kingdom, 1999, 355–362.
90. Metzger, D. A., Treatment of infertility associated with endometriosis, in *Endometriosis: Advanced Management and Surgical Techniques*, Nezhat, C. R. et al., Eds., Springer-Verlag, New York, 1995, 245–255.
91. Metzger, D. A., Scott, L., Nulsen, J. C. et al., Optimal use of human menopausal gonadotropin (hMG) superovulation combined with intrauterine insemination (IUI) as an adjunct to conservative laparoscopic surgery for the treatment of infertility associated with endometriosis, *Am. Assoc. Gynecol. Laparoscopists, 20th Ann Meet., Las Vegas, N. V., November 13–17, 1991.*
92. Jacobs, S. L., Metzger, D. A., Dodson, W. C., and Haney, A. F., Effect of age on response to human menopausal gonadotropin stimulation, *J. Clin. Endocrinol. Metab.*, 71, 1525–1530, 1990.
93. Matson, P. L. and Yovick, J. L., The treatment of infertility associated with endometriosis by *in vitro* fertilization, *Fertil. Steril.*, 46, 432–434, 1986.
94. Yovick, J. L., Matson, P. L., Richardson, P. A., and Hilliard, C., Hormonal profiles and embryo quality in women with severe endometriosis treated by *in vitro* fertilization and embryo transfer, *Fertil. Steril.*, 50, 308–313, 1988.
95. Chillik, C. F., Acosta, A. A., Garcia, J. E. et al., The role of *in vitro* fertilization in infertile patients with endometriosis, *Fertil. Steril.*, 44, 56–61, 1985.
96. Oehninger, S. and Rosenwaks, A., *In vitro* fertilization and embryo transfer: an established and successful therapy for endometriosis, *Prog. Clin. Biol. Res.*, 323, 319–335, 1990.
97. Damewood, M. D. and Rock, J. A., Treatment independent pregnancy with operative laparoscopy for endometriosis in an *in vitro* fertilization program, *Fertil. Steril.*, 50, 463–465, 1988.
98. March, C. M., Hysteroscopy and the uterine factor in infertility, in *Mishell's Textbook of Infertility, Contraception, and Reproductive Endocrinology*, 4th ed., Lobo, R. A., Mishell, D. R., Jr., Paulson, R. J., and Shoupe, D., Eds., Blackwell Science, Inc., Malden, MA, 1997, 580–603.
99. Wallach, E. E., Myomectomy, in *TeLinde's Operative Gynecology*, 7th ed., Thompson, J. D. and Rock, J. A., Eds., Lippincott, Philadelphia, PA, 1992, 647–62.
100. Verkauf, B. S., Myomectomy for fertility enhancement and preservation, *Fertil. Steril.*, 58, 1–15, 1992.
101. Katz, V. L., Dotters, D. J., and Droegemueller, W., Complications of uterine leiomyomas in pregnancy, *Obstet. Gynecol.*, 73, 593–596, 1989.
102. Lanouette, J. M. and Diamond, M. P., Pregnancy in women with uterine myoma uteri, *Infertil. Reprod. Med. N. Am.*, 7, 19–32, 1996.
103. Excoustos, C. and Rosati, P., Ultrasound diagnosis of uterine myomas and complications in pregnancy, *Obstet. Gynecol.*, 82, 97–101, 1993.
104. Vollenhoven, B. J., Lawrence, A. S., and Hely, D. L., Uterine fibroids: a clinical review, *Br. J. Obstet. Gynecol.*, 97, 285–298, 1990.
105. Deligdish, L. and Lowenthal, M., Endometrial changes associated with myomata of the uterus, *J. Clin. Pathol.*, 23, 676–680, 1970.
106. Settladge, D. S. F., Motoshima, M., and Tredway, D. R., Sperm transport from the external os to the fallopian tubes in women: a time and quantitation study, *Fertil. Steril.*, 24, 655–658, 1972.

107. Iosif, C. S. and Akerland, M., Fibromyomas and uterine activity, *Acta Obstet. Gynecol. Scand.*, 62, 165–167, 1983.
108. Goldzieher, J. W., Maqueo, M., Ricand, L. et al., Induction of degenerative changes in uterine myomas by high-dose progestin therapy, *Am. J. Obstet. Gynecol.*, 96, 1078–1087, 1966.
109. Murphy, A. A., Kettel, L. M., Morales, A. J. et al., Regression of uterine leiomyomata in response to the antiprogesterone RU486, *J. Clin. Endocrinol. Metab.*, 76, 513–517, 1993.
110. Letterie, G. S., Shawker, T. H., Coddington, C. C. et al., Efficacy of a gonadotropin-releasing hormone agonist in the treatment of uterine leiomyomata: long term follow-up, *Fertil. Steril.*, 51, 951–956, 1989.
111. Friedman, A. J., Rein, M. S., Harrison-Atlas, D. et al., A randomized, placebo-controlled, double blind study evaluating leuprolide acetate depot treatment before myomectomy, *Fertil. Steril.*, 52, 728–733, 1989.
112. Atlee, W. L., Case of a successful extirpation of a fibrous tumor of the peritoneal surface of the uterus by the large peritoneal section, *Am. J. Med. Sci.*, 9, 309–334, 1844.
113. Semm, K. and Mettler, L., New methods of pelviscopy for myomectomy, ovariectomy, tubectomy and adnexectomy, *Endoscopy*, 11, 85–93, 1979.
114. Nezhat, C., Nezhat, F., Silfen, S. L. et al., Laparoscopic myomectomy, *Int. J. Fertil.*, 36, 275–280, 1991.
115. Daniell, J. F. and Guerly, L. D., Laparoscopic treatment of clinically significant symptomatic uterine fibroids, *J. Gynecol. Surg.*, 7, 37–40, 1991.
116. Hasson, H. M., Rotman, C., Rana, N. et al., Laparoscopic myomectomy, *Obstet. Gynecol.*, 80, 884–888, 1992.
117. Dubuisson, J. B., Chapron, C., Mouly, M. et al., Laparoscopic myomectomy, *Gynaecol. Endosc.*, 2, 171–173, 1993.
118. Darai, E., Dechaud, H., Benifla, J.-L., Renolleau, C., Panel, P., and Madelenat, P., Fertility after laparoscopic myomectomy: preliminary results, *Hum. Reprod.*, 12, 1931–1934, 1997.
119. Berkeley, A. S., De Cherney, A. H., and Polan, M. L., Abdominal myomectomy and subsequent fertility, *Surg. Gynecol. Obstet.*, 156, 319–322, 1983.
120. Dubuisson, J. B., Chapron, C., Chavet, X. et al., Fertility after laparoscopic myomectomy of large intramural myomas: preliminary results, *Hum. Reprod.*, 11, 518–522, 1996.
121. Buttram, V. C. and Reiter, R. C., Uterine leiomyomata: etiology, symptomatology and management, *Fertil. Steril.*, 36, 433–435, 1981.
122. Goldenberg, M., Sivan, E., Sharabi, Z., Bider, D., Rabinovici, J., and Seidman, D., Outcome of hysteroscopic resection of submucous myomas for infertility, *Fertil. Steril.*, 64, 714–716, 1995.
123. Ubaldi, F., Tournaye, H., Camus, M., Van der Pas, H., Gepts, E., and Devroey, P., Fertility after hysteroscopic myomectomy, *Hum. Reprod.*, 1, 81–90, 1995.
124. Eldar-Geva, T., Meagher, S., Healy, D. L., MacLachlan, V., Breheny, S., and Wood, C., Effect of intramural, subserosal, and submucosal uterine fibroids on the outcome of assisted reproductive technology treatment, *Fertil. Steril.*, 70, 687–691, 1998.
125. Ramzy, A. M., Sattar, M., Amin, Y., Mansour, R. T., Serour, G. I., and Aboulghar, M. A., Uterine myomata and outcome of assisted reproduction, *Hum. Reprod.*, 13, 198–202, 1998.
126. Asherman, J. G., Amenorrhoea traumatica (atretica), *J. Obstet. Gynaecol.*, 55, 23–30, 1948.

127. Schlaff, W. D. and Hurst, B. S., Preoperative sonographic measurement of endometrial pattern predicts outcome of surgical repair in patients with severe Asherman's syndrome, *Fertil. Steril.*, 63, 410–413, 1995.

128. Schenker, J. G. and Margalioth, E. J., Intrauterine adhesions: an updated appraisal, *Fertil. Steril.*, 37, 593–610, 1982.

129. Shaffer, W., Role of uterine adhesions in the cause of multiple pregnancy losses, *Clin. Obstet. Gynecol.*, 29, 912–924, 1986.

130. Yaffe, H., Ron, M., and Polishuk, W. Z., Amenorrhea, hypomenorrhea and uterine fibrosis, *Am. J. Obstet. Gynecol.*, 130, 599–601, 1978.

131. Westendorp, I. C. D., Ankum, W. M., Mol, B. W. J., and Vonk, J., Prevalence of Asherman's syndrome after secondary removal of placental remnants or a repeat curettage for incomplete abortion, *Hum. Reprod.*, 13, 3347–3350, 1998.

132. Fayez, J. A., Mutie, G., and Schneider, P. J., The diagnostic value of hysterosalpingography and hysteroscopy in infertility investigation, *Am. J. Obstet. Gynecol.*, 156, 558–560, 1987.

133. Siegler, A. M. and Kontopoulos, V. G., Lysis of intrauterine adhesions under hysteroscopic control, *J. Reprod. Med.*, 26, 372–374, 1981.

134. McComb, P. F. and Wagner, B. L., Simplified therapy for Asherman's syndrome, *Fertil. Steril.*, 68, 1047–1050, 1997.

135. Wider, J. A. and Marshall, J. R., Hysterotomy and insertion of an intrauterine device for endometrial sclerosis: importance of long-term follow-up, *Fertil. Steril.*, 21, 240–243, 1970.

136. March, C. M. and Israel, R., Intrauterine adhesions secondary to elective abortion: hysteroscopic diagnosis and management, *Obstet. Gynecol.*, 48, 422–424, 1976.

137. Neuwirth, R. S., Hussein, A. R., Schiffman, B. M. et al., Hysteroscopic resection of intrauterine scars using a new technique, *Obstet. Gynecol.*, 60, 111–113, 1982.

138. Louros, N. C., Damezis, J. M., and Pontifix, G., Use of intrauterine devices in the treatment of intrauterine adhesions, *Fertil. Steril.*, 19, 509–528, 1968.

139. March, C. M. and Israel, R., Gestational outcome following hysteroscopic lysis of adhesions, *Fertil. Steril.*, 36, 455–459, 1981.

140. Valle, R. F. and Sciarra, J. J., Intrauterine adhesions: hysteroscopic diagnosis, classification, treatment, and reproductive outcome, *Am. J. Obstet. Gynecol.*, 158, 1459–1470, 1988.

141. Hatch, K. D. and Fu, Y. S., Cervical and vaginal cancer, in *Novak's Gynecology*, 12th ed., Berek, J. S. et al., Eds., Williams & Wilkins, Baltimore, MD, 32, 1111–1153, 1996.

142. Smith, O. W., Diethylstilbestrol in the prevention and treatment of complications of pregnancy, *Am. J. Obstet. Gynecol.*, 56, 821–834, 1948.

143. Dieckmann, W. J., Davis, M. E., Rynkiewicz, L. M., and Pottinger, R. E., Does the administration of diethylstilbestrol during pregnancy have therapeutic value?, *Am. J. Obstet. Gynecol.*, 66, 1062–1081, 1953.

144. Kaufman, R. H., Adam, E., Binder, G. L. et al., Upper genital tract changes and pregnancy outcome in offspring exposed *in utero* to diethylstilbestrol, *Am. J. Obstet. Gynecol.*, 137, 299–308, 1980.

145. DeCherney, A. H., Cholst, I., and Naftolin, F., Structure and function of the fallopian tubes following exposure to diethylstilbestrol (DES) during gestation, *Fertil. Steril.*, 36, 741, 1981.

146. Stillman, R. J., *In utero* exposure to diethylstilbestrol: adverse effects on the reproductive tract and reproductive performance of male and female offspring, *Am. J. Obstet. Gynecol.*, 142, 905–921, 1982.

147. Mottla, G. L. and Stillman, R. J., Considering the role of assisted reproduction in infertile patients exposed *in utero* to diethylstilbestrol, *Assist. Reprod. Rev.*, 2, 173–183, 1992.

148. Barnes, A. B., Colton, T., Gundersen, J., Noller, K. L., Tilley, B. C., Strama, T., Townsend, D. E., Hatab, P., and O'Brien, P. C., Fertility and outcome of pregnancy in women exposed *in utero* to diethylstilbestrol, *N. Engl. J. Med.*, 302, 609, 1980.

149. Herbst, A. L., Ulfelder, H., and Poskanzer, D. C., Adenocarcinoma of the vagina: association of maternal stilbestrol therapy with tumor appearance in young women, *N. Engl. J. Med.*, 284, 878, 1971.

150. Senekjian, E. K., Potkul, R. K., Frey, K. et al., Infertility among daughters either exposed or not exposed to diethylstilbestrol, *Am. J. Obstet. Gynecol.*, 158, 493, 1988.

151. Kaufman, R. H., Adam, E., Noller, K. et al., Upper genital tract changes and infertility in diethylstilbestrol-exposed women, *Am. J. Obstet. Gynecol.*, 154, 1352, 1986.

152. Karande, V. C., Lester, R. G., Muasher, S. J., Jones, D. L., Acosta, A. A., and Jones, H. W., Jr., Are implantation and pregnancy outcome impaired in diethylstilbestrol-exposed women after *in vitro* fertilization and embryo transfer?, *Fertil. Steril.*, 54, 287–291, 1990.

153. Salat Baroux, J., Recurrent spontaneous abortion, *Reprod. Nutr. Dev.*, 28, 1555–68, 1988.

154. Stirrat, G. M., Recurrent miscarriage 1: definitions and epidemiology, *Lancet*, 336, 673–75, 1990.

155. Stephenson, M. D., Frequency of factors associated with habitual abortion in 197 couples, *Fertil. Steril.*, 66, 24–9, 1996.

156. Goldstein, P., Berrier, J., Rosen, S., Sacks, H. S., and Chalmers, T. C., A meta-analysis of randomized control trials of progestational agents in pregnancy, *Obstet. Gynecol.*, 96, 25–274, 1989.

157. Balen, A. H., Tan, S. L., and Jacobs, H. S., Hypersecretion of luteinizing hormone: A significant cause of infertility and miscarriage, *Br. J. Obstet. Gynecol.*, 100, 1082–9, 1993.

158. Hatasaka, H. H., Recurrent miscarriages: epidemiologic factors, definitions, and incidence, *Clin. Obstet. Gynecol.*, 37, 625–634, 1994.

159. Diedrich, U., Hansmann, I., Janke, D. et al., Chromosome antibodies in 136 couples with a history of recurrent abortions, *Human Genet.*, 65, 48–52, 1983.

160. Stray-Pedersen, B. and Lorentzen-Stry, A., Uterine toxoplasma infections and repeated abortion, *Am. J. Obstet. Gynecol.*, 128, 716–721, 1977.

161. Branch, D. W., Immunologic disease and fetal death, *Clin. Obstet. Gynecol.*, 30, 295–311, 1987.

162. Hill, J., Sporadic and recurrent spontaneous abortion, *Curr. Probl. Obstet. Gynecol. Fertil.*, XVII, 4, 113–164, 1994.

163. Correras, L. O., Vermylen, J., Spitz, B. et al., Lupus anticoagulant and inhibition of prostacyclin formation in patients with repeated abortion, intrauterine growth retardation and intrauterine death, *Br. J. Obstet. Gynecol.*, 88, 890, 1981.

164. Coriou, R., Tolelen, G., Soria, C. et al., Inhibition of protein C activation by endothelial cells in the presence of lupus anticoagulant, *N. Engl. J. Med.*, 314, 1193, 1986.

165. Lyden, T. W., Ng, A. K., and Rote, N. J., Modulation of phosphatidyl-serine epitope expression on Be Wo cells during forskolin treatment, *Am. J. Reprod. Immunol.*, 27, 24, 1992.

166. Silver, R. M. and Branch, D. W., Recurrent miscarriage: Autoimmune considerations, *Clin. Obstet. Gynecol.*, 37, 745–760, 1994.

167. Stagnaro-Green, A., Roman, S. H., Cobin, R. H., El-Horazy, E., Alvarez-Marfany, M., and Davies, T. F., Detection of at-risk pregnancy by means of highly sensitive assays for thyroid autoantibodies, *JAMA*, 264, 1422–5, 1990.

168. Scott, J. A. and Branch, D. W., Potential alloimmune factors and immunotherapy in recurrent miscarriage, *Clin. Obstet. Gynecol.*, 37, 761–67, 1994.

169. Aoki, K., Kajiura S., and Matsumoto, Y., Preconceptional natural-killer cell activity as a predictor of miscarriage, *Lancet*, 345, 1340–42, 1995.

170. Higuchi, K., Aoki, K., Kimbara, T., Hosoi, N., Yamamato, T., and Okada, H., Suppression of natural killer cell activity by monocytes following immunotherapy for recurrent spontaneous aborters, *Am. J. Reprod. Immunol.*, 33, 221–27, 1995.

171. Scott, R. J., Adler, R. R., Mack, R. et al., Peripheral natural killer (NK) cell levels and other peripheral lymphocyte subsets (reproductive immunophenotype) do not prognosticate IVF implantation rates, pregnancy rates, or pregnancy outcome, *Fertil. Steril.*, (Abst) 0–54, 521, (suppl) 1998.

172. Hill, J. A., Polyer, K., Harlow, B., and Anderson, D. J., Evidence of embryo and trophoblast-toxic cellular immune response(s) in women with recurrent spontaneous abortion, *Am. J. Obstet. Gynecol.*, 166, 1044–52, 1992.

173. Branch, D. W., Silver, R., Pierangeli, S., Van Leevwen, I., and Harris, E. N., Antiphospholipid antibodies other than lupus anticoagulant and anticardiolipin antibodies in women with recurrent pregnancy loss, fertile controls, and antiphospholipid syndrome, *Obstet. Gynecol.*, 89, 549–55, 1997.

174. Quinn, P. A. et al., Efficacy of antibiotic therapy in preventing spontaneous pregnancy loss among couples colonized with genital mycoplasmas, *Am. J. Obstet. Gynecol.*, 145, 239, 1983.

175. Kutteh, W. H., Antiphospholipid antibody associated recurrent pregnancy loss: treatment with heparin and low-dose aspirin is superior to low dose aspirin alone, *Am. J. Obstet. Gynecol.*, 174, 1584–9, 1996.

176. Coulam, C. B., Clark, D. A., Collins, J. et al., Worldwide collaborative observational study and meta-analysis on allogenic leukocyte immunotherapy for recurrent abortion, *Am. J. Reprod. Immunol.*, 32, 55–72, 1994.

177. Hewe, O. and Mueller-Eckhardt, C., Intravenous immune golobulin in recurrent abortion, *Clin. Exp. Immunol.*, 97 (Suppl. 1), 39–42, 1994.

178. Coulam, C. B., Alternative treatment to leukocyte immunization for treatment of recurrent spontaneous abortion. Immunotherapy with intravenous immunoglobulin for treatment of recurrent pregnancy loss: American experience, *Am. J. Reprod. Immunol.*, 32, 286–289, 1994.

179. Sher, G., Feinman, M., Zouves, C. et al., High fecundity rates following *in vitro* fertilizaton and embryo transfer in antiphospholipid antibody seropositive women treated with heparin and aspirin, *Hum. Reprod.*, 9, 2278–2283, 1994.

180. Nip, M., Taylor, P. V., Rutherford, A. J., and Hancock, K. W., Autoantibodies and antisperm antibodies in sera and follicular fluids of infertile patients; relation to reproductive outcome after *in vitro* fertilization, *Hum. Reprod.*, 10, 2564–2569, 1995.

181. Geva, E., Amit, A., Lerner-Geva, L. et al., Autoimmune disorders: another possible cause for *in vitro* fertilization and embryo transfer failure, *Hum. Reprod.*, 10, 2566–63, 1995.

182. Kutteh, W. H., Yetman, D. L., Chantilis, S. J., and Crain, J., Effect of antiphospholipid antibodies in women undergoing *in vitro* fertilization: role of heparin and aspirin, *Hum. Reprod.*, 12, 1171–75, 1997.

183. Crosignani, P. G., Collins, J., Cooke, I. D., Duzfalvsky, E., and Rubin, B., Unexplained infertility, *Hum. Reprod.*, 8, 977, 1993.

184. Collins, J. A., Unexplained infertility: a review of diagnosis, prognosis, treatment efficacy and management, *Int. J. Gynecol. Obstet.*, 39, 267–75, 1992.
185. Klentzeris, L. D., Bulmer, J. N., Trejosiewicz, L. K., Morrison, L., and Cooke, I. D., Beta-1 integrin cell adhesion molecules in the endometrium of fertile and infertile women, *Hum. Reprod.*, 8, 1223–1230, 1993.
186. Klentzeris, L. D., Bulmer, J. N., Warren, M. A., Morrison, L., Li, J. C., and Cooke, I. D., Endometrial lymphoid tissue in the timed endometrial biopsy: morphometric and immunohistochemical aspects, *Am. J. Obstet. Gynecol.*, 167, 667–674, 1992.
187. Blacker, C. M., Ginsburg, K. A., Leach, R. E., Randolph, J., and Moghissi, K. S., Unexplained infertility: evaluation of the luteal phase; results of the National Center for Infertility Research at Michigan, *Fertil. Steril.*, 67, 437–42, 1997.
188. Asch, R., Simerly, C., Ord, T. et al., The stages at which human fertilization arrests; microtubule and chromosome configuration in inseminated oocytes which failed to complete fertilization and development in human, *Mol. Hum. Reprod.*, 10, 1897–1906, 1995.
189. Khorram, O., Hewitson, L., Simerly, C., and Schatten, G., Novel insights into fertilization and its failures, *Assisted Reprod. Rev.*, in press.
190. Zainul Rashid, M. K., Fishel, S. B., Tornton, S., Hall, J. A. et al., The predictive value of the zona-free hamster egg penetration test in relation to *in vitro* fertilization at various insemination concentrations, *Hum. Reprod.*, 13, 624–629, 1998.
191. Navarra, C. S., First, N. L., and Schatten, G., Phenotypic variations among paternal centrosomes expressed within the zygote as disparate microtubule lengths and sperm aster organization: correlation between centrosome activity and developmental success, *Proc. Natl. Acad. Sci. USA*, 93, 5384–5388, 1996.
192. Guzick, D. S., Carson, S. A., Coutifaris, C. et al., Efficacy of superovulation and intrauterine insemination in the treatment of infertility, *N. Engl. J. Med.*, 340, 177–183, 1999.
193. Dodson, W. C., Whitesider, D. B., Hughs, C. L., Easley, H. A., III, and Haney, A. F., Superovulation with intrauterine insemination in the treatment of infertility: a possible alternative to gamete intrafallopian transfer and *in vitro* fertilization, *Fertil. Steril.*, 48, 441, 1987.
194. Debroey, P., Van Steirteghem, A., Mannaerts, B., and Coelingh Bennink, H., First singleton term birth after superovulation with recombinant human follicle stimulating hormone, *Lancet*, 340, 1108, 1992.
195. Milki, A. A., Fisch, J. D., and Behr, B., Two-blastocyst transfer has similar pregnancy rates and a decreased multiple gestation rate compared with three-blastocyst transfer, *Fertil. Steril.*, 72, 225–228, 1999.
196. Gardner, D. K., Schoolcraft, W. B., Wagley, L., Schenker, T., Stevens, J., and Hesla, J., A prospective randomized trial of blastocyst culture and transfer in *in vitro* fertilization, *Hum. Reprod.*, 13, 3434–3440, 1998.

6 Ovarian Stimulation and Ovulation Induction

Victoria M. Maclin

CONTENTS

I. INTRODUCTION

Over the past 20 years, the benefits of ovarian stimulation have transformed the field of reproductive endocrinology as it pertains to the treatment of infertility. While previously considered appropriate only for treatment of anovulation, ovarian stimulation with gonadotropins[1–5] and/or clomiphene citrate[6] for ovulation induction now plays a major role in the management of other disorders affecting fertility such as unexplained infertility,[1,2] endometriosis,[3,4] male factor,[1] and cervical factor infertility.[5] Proposed mechanisms by which ovarian stimulation improves fecundity include normalization of abnormal gonadotropin patterns,[7] improved folliculogenesis,[7] improved endometrial receptivity,[7] increased availability of fertilizable oocytes,[8] increased preovulatory estradiol (E2) levels,[9] and correction of occult ovulatory dysfunction.[10] Ovarian stimulation in combination with intrauterine insemination for the treatment of unexplained infertility, male factor, and minimal/mild endometriosis shows an efficacy three to five times greater than no treatment.[1,3,11] In addition, ovarian stimulation has improved *in vitro* fertilization (IVF) outcomes by enabling the development of multiple embryos and a choice of the best embryos for transfer.[12]

In this chapter, the dynamics of the menstrual cycle will be reviewed with emphasis on ovarian follicular growth and selection. This will serve as a basis for understanding the various approaches to ovarian stimulation and luteal phase support that will be described. The chapter reviews drugs of choice with respect to their mechanisms of action, metabolism, contraindications, side effects, and adverse effects. Several approaches to patient screening will be discussed to help the reader identify the candidates most likely to benefit from ovarian stimulation and the protocol most likely to benefit a particular candidate.

II. OVARIAN FOLLICULAR GROWTH, SELECTION, AND OVULATION

At birth, each ovary contains approximately one million primordial follicles. Through an ongoing process of apoptosis, the majority of primordial follicles become atretic such that by menarche, only 500,000 remain. From menarche until menopause, follicular loss takes place at an average rate of approximately 1000 per month. Indeed, only about 400 follicles actually achieve maturity and ovulation in a reproductive lifetime.[13]

Growth of primordial follicles initiates at random and by unknown factors.[13,14] Furthermore, follicular growth from the primordial through the early antral stage is gonadotropin independent.[13,14] Follicular development from the primordial through the pre-antral stage can take as long as 300 days due to the slow rate of granulosa cell doubling (~250 hours).[15] When primordial follicles enter the growth phase, the oocyte enlarges and the surrounding layer of granulosa cells begins proliferation, thus forming the primary follicle. Transition to the secondary follicle occurs with alignment of stroma cells around the basal lamina and establishment of independent blood supply. Stromal cells then differentiate into theca interna and externa.[13] Follicle stimulating hormone (FSH) and luteinizing hormone (LH) receptors develop on the pre-antral granulosa and theca cells, respectively. When the pre-antral follicle becomes 100 to 200 μm in diameter, follicular fluid accumulates, forming an antral cavity. Antral follicular growth does not become gonadotropin dependent until it reaches a diameter of 2 to 5 mm. Follicles exist within the ovary at various stages of development and may also undergo atresia at any stage.[13]

Ovarian steroid production and follicular maturation are coordinated through a two cell, two-gonadotropin mechanism that is modulated by autocrine and paracrine factors. A cohort of 2 to 5 mm follicles becomes sensitive to gonadotropin stimulation during the FSH rise at the menstrual cycle luteo-follicular shift. FSH up regulates thecal P450c17α mRNA through granulosa-on-theca paracrine signalling[16] via modulators such as inhibin. Inhibin potentiates LH induced thecal androgen production. FSH also induces aromatase activity in the granulosa cells.[16,17] The result is thecal production of androgens, which are aromatized within the granulosa to estrogens. The granulosa cells of these cohort follicles exhibit accelerated mitosis possibly initiated by luteolysis[14] and sustained by the rise in FSH. In the early follicular phase, one follicle attains dominance by acquiring enhanced FSH sensitivity and increased intrafollicular levels of FSH. The mechanism that favors this chosen follicle over others in the cohort is not well understood, but likely is effected by intrafollicular autocrine and paracrine factors. As the dominant follicle grows rapidly, its increased production of inhibin B and estrogen causes decreased pituitary FSH.[13] The other less sensitive cohort follicles undergo mitotic arrest and apoptosis as FSH decreases. Nondominant follicles usually do not attain a diameter of greater than 9 mm. The dominant follicle, on the other hand, progresses to a pre-ovulatory diameter of 18 to 25 mm and produces peak levels of estradiol, which through positive feedback induce an LH surge. This LH surge initiates resumption of meiosis in the oocyte and works in concert with an FSH surge to release the oocyte from its follicular attachments. These gonadotropin surges also stimulate the granulosa and thecal cells to produce plasminogen activators, which ultimately lead to the production of collagenase, which digests the follicular wall. Follicular rupture is followed by release of the oocyte.[17]

III. THE MENSTRUAL CYCLE

The period of gonadotropin dependent follicular growth that leads up to ovulation is referred to as the follicular phase of the menstrual cycle. Estradiol produced during the follicular phase stimulates the uterine endometrium to proliferate. After ovulation, the granulosa and thecal cells of the collapsed dominant follicle transform into the corpus luteum. Accordingly, the quality of corpus luteum development and function is affected by the quality of follicular development. Normal luteal function requires optimal preovulatory follicular development.[17] The corpus luteum produces estradiol and progesterone which coordinate endometrial secretory changes, preparing the endometrium for possible implantation of an early embryo. If implantation does not occur by midluteal phase, the corpus luteum regresses, estradiol and progesterone levels fall, and menstruation ensues with the beginning of the next follicular phase.[17]

IV. THE PHYSIOLOGIC BASIS FOR OVARIAN STIMULATION: THE THRESHOLD AND WINDOW HYPOTHESES

In 1975, McNatty and co-workers reported that intrafollicular FSH levels were higher in dominant follicles than in nondominant or atretic follicles.[18] A few years later, Brown reported that an "FSH threshold" needed to be exceeded to stimulate follicular growth.[19] The range of serum FSH levels consistent with this threshold has been reported to be between 5.7 and 12 IU/L,[20,21] though individual follicular threshold levels may vary depending on follicle size, stage of growth, and dynamic changes of intrafollicular paracrine and autocrine factors.[13] Ovarian stimulation rests on the concept that increased circulating FSH levels sustain the growth of additional cohort follicles by raising their intrafollicular FSH above the critical threshold, thereby rescuing them from atresia. This rescuing of additional follicles from the cohort is referred to as *recruitment*. The size of the recruitable cohort is proportional to the ovarian reserve of follicles.[13]

In the early follicular phase, cohort follicles are morphologically similar, ranging in diameter from 4 to 8 mm.[13,14] The dominant follicle is not selected until day 5. Therefore, ovarian stimulation initiated prior to day 5 overrides dominant follicle selection, resulting in multifollicular recruitment. Both the magnitude and duration of FSH dose determine ongoing multifollicular development. When stimulated follicles reach a diameter of greater than 12 mm, their sensitivity to FSH increases. Accordingly, FSH levels must be maintained above the threshold until the leading follicle reaches a diameter of 12 mm.[20,21] Once this is achieved, the dose should be decreased to avoid excessive stimulation. Conversely, decreasing the dose of FSH before the leading follicle has achieved a diameter of 12 mm may result in arrest and atresia. The "window concept" refers to the duration that suprathreshold levels must be maintained to sustain follicular growth before increased FSH sensitivity enables reduced dosing.[22] Differences in extent of pharmacological manipulation of the threshold and the window depend upon whether one intends to achieve modest numbers of mature follicles (1 to 2) for ovulation induction or to effect controlled ovarian hyperstimulation (10 to 12 mature follicles) for oocyte retrieval in conjunction with *in vitro* fertilization and related techniques. Pharmacological intervention for these dissimilar goals is quite different, as will be evident with review of the various ovarian stimulation protocols.

V. PRELIMINARY PATIENT EVALUATION

All women should undergo a thorough work-up prior to drug therapy. This work-up should include baseline hormonal assessments consisting of day 3 FSH, LH, estradiol, TSH, and prolactin. These assessments serve to (1) screen ovarian reserve, (2) determine status of thyroid function, and (3) rule out one of the more common causes of ovarian dysfunction, hyperprolactinemia. Androgen levels should be measured in women with signs of hyperandrogenemia. Ovulatory status should be known and an assessment of tubal patency should be done. Finally, no woman should be treated with ovarian stimulation before the status of male factor is known. No oocyte can be fertilized without an able sperm cell.

VI. DRUGS COMMONLY USED FOR OVARIAN STIMULATION

Clomiphene citrate, human chorionic gonadotropin, human menopausal gonadotropins (HMG), and subsequent generations of gonadotropins comprise the main medications used for ovarian stimulation. Gonadotropin releasing hormone agonists (GnRHa) are adjuvants to gonadotropin treatment which may enhance control of the ovarian response. Proper use of all of these agents requires an exquisite understanding of their mechanisms of action, contraindications, adverse effects and potential complications.

One issue deserves special mention before detailed discussion of the individual medications. A link between the occurrence of epithelial ovarian cancer and the use of fertility drugs has been suggested[23,24] and supported by several case reports and epidemiological studies.[25–28] However, other evidence suggests that the association between ovarian stimulation and ovarian cancer is not causal.[29] Infertility is an independent risk factor for ovarian cancer, as is nulliparity. Mosgaard et al.[30] reported that nulliparous women have a 1.5 to 2-fold increased risk for ovarian cancer when compared to parous women. In addition, their data demonstrated that infertility without drug therapy increases the risk further. Among both parous and nulliparous women, treatment with fertility drugs did not increase the ovarian cancer risk compared to nontreated infertile women. It appears that fertility medications are an *associated factor* because they are apt to be used by women who may have a pre-existing high risk for ovarian cancer. This also has been confirmed by a recent long term historic-prospective study[31] which found that the incidence of ovarian cancer in women treated with fertility drugs was not different from the rate in those not exposed or in the general population.

A. CLOMIPHENE CITRATE (CLOMID™, SEROPHENE™)

Clomiphene citrate is an antiestrogen with weak estrogenic effects because of its structural similarity to estrogen. It is a racemic mixture of the geometric isomers zuclomiphene and enclomiphene.[12] Its mechanism of action is through its prolonged binding to estrogen receptors. Clomiphene binds estrogen receptors longer than estrogen. In the hypothalmus and pituitary, this prolonged binding decreases the rate of estrogen receptor turnover, creating a false feedback signal suggesting that estrogen levels are low. In response to this feedback signal, the hypothalamus releases more gonadotropin releasing hormone, which in turn causes release of more FSH and LH. FSH and LH stimulate ovarian steroidogenesis, follicle maturation, and ovulation and effect corpus luteum development. Clomiphene citrate indirectly affects ovarian stimulation and ovulation induction by enhancing the hormonal events that normally control the menstrual cycle. Clomiphene citrate is administered orally, metabolized by the liver, and excreted in the feces via biliary elimination. Fifty percent is eliminated within 5 days, but drug may be detectable in the feces for up to 6 weeks.[12]

Indications for use are infertility associated with anovulation, ovulatory ovarian dysfunction, luteal insufficiency, unexplained infertility, male factor infertility, minimal and mild endometriosis, and ovarian stimulation in preparation for oocyte retrieval. Contraindications include impaired liver function, undiagnosed abnormal uterine bleeding, pregnancy, ovarian cysts, uncontrolled thyroid or adrenal dysfunction, intracranial lesion, and hypo- or hypergonadotrophic hypogonadism. The most common adverse effect is hot flushes, occurring in 11% of patients.[32] Ovarian enlargement and abdominal discomfort also occur commonly. Other effects include breast tenderness, nausea, visual changes, headache, depression, vaginal dryness, increased appetite, skin rash, dizziness, nervousness, weight gain, insomnia, polyuria, irritability, and hair loss. The multiple gestation rate is 7 to 8% consisting most often of twins. Ovarian hyperstimulation syndrome (OHSS) occurs rarely (see below). Normal endogenous feedback mechanisms limit excessive ovarian response to clomiphene, making high order multiple gestation (triplets or more) and ovarian hyperstimulation unlikely.

Clomiphene citrate may have an antiestrogenic effect on the endometrium, resulting in a luteal phase defect, implantation failure, and early pregnancy loss.[12] Bonhoff and co-workers found a high incidence of irregular endometrial development in midluteal phase endometrial biopsies of women treated with clomiphene. These irregularities include decreased glandular height and number.[33] This may explain the ultrasound findings of thin endometrial thickness with homogenous pattern in some women after clomiphene treatment.[34] There is no increased risk of congenital abnormalities with clomiphene use.[12]

B. HUMAN MENOPAUSAL GONADOTROPINS
(HMG; PERGONAL™, HUMAGON™, REPRONEX™)

Human menopausal gonadotropins are derived from the urine of postmenopausal women. This urine is passed over a Sepharose column and then high and low molecular weight impurities are removed via chromatography. The eluate consists of 3% FSH and LH and 97% nonspecific urinary proteins.[12] HMG is biologically standardized for 1:1 FSH and LH activities as per the 2nd International Reference Preparation for Human Menopausal Gonadotropins. Because the LH bioactivity in normal postmenopausal urine is usually one third that of FSH, the 1:1 standard is often achieved by the addition of human chorionic gonadotropin (HCG)[35] which is structurally and biologically similar to LH. (HCG is purified from the urine of pregnant women.) HMG's mechanism of action is direct stimulation of the granulosa and theca by binding to FSH and LH receptors. This results in follicular growth, maturation, and steroidogenesis.

HMG is given by intramuscular (IM) injection. It is indicated for ovarian stimulation in women with tubal patency and clomiphene resistant anovulation, poor endometrial response to clomiphene, hypogonadotrophic hypogonadism, infertility related to ovulatory dysfunction, unexplained infertility, male factor, cervical factor, endometriosis, and ovarian stimulation in preparation for oocyte retrieval. Treatment with HMG usually results only in follicular growth and maturation. Ovulation is usually induced by the administration of HCG (also given by IM injection) at the end of HMG treatment. Contraindications are hypergonadotrophic hypogonadism, overt thyroid or adrenal dysfunction, pituitary tumor, abnormal uterine bleeding of undetermined etiology, ovarian cysts unrelated to polycystic ovarian disease, and pregnancy. The most salient potential adverse effects are OHSS, pulmonary and vascular complications (related or unrelated to OHSS), and multiple gestation. Other potential adverse effects include hemoperitoneum, adnexal torsion, abdominal pain, ovarian enlargement, hypersensitivity, nausea, vomiting, diarrhea, bloating, dizziness, and tachycardia.[35]

OHSS is characterized by bilateral ovarian enlargement which may be accompanied by peritoneal irritation with ascites, hemoconcentration, electrolyte imbalance, oliguria, pleural and/or pericardial effusion, and hypercoagulability. OHSS falls into three categories, mild, moderate, and severe. Mild OHSS is characterized by estradiol levels exceeding 2000 pg/ml, abdominal discomfort, and ovarian enlargement ≤5 cm in diameter. This classification is of limited clinical value because its incidence is hard to quantify. Most patients stimulated respond with ovarian enlargement and some abdominal discomfort without becoming debilitated. Moderate OHSS is characterized by increased abdominal discomfort with nausea, vomiting, and/or diarrhea. Weight gain and ovarian enlargement up to 12 cm can also accompany this. This occurs in 6% of HMG treated patients. Severe OHSS is characterized by ascites, electrolyte imbalance, hypovolemia, hemoconcentration, increased blood viscosity, and hypercoagulability. As a result of the latter, thromboembolic phenomena can occur. Pleural and pericardial effusion also may occur. Ovarian enlargement is >12 cm. This occurs in 2 to 3% of HMG treated patients. A subgroup of severe OHSS patients have what has been described as "critical

OHSS." This can include in addition to severe ascites, critical conditions such as adult respiratory distress syndrome (ARDS), acute renal failure, leukocytosis > 25,000, and thromboembolism.[36]

The pathogenesis of OHSS relates to vasoactive factors that enhance arteriolar dilatation and increase capillary permeability. The renin-angiotensin system,[37,38] prostaglandins,[39] and histamine[40] have been proposed as pathogenic factors, but their causal role has been disputed.[41-43] Increasing evidence suggests that the salient vasoactive factor of systemic origin may be vascular endothelial growth factor (VEGF).[44-47]

Multiple gestation occurs in 20% of all patients treated with HMG. Overall, 80% of pregnancies are single gestations, 15% are twins, and 5% are triplets or more. There is no increased risk of congenital abnormalities after treatment with HMG or any of the subsequent generation gonadotropins.[35]

Management of HMG therapy requires an exquisite understanding of its narrow therapeutic window. Serum estradiol and sonographic measurement of ovarian size and follicular diameters should be followed closely to ensure appropriate dose adjustment so that the risks of ovarian hyperstimulation and multiple gestation are minimized. The novice is strongly encouraged to defer candidates for this therapy to those with special expertise.

C. Urofollitropin (Purified FSH; Metrodin™)

Urofollitropin is a second-generation urinary gonadotropin. LH and high and low molecular weight impurities are removed from postmenopausal urine by a process involving immunochromatography. One ampule of the final product contains FSH 75 IU and LH 1 IU. However, only 2% of the final protein content is FSH. The other 98% contains unspecified urinary proteins. Mechanism of action, indications for use, dosage, administration, adverse effects, contraindications, and risks are the same as for HMG. This drug was intended to more appropriately treat patients with polycystic ovarian disease. Because of the high levels of LH in this group of patients, it was believed that better quality of response with less hyperstimulation would result. However, clinical studies in these patients have demonstrated that purified FSH does not improve ovulation rates[48] and does not reduce OHSS[48,49] when compared to comparable HMG dosing regimens.[12] Purified FSH has been replaced by the third-generation urinary gonadotropin, highly purified follicle stimulating hormone(FSH-HP).

D. Highly Purified Follicle Stimulating Hormone (FSH-HP; Fertinex™, Metrodin-HP™)

Menotropins pass over an immunoaffinity column with monoclonal antibodies to FSH. FSH is retained on the column. The FSH is then eluted from the column in a highly basic solution and crystallized. FSH comprises 90% of the protein of the final product. The mechanism of action, indications for use, dosing, adverse effects, contraindications, and risks are the same as for HMG and purified FSH. Its main advantage is that it can be administered subcutaneously rather than IM because of its purity. FSH-HP will likely be replaced by the fourth-generation gonadotropin, recombinant FSH.[50]

E. RECOMBINANT HUMAN FSH (rhFSH; FOLLISTIM™, GONAL-F™)

Recombinant FSH is produced using recombinant DNA technology. FSH must be glycosylated for biological activity. This glycosylation can only be done correctly by a mammalian cell, so clinicians use Chinese hamster ovary (CHO) cell to produce rhFSH. The CHO cell is transfected with a vector carrying the genes coding for the alpha and beta subunits of FSH.[51] Through a complex process, the properly glycosylated FSH is collected from the cells and highly purified. The resulting product has a specific activity > 10,000 IU FSH/mg protein.[52] rhFSH has no LH activity.

Mechanism of action, indications for use (with the exception of LH deficient women), dosing, adverse effects, contraindications, and risks are similar to those of HMG, purified FSH, and FSH-HP. Advantages of rhFSH are route of administration,[53] bioactivity superior to that of urinary gonadotropins,[53] high availability and batch to batch consistency previously impossible with urinary products.[52,53]

F. HUMAN CHORIONIC GONADOTROPIN (HCG; PROFASI™, PREGNYL™)

The human placenta produces HCG. It is excreted in large quantities in the urine of pregnant women from which it is processed for commercial use.[12,54] Mechanism of action is through binding of LH receptors. HCG has biologic and structural similarity to LH and may be used to simulate the LH surge. It is indicated for induction of ovulation at the end of gonadotropin stimulated follicular growth and maturation. It also is indicated for luteal phase support. HCG is given by intramuscular injection and is relatively contraindicated in patients with seizure disorder, migraine headaches, asthma, cardiac and renal disease because it may cause fluid retention. HCG has a longer half-life than LH (>24 hours vs. 1 hour, respectively) and therefore may cause a more exaggerated stimulation of corpus luteum activity than LH.[12] Higher luteal levels of estradiol and progesterone may result. Adverse effects include headache, irritabilty, depression, fatigue, edema, breast tenderness, pain at the injection site, and exacerbation of OHSS.[54]

G. GONADOTROPIN RELEASING HORMONE AGONISTS (GNRHA; LUPRON™, LUPRON-DEPOT™, SYNAREL™)

Gonadotropin releasing hormone is a 10 amino acid peptide hormone. A D-amino acid substitution at position 6 with an ethylamide group instead of the C-terminal glycinamide residue leads to increased potency and biological activity. GnRHa also occurs with substitutions at both positions 6 and 10. Administration of a GnRHa causes a biphasic pattern of gonadotropin secretion. Initially, a 48 hour stimulatory phase occurs (also referred to as a flare response) during which FSH and LH are released from the pituitary. This is followed by an inhibitory phase, during which the pituitary is desensitized due to GnRH receptor down regulation and intracellular uncoupling. A progressive reduction in gonadotropin synthesis occurs, which is maintained during GnRH administration. The inhibition phase affords increased ability to manipulate the hormonal control of the menstrual cycle. This enhanced cycle control has improved the success of assisted reproduction, affording (1) better timing of ovarian stimulation cycles, (2) synchronization of the follicular cohort with greater homogeneity and improvement of follicular response to stimulation, (3) prevention of endogenous LH surge, (4) decreased cycle cancellation, (5) improved numbers of harvested oocytes and numbers of total embryos obtained, and (6) improved implantation rate after IVF.[55]

GnRHa is available in short-acting forms (which can be given by daily intranasal or subcutaneous administration) and long-acting forms (which can be given by monthly or trimonthly IM injection). GnRHa works in short and long protocols. Long protocols are used when the inhibition phase is desired prior to ovarian stimulation. Long protocols begin either in the midluteal phase or in the follicular phase of the cycle preceding the ovarian stimulation cycle. Short protocols typically are used to take advantage of the flare effect. The endogenous gonadotropin flare response to GnRHa augments ovarian stimulation in women with diminished ovarian responsiveness (see Protocols for the Low Responder). In short protocols, GnRHa is started in the follicular phase concurrently with gonadotropins.

Adverse effects of GnRHa are lowered ovarian sensitivity to gonadotropins and possibly a deleterious effect on oocyte and embryo quality.[55] A higher incidence of diploid oocytes and prematurely condensed chromosomes has been reported suggesting impairment of nuclear and cytoplasmic maturation processes.[56] An increase in triploid embryos also has been observed[57] with a tendency toward more chromosomally abnormal oocytes.

Leuprolide acetate, a GnRH agonist commonly used as an adjuvant to gonadotropin therapy, is in Pregnancy Category X, meaning that it is contraindicated for women who are or may become pregnant while receiving the drug. This is based upon studies done in rabbits that demonstrated a dose-related increase in fetal abnormalities at 1/600 to 1/6 the human dose. Similar studies in rats failed to demonstrate an increase in fetal abnormalities.[58]

VII. ASSESSMENT OF OVARIAN RESERVE: THE KEY TO CHOOSING THE RIGHT STIMULATION PROTOCOL

Reproductive potential is defined as the ability of a woman to conceive in the absence of specific pathophysiologic changes in her reproductive system.[59] A woman's reproductive potential is directly related to her follicular supply and oocyte quality. The age-related decline in follicle number and oocyte quality is referred to as diminished ovarian reserve. Ovarian reserve affects ovarian response to stimulation. Therefore, one must understand each patient's level of ovarian responsiveness in order to select the correct therapeutic regimen. Three categories of response, low, normal, and high, have been defined as they pertain to response to *conventional* controlled ovarian hyperstimulation in preparation for IVF. Low response indicates a peak E2 of ≦500 pg/ml and/or mature follicle number ≦4. This category generally carries poor prognosis with respect to pregnancy outcome either because of low number or poor quality of transferable embryos. Normal response is characterized by a peak E2 of 500 to 2999 pg/ml and mature follicle number ≥ 4 and <15. This category corresponds to the best pregnancy outcome. High response is characterized by peak E2 >3000 pg/ml. The latter category carries a high risk for complications such as severe OHSS and multiple gestation. This response pattern typically appears in patients with polycystic ovarian syndrome, for which the clinical and laboratory signs are easily identified. Distinguishing between low and normal responders can be challenging, particularly among women less than 40 years of age. Fortunately, tests of ovarian reserve assist in predicting ovarian responsiveness so that appropriate therapeutic regimens can be selected.

Several tests of ovarian reserve have been described. These include day 3 FSH with or without day 3 E2, FSH:LH ratio, the GnRH stimulation test, the basal antral follicle count, and the clomiphene citrate challenge test.

The day 3 FSH level and the parameters for its interpretation were first described a decade ago by the Norfolk group.[60] High, moderate, and low responders were characterized by basal FSH levels <15, 15 to 24.9, and ≥ 25 mIU/ml, respectively.[60] FSH was measured by radioimmunoassay (RIA) [Binax, S. Portland, ME (formerly Leeco Diagnostics, Southfield, MI)]. After further analysis of their database, Norfolk later redefined the upper limit of normal as 15 mIU/ml by the same RIA, considering an FSH <15 mIU/ml normal and >15 mIU/ml indicative of diminished ovarian reserve (J. Ramey, personal communication). With the advent of widespread use of the immunometric assay (MEIA; Abbott Laboratories, IL) for FSH and LH, the Norfolk investigators sought to compare the Binax RIA to the Abbott MEIA assay. They found that an FSH value of 9.5 mIU/ml by MEIA corresponds to the 15 mIU/ml value by Leeco RIA.[61] As a result of this work, basal FSH ≥ 10 mIU/ml by MEIA suggests diminished ovarian reserve.

Basal FSH is an indirect measure of ovarian reserve as it correlates negatively with basal serum inhibin-B production by the granulosa cells of antral follicles.[62,63] Normal basal FSH levels, on the other hand, can be misleading when they are found in women with greater intercycle FSH variability[64]. Concurrent measurements of basal E2 help to distinguish between normal and low responders with normal basal FSH.[65–67] The upper limit of basal E2 associated with normal response and favorable outcome ranges from 60 to 80 pg/ml.[65–67] Basal E2 levels in excess of this range suggest diminished ovarian reserve regardless of FSH level.

The FSH:LH ratio was described by Mukherjee et al.[68] These investigators associated an FSH:LH ratio of >3.6 with a poor prognosis and contended that the ratio may be more useful than FSH alone since the ratio may increase before an increase in FSH is observed. Unfortunately, the reliability of the ratio might be altered by intercycle variability of basal FSH.

The GnRH stimulation test was first described by Padilla et al.[69] and later modified by Winslow et al.[70] This test utilizes the magnitude of change in E2 from day 2 to day 3 and the pattern of E2 response after a single dose of leuprolide acetate 1 mg on day 2. Winslow et al. contended that the GnRH stimulation test was a more sensitive predictor of response to stimulation than both day 3 FSH and age. They demonstrated that magnitude of change in E2 predicted number of mature oocytes retrieved and pregnancy rate. Pattern of E2 response predicted duration and number of ampules required for stimulation. The authors argued that while this test depended on the pituitary's production of gonadotropins, it was a direct indicator of the ovarian response to gonadotropin stimulation. This is in contrast to basal FSH, which is an indirect indicator of ovarian response. Recently, investigators from the U.K. reported that the E2 response to GnRH stimulation considered simultaneously with basal FSH provided improved prediction of ovarian reserve compared to either assessment alone.[71] However, several limitations to the usefulness of this test remain. The extent to which it may have intercycle variability has not been evaluated, and its predictive value has only been determined in the context of IVF outcome. Furthermore, its applicability to the general infertility population has not been determined.

The basal antral follicle count as determined by transvaginal ultrasound examination on cycle day 2 has been described by two groups of investigators and correlates positively with various measures of outcome after ovarian stimulation. In general, women with less than four or five 2 to 5 mm follicles have poor outcome.[72-74] Chang et al. reported a high IVF cycle cancellation rate (68.8%)[72] and no IVF pregnancies in this group of patients.[72,74] Counts of 5 to 15 correlated with normal response and greater than 15 was associated with high response and increased risk of OHSS.[73] Antral follicle count correlated significantly with day 3 FSH, use of gonadotropins, peak E2 levels, number of dominant follicles, number of oocytes retrieved, number of embryos transferred, and pregnancy rates.[72] As with the GnRH stimulation test, this test of ovarian reserve is considered a direct assessment of ovarian potential. However, its usefulness needs additional verification with larger studies. The influence of intercycle and interobserver variability also needs to be determined, and its applicability to the general infertility population should be evaluated.

The clomiphene citrate challenge test (CCCT) is the most extensively evaluated assessment of ovarian reserve.[59] It is superior to a basal FSH because the clomiphene-stimulated FSH is not hampered by intercycle variability.[75] The physiologic basis for the CCCT is diminished inhibin-B production by granulosa cells of cohort follicles.[63] Women with an exaggerated FSH response to clomiphene stimulation have insufficient inhibin-B to suppress FSH to basal levels. Researchers hypothesize that these follicles, which are fewer, are also of inferior quality by virtue of functionally compromised oocytes and granulosa cells.[63] The CCCT consists of serum FSH levels before (day 3) and after (day 10) taking clomiphene citrate 100 mg on days 5 through 9 of the of the menstrual cycle.[76] Criteria for normal vs. abnormal results vary from study to study, depending upon the particular FSH assay and the normal threshold values in the given population (usually determined by the mean clomiphene-stimulated (day 10) FSH level for normal fertile women + 2 standard deviations).[76] In general, day 10 levels should be comparable to day 3 levels. Elevation of either value above the normal threshold indicates abnormality and predicts diminished ovarian reserve. At University of Nebraska Medical Center, we use the Abbott MEIA to measure FSH. Accordingly, a basal or clomiphene-stimulated FSH ≥ 10 mIU/ml is considered abnormal.

Several authors have reported on the usefulness of the CCCT for predicting prognosis with fertility treatment.[75-78] Navot et al. reported a significantly higher conception rate after fertility treatment (timed intercourse, intrauterine insemination with or without ovulation induction) in women with a normal CCCT (42%) than in women with an abnormal CCCT (5%).[76] Loumaye et al. reported poor response to ovarian stimulation and no pregnancies among women with an abnormal CCCT undergoing IVF.[77] Tanbo et al. reported that clomiphene-stimulated FSH levels (days 9 through 11) correlated better than basal FSH (days 2 through 3) with subsequent response to ovarian stimulation for IVF.[75] They also reported no pregnancies in the abnormal CCCT group. Scott et al. prospectively evaluated the CCCT in the general infertility population.[78] They found that approximately 10% of patients in the general infertility population had an abnormal CCCT. In addition, they found that abnormal results increase with age beginning in the early 30s, and prognosticate decreased long term pregnancy rates. Most interestingly, they found that 52% of patients with abnormal CCCT had unexplained infertility. They recommend routine screening of all women age 30 or older and all women with unexplained infertility. These criteria were later expanded to include women with one ovary and poor response to HMG.[79] The same group of investigators in another study used life table analysis to examine the effects of age and abnormal CCCT on pregnancy rates in a general infertility population.[80] They reported that an abnormal CCCT predicts uniformly poor pregnancy rates, regardless of age. However, patients with a normal CCCT have a significant age-related decline in pregnancy rate. In fact, a normal CCCT has a poor predictive value in women over 40.[59,80] The test is not sensitive to the diminished oocyte quality in these older patients. It seems questionable under these circumstances that diminished granulosa cells go hand in hand with impaired oocytes, since sufficient inhibin-B appears in the granulosa of some older women with normal CCCT and poor pregnancy rates. The possibility exists that the CCCT reflects residual follicle quantity rather than oocyte quality. Lim and Tsakok suggested that oocyte quality played a more significant role in the age-related decline in fertility than oocyte quantity.[81] They reported that diminished oocyte quality with advancing age might be due to an increased incidence of oocyte chromosome degeneration. Theirs is one of many proposed mechanisms of functional deterioration. Different investigators cite other nuclear and cytoplasmic abnormalities underlying the age-related decline in fertility.[57,82–84]

A limitation of the studies evaluating or applying the CCCT is an inherent bias in the methods and outcome measures. Oocyte number, number of embryos transferred, and pregnancy are outcome measures that, in part, depend on the type of stimulation used. In both of the studies of IVF outcome relative to CCCT results, the same conservative stimulation protocols designed for normal responders were used for patients with diminished ovarian reserve. One cannot be surprised that these poor responders did not respond well under these circumstances. Similarly, Scott et al.[80] in their general infertility population study state in materials and methods that abnormal CCCT results did not influence their approach to treatment.[80] Specifically, they wrote, "... therapeutic interventions as indicated for the various diagnoses were not affected by these results or by the patients' participation in this study." Certainly this approach is necessary to minimize confounding variables, but it also alters the implications of the study. What we conclude is that patients with diminished ovarian reserve do not respond well to routine approaches to treatment. But, we cannot state fairly that they will not respond well to any intervention without first submitting them to interventions designed for low responders. Hanoch et al.[85] recently reported that young low responders might be protected from the untoward effects of reduced ovarian response.[85] In women between the ages of 20 and 30 with a peak E2 of 688.3 ± 178.5 after stimulation with a GnRH flare—HMG protocol—a relatively low number of oocytes (5.0 ± 3.7), a low mean number of fertilized oocytes (2.9 ± 2.2), and a clinical pregnancy rate of 19.3% occurred. This suggests that in younger patients with evidence of diminished ovarian reserve, adequate oocyte quality may prevail in spite of decreased follicular quantity. Not surprisingly, a stimulation protocol designed for low responders was utilized in this study.

Ovarian reserve screening should be used as a means of determining appropriate protocols. While some patients with diminished ovarian reserve require nothing short of oocyte donation or adoption, there are others, particularly those under age 40, who deserve the benefit of the doubt. Patients with normal ovarian reserve screening should receive protocols suited to normal responders. Patients with diminished ovarian reserve should receive protocols designed for low responders. High responders should be approached with caution, stimulating them with considerably less medication than the normal responder.

In summary, ovarian reserve screening can improve diagnostic acumen and assist in designing the most appropriate therapeutic regimens for ovarian stimulation. The most useful tests are basal FSH in combination with basal E2 and the clomiphene citrate challenge test (CCCT). Normal values for basal FSH and E2 are <10 mIU/ml (by immunometric assay) and <80 pg/ml, respectively. For the CCCT, the normal value for both basal and stimulated FSH is 10 mIU/ml. FSH or E2 levels exceeding these values are consistent with diminished ovarian reserve. Women less than age 40 with diminished ovarian reserve or over 40 with normal reserve should be treated with protocols designed for low responders (see below). Women over 40 with diminished reserve should consider oocyte donation or adoption. Women with normal ovarian reserve should be treated with protocols designed for normal responders, and high responders should be treated with protocols modified to minimize the risk of OHSS.

VIII. OVARIAN STIMULATION PROTOCOLS

A. Ovulation Induction for Normal Responders

1. Clomiphene Citrate (CC)

The goal of ovarian stimulation for ovulation induction is to produce ≦ 4 mature follicles. In patients never before treated with ovarian stimulation, the first therapeutic choice should be CC. Seventy-five to eighty percent of anovulatory women will ovulate and 50% will conceive after treatment with CC.[86,87] CC has been shown to effectively treat subtle disorders of ovulation in patients with otherwise unexplained infertility.[2,6] Furthermore, retrospective analyses shows CC + intrauterine insemination (IUI) to be the first line of treatment in a cost-effective infertility treatment algorithm.[2,88] This is due to the relatively low cost of the drug, limited requirements for monitoring, and low risk of multiple gestation and other complications. At University of Nebraska Medical Center, we recommend combining CC with IUI regardless of the presence of male factor because the pregnancy rate per initiated cycle is twice that of CC alone.[2] This approach also circumvents the problem of unfavorable cervical mucus often induced with CC. We prescribe human chorionic gonadotropin (HCG) to trigger ovulation to ensure the most precise coordination with a single IUI. While ovulation predictor kits may be useful for timed intercourse in minimally monitored cycles, using them to time IUI is inconvenient and somewhat disruptive to clinic and andrology laboratory schedules. In addition, their use circumvents the advantages of monitoring the response to CC.

Monitoring is aimed at measuring the E2 response to CC as well as the endometrial response. The E2 response reflects the quality of follicular maturation. An E2 level of $\geq$ 250 pg/ml per mature follicle is desired.[89] The endometrial thickness and pattern is evaluated by transvaginal ultrasound (TVUS). Thickness is determined by measuring the greatest antero-posterior endometrial dimension from basalis to basalis.[90] The echogenicity pattern appears either homogenous or trilaminar. A homogenous pattern consists of a single hyperechoic layer. A trilaminar pattern consists of a hypoechoic layer with a central hyperechoic line. An 8 mm endometrial thickness is usually desired, though a thickness as low as 5 mm may be acceptable as long as the pattern is trilaminar.[34,90] Some investigators have shown that a trilaminar pattern is more important than thickness.[34,90–92] A thick ($\geq$ 8 mm) but homogenous endometrium is associated with poor implantation and pregnancy rates.[34,90,91] Impaired endometrial development is a known adverse effect of CC treatment.[3,34,93] In general, a finding of thin, homogenous endometrium in the late follicular phase corresponds to poor pregnancy rates and contraindicates CC treatment.

Protocol: CC/HCG + IUI

1. CC 50 mg by mouth on days 5 through 9 of the menstrual cycle. Monitoring with E2, LH, and transvaginal ultrasound (TVUS) starting 4 days after the last dose of CC. By this time, most patients are within 1 to 2 days of preovulatory follicular development.
2. HCG 5000 to 10000 IU IM should be given when the leading follicle is 20 mm in mean diameter, 24–36 hours prior to a single IUI. If LH surge is detected, IUI should be done the next day. Dosage: 50 to 150* mg
   *(We have seen no improvement in response at doses greater than 150 mg.)

Notes: *Dosage should be increased in increments of 50 mg with consecutive cycles if*

   a. E2 per mature follicle ($\geq$ 20 mm) is less than 250 pg/ml, or
   b. there is no dominant follicle recruitment.

Notes: *Dosage should not be increased in the presence of an adequate follicular response if*

   a. the patient does not conceive, or
   b. the endometrium is poor.

Adequate follicular and endometrial response are the only outcome measures that should effect dosage adjustment. *Dose should not be increased because a patient failed to conceive in a given cycle of treatment.* Failure to conceive during any single treatment cycle in the presence of an adequate follicular and endometrial response is consistent with reasonable probability of conception. Fecundability per cycle after treatment with CC/IUI is 16% at the University of Nebraska Medical Center, but may be as low as 8.3%.[2] Most patients conceive within the first 3 to 6 cycles of treatment. Therefore, treatment should begin with a dose that renders a normal response for a maximum of 6 cycles before it increases to more aggressive protocols. *Dose should not be increased to improve inadequate endometrial response.* Increasing the dose of CC will not improve endometrial quality, particularly if the poor endometrium is associated with adequate estradiol levels. Women with poor endometrial response to clomiphene should be treated with gonadotropins.

2. Clomiphene Citrate plus Human Menopausal Gonadotropin (CC + HMG)

Two benefits result from combining CC and HMG for ovulation induction: (1) it augments inadequate follicular response to CC alone, and (2) it reduces the amount of HMG needed for stimulation. For patients in whom CC enhances follicular recruitment, but fails to sustain follicular growth to maturity, adding HMG at the end of CC may be useful.

Protocol: CC + HMG/HCG + IUI

1. CC 100 to 150 mg by mouth on days 5 through 9 of the menstrual cycle.
2. HMG 75 to 150 IU daily by IM injection starting day 10.
3. Monitoring with serum E2, LH, and TVUS starting on cycle day 12. Daily dosage should be decreased to or maintained at 75 IU daily when the leading follicle is >12 mm in mean diameter.
4. HCG 5000 to 10000 IU should be given when the leading follicle is 20 mm in mean diameter, 24 to 36 hours prior to a single IUI.

Another approach to combining CC and HMG, referred to as the *minimal stimulation* protocol, has been reported by the Mayo group.[94] It will be referred to here as CC + HMGms.

Protocol: CC + HMGms/HCG + IUI

1. CC 100 mg by mouth on cycle days 3 through 7 of the menstrual cycle.
2. A single dose of HMG 150 IU IM is given on cycle day 9.
3. Monitoring with TVUS on cycle day 12 to assess follicle development.
4. HCG 5000 to 10000 IU IM is given when the leading follicle mean diameter is 20 mm. If follicle diameter is not 20 mm on day 12, HCG is given when the diameter is projected to be 20 mm assuming 1 to 2 mm growth per day.

The Mayo group reported that this protocol is as effective as HMG alone. The cited benefits were comparable pregnancy rate to that of HMG as well as decreased medication cost because of reduced requirements for HMG. A contraindication to CC + HMG protocols is poor endometrial response to CC alone. Adding HMG to CC does not prevent the deleterious effect of CC on the endometrium.[91]

3. Urinary Gonadotropins (HMG, Purified FSH, FSH-HP)

Ovulation induction with gonadotropins requires close monitoring because ovarian response is not limited by endogenous feedback mechanisms. Multifollicular growth of high order (>4 follicles) can be limited only by decreasing the dose at the appropriate time. The goal of therapy is to raise the level of FSH just above the threshold necessary to stimulate follicular growth. Once 2 to 4 leading follicles have reached a mean diameter of >12 mm, the dose should be decreased to sustain growth to maturity, assuming that the leading follicles have achieved increased gonadotropin sensitivity. Dose for dose, the different generations of urinary gonadotropins have similar effects and can be used interchangeably.[95] The following protocol for use of HMG will serve for any of the urinary gonadotropins. Once again, these protocols will include IUI. As with CC ovulation induction, fecundability per treatment cycle doubles with addition of IUI.[1,2]

Protocol: HMG/HCG + IUI

1. Baseline TVUS should be done after onset of menses and before initiation of stimulation to measure basal follicle number and size and to rule out residual cysts >12 mm.
2. Start HMG 75 to 150 IU IM on cycle day 3 through 5.
3. Monitoring should begin on the 4th day of stimulation with serial TVUS, serum E2, and LH to measure interval follicular development, magnitude of E2 rise, and basal LH (which can be used comparatively to recognize an LH surge). These assessments should be repeated every 2 to 3 days.
4. Dosage should be adjusted to maintain progressive follicular growth and E2 doubling every other day. Dosage should be decreased when the leading follicle mean diameter is >12 mm.
5. HCG 5000 to 10000 IU IM is given when the leading follicle has a mean diameter of 18 mm, 24 to 36 hours prior to IUI.

4. Recombinant Human FSH

Recombinant human FSH (rhFSH) appears to have greater potency than urinary gonadotropins and therefore greater efficiency in both ovulatory[53,96] and anovulatory women.[97] When using it for ovulation induction and IUI, the same guidelines described above apply for HMG (except that rhFSH may be given by subcutaneous injection), bearing in mind that criteria for decreasing dosage may be met sooner than with HMG. One must assess interval response by day 4 of stimulation to avoid excessive stimulation.

5. Gonadotropin Releasing Hormone Agonists (GnRHa) plus Gonadotropins

GnRHa is a useful adjuvant for ovulation induction in normal responders with premature LH surge. A variety of protocols utilize GnRHa in combination with gonadotropins. Depending on when GnRHa is initiated, one can take advantage of the stimulatory and/or inhibitory phases of gonadotropin secretion. Short GnRHa protocols benefit from the stimulatory phase while long protocols exploit the inhibitory phase. One of the many advantages of long protocols is LH surge prevention in the subsequent stimulation cycle. This enables stimulation to continue until follicles have achieved maturity and meet criteria for HCG administration. The most frequently used long protocol involves initiation of the GnRHa in the midluteal phase of the cycle preceding stimulation. The following protocol may be used with either urinary or recombinant gonadotropin.

Protocol: Long GnRHa + HMG/HCG + IUI

1. Leuprolide acetate 0.5 mg subcutaneous injection is started on day 21 of the cycle preceding the stimulation cycle.
2. After onset of menses, serum estradiol should be less 50 pg/ml to ensure adequate ovarian suppression.
3. Baseline TVUS should demonstrate no residual ovarian cysts >12 mm.
4. On cycle day 3, start HMG 150 IU IM daily.
5. Monitor every 2 to 3 days starting on the 4th day of stimulation (cycle day 6) with TVUS and serum E2.
6. Dosage should be adjusted to maintain progressive follicular growth and E2 rise. (If recombinant FSH is used, E2 levels should not be expected to double during the early and mid follicular phase. E2 levels may not rise significantly until the late follicular phase because of decreased levels of LH. As long as follicular growth is observed, dosage should be maintained.) Dosage should be decreased to 75 IU when the leading follicle mean diameter is >12 mm.
7. HCG 5000 to 10000 IUIM should be administered when the leading follicle is 18 mm in mean diameter, 24 to 36 hours prior to IUI.

B. OVULATION INDUCTION FOR HIGH RESPONDERS

High responders are most predictably women with World Health Organization (WHO) group II anovulation. This group is characterized by evidence of endogenous estrogen activity and a gonadotropin pattern with an elevated LH:FSH ratio. Most of these women have polycystic ovarian syndrome and are clomiphene citrate resistant.[96,97] These patients are difficult to stimulate without inducing multifollicular development and are at higher risk for spontaneous abortion and developing OHSS. Priorities for stimulation protocols include monofollicular development, follicular phase LH level suppression, and OHSS prevention. Three protocols for ovulation induction in the high responder will be described.

1. Monofollicular Development

The first protocol is the Low Dose HMG Step-Up. This protocol works with either urinary or recombinant gonadotropins and is designed to promote monofollicular development.[87,96,97]

Protocol: Low Dose HMG Step-Up/HCG + IUI

1. Baseline TVUS to rule out ovarian cysts.
2. HMG 75 IU IM daily for 7 days.
3. Repeat TVUS, serum E2, and LH on stimulation day 8. If there are no follicles >12 mm, dose is increased by weekly increments of 37.5 IU. When the leading follicle is >12 mm, daily dosage is maintained.
4. HCG 5000 to 10000 IU IM is given when the leading follicle is 18 mm in mean diameter, 24 to 36 hours prior to IUI.

2. High Endogenous LH Suppression

The next protocol is aimed at decreasing follicular phase LH levels, which have been associated with an increased rate of spontaneous abortion.[98–100] GnRHa + HMG ovarian stimulation has been shown to significantly decrease spontaneous abortion rate in women with PCOS when compared to stimulation with HMG alone. Oral contraceptive pills (OCPs) are used in anovulatory women in the cycle preceding stimulation to ensure adequate endometrial withdrawal bleeding prior to stimulation.

Protocol: OCPs + Long GnRHa + HMG/HCG + IUI

1. Oral contraceptive pills for 21 days starting on day 3 of spontaneous or induced menses.
2. Leuprolide acetate 0.5 mg subcutaneously daily starting on OCP day 15 and continued until day 2 of menses.
3. Baseline TVUS to rule out ovarian cysts >12 mm.
4. On day 3 of menses, decrease leuprolide acetate to 0.25 mg and start HMG 75 IU IM daily.
5. Monitor every 2 to 3 days with TVUS and E2.
6. Dose is increased every 5 to 7 days by increments of 75 IU until follicle growth and E2 elevation is observed. When the leading follicle is >12 mm, the dose is maintained.
7. HCG 5000 IU IM is administered when the leading follicle is 18 mm in mean diameter, 24 to 36 hours prior to IUI.

3. OHSS Prevention

OHSS usually results from HCG administration to trigger ovulation in a woman who has been hyperstimulated with gonadotropins. HCG is given to simulate an LH surge. While it is structurally similar to LH, its half-life is longer (>24 hours) than that of LH (60 minutes). Investigators have shown that an LH surge triggered by administration of a GnRHa successfully induces ovulation and without causing OHSS.[101–103]

Protocol: HMG + GnRHa Ovulation Induction + IUI

1. See HMG simulation protocol above.
2. When the leading follicle is 18 mm in mean diameter, administer leuprolide acetate 1 mg, 24–36 hours prior to IUI.

C. OVULATION INDUCTION FOR LOW RESPONDERS

Low responders have diminished quantity or quality of residual follicles, manifested by a smaller recruitable cohort. Optimal follicular recruitment in these women requires higher levels of gonadotropins than in women with normal reserve. Increasing the dose of exogenous gonadotropin seems a likely solution, but high dose gonadotropin therapy beyond a dose of 450 IU (6 ampules) has limited value.[104,105] Protocols that promote synergistic ovarian stimulation by both endogenous and exogenous gonadotropins achieve the best response. Indeed, induced secretion of endogenous gonadotropin may have a more potent affect on recruitment than high dose HMG. The Norfolk group reported that magnitude of change in E2 after HMG/FSH 450 IU was less predictive of ovarian responsiveness than change in E2 after leuprolide acetate 1 mg.[70] They argued that high dose exogenous gonadotropins may be less potent than endogenous gonadotropins and/or that the former fails to provide the threshold levels necessary to express the recruitable cohort maximally. They supported the latter with their finding that FSH and LH levels sixteen hours after IM administration of HMG/FSH 450 IU vs. leuprolide acetate 1 mg are 17 and 16 mIU/ml and 54 and 108 mIU/ml, respectively.[70] The following protocols are effective in low responders because of increased endogenous and/or exogenous gonadotropin activity.

1. GnRHa Flare

GnRHa flare protocols take advantage of the stimulatory phase of GnRHa induced secretion of FSH and LH, while maintaining the benefit of LH surge prevention. These protocols are referred to as short or ultrashort depending on the duration of GnRH administration. In the short protocol, GnRHa begins on day 1 to 3 of the stimulation cycle and continues daily until administration of HCG. In the ultrashort protocol, GnRHa starts on days 1 to 3 of the stimulation cycle and continues for only 3 to 5 days. Ultrashort protocols result in a more profound decrease in LH after discontinuation of GnRHa, perhaps because of decreased endogenous GnRH secretion resulting from ultrashort feedback of GnRHa in the hypothalmus.[106] This decrease in LH is associated with decreased E2 production which may confound interpretation of cycle progress.[106] Interestingly, this decrease in LH is not observed when GnRHa is continued until HCG stimulation. The short protocol will be described below. In order to achieve the best results with this protocol, one must be certain that no residual corpus luteum activity occurs. This can be ascertained by either follicular phase progesterone (P) levels <1 ng/ml or pretreatment with OCPs in the cycle preceding stimulation.

Protocol: Short GnRHa Flare + HMG + HCG + IUI

1. Baseline TVUS to rule out follicular cysts >12 mm.
2. Start leuprolide acetate 0.25 to 1.0 mg subcutaneously on cycle day 2.
3. Start HMG or FSH 150 to 225 IU IM daily on cycle day 3.
4. On the 4th day of stimulation, start monitoring with serial TVUS, E2, and LH levels. Adjust the dose to maintain progressive follicular development and E2 rise.
5. When the leading follicle reaches >12 mm, decrease the dose by one ampule.
6. Administer HCG 5000 to 10000 IU IM when the leading follicle reaches a mean diameter of 18 mm, 24 to 36 hours prior to IUI.

2. Microdose GnRHa Flare

One disadvantage of the short GnRHa flare protocol is untoward rises in circulating LH, testosterone (T), or P levels.[107] While pretreatment with OCPs may eliminate rises in P, rises in LH and T may still remain a problem. Premature luteinization and increased follicular androgen production might adversely impact oocyte maturation and function.[108] The microdose GnRHa flare protocol enhances release of FSH without concomitant elevation of LH and T.[107] This protocol results in higher endogenous FSH release, multifollicular recruitment, and premature LH surge suppression.[107,109] Furthermore, cost of stimulation is decreased by lesser requirements for leuprolide acetate as well as gonadotropins.[109] Schoolcraft et al.[110] reported on the efficacy of a microdose GnRHa flare in combination with HMG/FSH and growth hormone. However, the value of growth hormone has been questioned[111] and is not recommended as an adjuvant for ovulation induction.

Protocol: Microdose GnRHa Flare + HMG + HCG + IUI

1. OCPs for 21 days starting on day 3 of the preceding cycle.
2. Baseline TVUS on day 1 to 2 of post-pill menses.
3. Start leuprolide acetate 50 mcg b.i.d. on day 2 of post-pill menses (cycle day 2).
4. Start HMG 150 to 300 IU IM on cycle day 3.
5. Start monitoring on the 4th day of stimulation with serial TVUS, serum E2, and LH and repeat every 2 to 3 days.
6. Adjust dose of medication according to follicular and E2 response.
7. When the leading follicle is >12 mm, decrease the dose by 75 IU.
8. Administer HCG 5000 to 10000 IU IM when the leading follicle is 18 mm in mean diameter, 24 to 36 hours before IUI.

3. Clomiphene Citrate and Gonadotropins

Clomiphene citrate and HMG (CC + HMG) is an alternative for low responders who do not have a poor endometrial response to CC.

Protocol: CC + HMG + HCG + IUI

1. Baseline TVUS on cycle day 1 to 3.
2. CC 100 mg on days 3 through 7.
3. Start HMG 150 to 300 IU IM daily on cycle day 5.
4. Start monitoring on the 4th day of HMG stimulation with serial serum E2, LH, and TVUS and repeat every 2 to 3 days.
5. Adjust dose of HMG to maintain progressive follicular growth and doubling of E2 every other day.
6. When the leading follicle reaches a mean diameter of >12 mm, decrease the dose of HMG by 75 IU.
7. Administer HCG 5000 to 10000 IU IM when the leading follicle reaches a mean diameter of 18 mm, 24 to 36 hours prior to IUI.

D. CONTROLLED OVARIAN HYPERSTIMULATION FOR NORMAL RESPONDERS

The goal of controlled ovarian hyperstimulation (COH) is to recruit and mature multiple follicles that may yield mature oocytes, without inducing moderate to severe OHSS. In general, a lower limit of 4 and an upper limit of 12 to 14 follicles characterize an acceptable response. Fifteen or greater is considered a high response.[73] Historically, COH was accomplished with combinations of CC and HMG or with HMG alone. As much as 15 to 30% cycle cancellation due to LH surge made these protocols less than ideal.[112] In the mid to late 1980s, stimulation regimens incorporated GnRHa and improved outcomes (see Drugs Commonly Used for Ovarian Stimulation above). The long protocols with midluteal phase vs. follicular phase GnRHa start have been compared in prospective, randomized trials.[113–115] Two of the larger trials found that down regulation occurs more rapidly with the midluteal phase start and corresponds to better pregnancy and live birth rates.[113,114] Others have reported no difference in efficacy with either approach.[115] Currently, the long GnRHa + gonadotropin protocol with GnRHa started in the midluteal phase of the preceding cycle is the most commonly used protocol for COH in normal responders and is presented below.

Protocol: Long GnRHa + HMG/HCG

1. Leuprolide acetate 0.5 mg subcutaneous injection is started on day 21 of the cycle preceding the stimulation cycle.
2. After onset of menses, serum estradiol should be less 50 pg/ml to ensure adequate ovarian suppression.

3. Baseline TVUS should demonstrate no residual ovarian cysts >12 mm.
4. On cycle day 3, start HMG 225 to 300 IU IM daily as a single evening dose. Concurrently, leuprolide acetate should be decreased to 0.25 mg daily and continued until the day of HCG.
5. Monitor every 2 to 3 days starting on the 4th day of stimulation (cycle day 6) with TVUS and serum E2.
6. Dosage should be adjusted to maintain progressive follicular growth and E2 rise. (If recombinant FSH is used, E2 levels should not be expected to double during the early and mid follicular phase. E2 levels may not rise significantly until the late follicular phase because of decreased levels of LH. As long as follicular growth is observed, dosage should be maintained.) Dosage should be decreased by 75 to 150 IU when four leading follicles have a mean diameter of >12 mm.
7. HCG 5000 to 10000 IU IM should be administered when four leading follicles are 18 mm in mean diameter, 36 hours prior to oocyte retrieval.

Researchers have shown interest in the use of long-acting GnRHa (leuprolide acetate depot 3.75 mg, single IM dose lasting 4 weeks). Its usefulness for short term (3 weeks)[116] as well as long term (4 months)[117] down regulation has been evaluated in prospective randomized trials. Long acting GnRHa was found to be associated with more profound ovarian suppression resulting in higher requirements for gonado-tropins. Furthermore, Devreker et al. reported that decreased implantation and preg-nancy rates may occur with long acting formulations due to diminished embryo quality or impaired endometrial receptivity.[116] Fabregues et al. reported no improve-ment in pregnancy rates with long term down regulation.[117]

E. CONTROLLED OVARIAN HYPERSTIMULATION FOR HIGH RESPONDERS

High responders, as discussed previously, are at high risk for OHSS. In addition they may be at higher risk for implantation failure because of a deleterious affect of high E2 levels on endometrial receptivity. Simon et al. reported in a prospective controlled study that an accelerated step down protocol aimed at reducing stimulated E2 levels resulted in a markedly improved pregnancy and implantation rates when compared to a standard step-down protocol (64.2 and 29.3% vs. 24.2 and 8.5%, respectively).[118] The accelerated step-down regimen included down regulation with leuprolide acetate 1 mg started in the midluteal phase of the preceding cycle followed by FSH 300 IU IM on stimulation day 1 followed by 225 IU, 150 IU, 150 IU, and 112.5 IU on stimulation days 2, 3, 4, and 5, respectively. Stimulation until criteria were met for HCG was adjusted on an individual basis according to serum E2 and TVUS. The standard protocol involved GnRHa down regulation with leuprolide acetate starting in the midluteal phase of the cycle preceding stimulation. Stimulation started with FSH/HMG 300 IU on stimulation days 1 and 2, decreasing to 150 IU on days 3, 4, and 5 with individual adjustment thereafter. Peak E2 levels with the standard protocol were >5000 pg/ml while the mean level after accelerated step-down was 1919 ± 477 pg/ml. The cancellation rate was 17.5% with the accelerated step-down because some patients failed to reach threshold before the dose was tapered. This is not surprising considering the wide range of threshold levels for different patients.[19]

1. Modified Step-Down

No correct answer to the controlled ovarian hyperstimulation of high responders exists. This author recommends abiding by the principles of identifying a threshold level to initiate follicular growth, maintaining that level of stimulation until at least 4 follicles are greater than 12 mm, then reducing the dose by increments individually adjusted to sustain growth of at least 4 follicles to a size consistent with maturity. Every women is unique, therefore, individualizing the approach to stimulation, while abiding to the above-mentioned principles, will likely yield the best results. Since these patients are often anovulatory, a protocol using pretreatment with OCPs ensures better down regulation and endometrial withdrawal bleeding prior to stimulation.

Protocol: OCPs + Long GnRHa + FSH + HCG

1. Take OCPs for 21 days starting on day 3 of the preceding cycle.
2. Start leuprolide acetate 0.5 mg subcutaneously daily on OCP day 15 and continue concurrently with OCPs.
3. After onset of menses, baseline TVUS to rule out ovarian cysts >12 mm.
4. Start stimulation on cycle day 3 with FSH 150 to 300 IU IM daily in a single evening dose. Concurrently, leuprolide acetate dose is decreased to 0.25 mg daily and continued until day of HCG.
5. On the 4th day of stimulation, start monitoring with serial serum E2 and TVUS every 2 to 3 days, with adjustment of dose to sustain follicular growth and/or E2 rise.
6. When 4 follicles reach a mean diameter of >12 mm, the dose should be decreased by 75 to 150 IU to continue growth.
7. HCG 5000 IU IM should be administered when at least 4 follicles have a mean diameter of 18 mm, 36 hours prior to oocyte retrieval.

2. Coasting

One cannot always avoid overstimulation with E2 levels greater than 3000 pg/ml before the follicles reach criteria for HCG. In the interest of decreasing morbidity associated with OHSS, coasting has been recommended to troubleshoot the overstimulated response. Tortoriello et al. retrospectively compared high responders treated with and without coasting.[119] Patients with an E2 of >3000 pg/ml at the time of reaching criteria for HCG were given a choice of receiving HCG or withholding HCG while continuing daily GnRHa until E2 levels fell below 3000 pg/ml, at which time they would receive HCG. These investigators found that for patients who achieved a peak E2 of 3000 to 3999 pg/ml, coasting did not adversely affect cycle outcome and did not increase their rate of OHSS. For patients who had E2 >4000 pg/ml, coasting did not prevent OHSS. Those with E2 >4000 pg/ml also had longer coast intervals which might have impacted negatively on implantation.

3. Embryo Cryopreservation with Transfer in a Nonstimulated Cycle

Another option for high responders who achieve peak E2 levels > 3000 pg/ml is to cryopreserve embryos and transfer in a later cycle after hormone replacement.[120] This may not avoid early OHSS induced by the administration of exogenous HCG, but late OHSS exacerbated by pregnancy-induced HCG elevation may be prevented.[121] Endometrial receptivity is better in cycles prepared with hormone replacement than in cycles with COH.[122] Of course, this option is only reasonable if one has access to an embryo cryopreservation program with good pregnancy and livebirth rates per transfer.

F. Controlled Ovarian Stimulation for Low Responders

As described previously, ovarian stimulation protocols for low responders include those that utilize the concept of endogenous and exogenous gonadotropin synergy to render a greater number of mature follicles. The following protocols help mitigate endogenous gonadotropin suppression with down regulation, or increased endogenous gonadotropin secretion.

1. Discontinuous Long GnRHa + HMG/HCG

GnRHa may inhibit ovarian steroidogenesis.[123] In the interest of maximizing endogenous gonadotropin action, suppressive adjuvants should be reduced or avoided entirely. The discontinuous long GnRHa protocol was first described by Corson et al. as an alternative to the long GnRHa protocol.[124] It entails discontinuing the GnRHa upon initiation of gonadotropin stimulation, allowing gonadotropin stimulation to proceed without concurrent GNRHa. The discontinuous long GnRHa protocol has been shown in two prospective randomized trials to be as effective as the long GnRHa protocol for prevention of premature luteinization[125] and premature LH surge.[124,125] In normal responders, number of ampules of HMG/FSH required is comparable[124] as are pregnancy rates.[124,125] Cancellation rates also are similar. One group was unable to confirm these findings.[126] At University of Nebraska Medical Center, we have replaced the long GnRHa protocol with the discontinuous long protocol to treat both normal and selected low responders with excellent results. Recently, the Norfolk group[127] reported a 32% IVF pregnancy rate in low responders with use of the discontinuous long GnRHa protocol in combination with high dose gonadotropin. They defined low responders as women with a day 3 FSH of ≧9 mIU/ml or previous poor response to controlled ovarian hyperstimulation (peak E2 <600 pg/ml).

Protocol: Discontinuous Long GnRHa + HMG/HCG

1. Leuprolide acetate 0.5 mg subcutaneous injection is started on day 21 of the cycle preceding the stimulation cycle.
2. After onset of menses, serum estradiol should be less 50 pg/ml to ensure adequate ovarian suppression.
3. Baseline TVUS should demonstrate no residual ovarian cysts >12 mm.
4. On cycle day 3, discontinue GnRHa and start HMG 450 to 600 IU IM daily.
5. Monitor every 2 to 3 days starting on the 4th day of stimulation (cycle day 6) with TVUS and serum E2. Adjust dose to maintain progressive follicular development and E2 rise. Dose can be decreased when 4 or more leading follicles reach a mean diameter >12 mm.
6. HCG 5000 to 10000 IU IM should be administered when 4 or more leading follicles are 18 mm in mean diameter, 36 hours prior to oocyte retrieval.

2. Short GnRHa Flare

For women who have a poor response to the discontinuous long GnRHa protocol, flare protocols are the better option. The protocol described below differs from that described above for ovulation induction in that higher doses of gonadotropins are utilized to effect the higher yield of follicles needed for ART.

Protocol: Short GnRHa Flare + HMG + HCG

1. Start OCPs on day 3 of the cycle preceding stimulation and continue for 21 days.
2. On day 1 to 2 of post-pill menses, baseline TVUS to rule out follicular cysts >12 mm.
3. Start leuprolide acetate 0.25 to 1.0 mg subcutaneously on cycle day 2.
4. Start HMG or FSH 300 to 450 IU IM daily on cycle day 3.
5. On the 4th day of stimulation, start monitoring with serial TVUS, E2, and LH levels. Adjust the dose to maintain progressive follicular development and E2 rise.
6. When 4 or more leading follicles reach >12 mm, decrease the dose by 75 to 150 IU.
7. Administer HCG 5000 to 10000 IU IM when 4 leading follicles reach a mean diameter of 18 mm, 36 hours prior to oocyte retrieval.

3. Microdose GnRHa Flare

The advantages of the microdose flare protocol over that of the short protocol are indicated above under Ovulation Induction for Low Responders. The protocol described below differs from that described above for ovulation induction in that the dose is increased to effect the higher yield of follicles needed for ART.

Protocol: Microdose GnRHa Flare + HMG + HCG + IUI

1. OCPs for 21 days starting on day 3 of the preceding cycle.
2. Baseline TVUS on day 1 to 2 of post-pill menses.
3. Start leuprolide acetate 50 mcg b.i.d. on day 2 of post-pill menses (cycle day 2).
4. Start HMG 300 to 450 IU IM on cycle day 3.
5. Start monitoring on the 4th day of stimulation with serial TVUS, serum E2, and LH and repeat every 2 to 3 days.
6. Adjust dose of medication according to follicular and E2 response.
7. When at least 4 leading follicles are > 12 mm, decrease the dose by 75 to 150 IU.
8. Administer HCG 5000 to 10000 IU IM when at least 4 leading follicles are 18 mm in mean diameter, 36 hours before oocyte retrieval.

4. Clomiphene Citrate and Gonadotropins

CC + HMG is a last alternative for women who fail to respond to GnRHa + HMG protocols. CC induces a flare of endogenous gonadotropins, but does not prevent a subsequent LH surge. No prospective randomized trials compare CC + HMG to microdose GnRHa flare + HMG, so it is uncertain whether one is superior to the other with respect to follicular recruitment. However, in view of the fact that cancellation rate with CC + HMG may be as high as 15 to 30%, in addition to possible untoward endometrial effects, CC + HMG is a reasonable alternative only if microdose GnRHa flare + HMG fails to render a satisfactory response. Benadiva et al. reported a 26.2% delivery rate/transfer in patients treated with CC + HMG who had previously failed IVF attempts after stimulation with gonadotropins with or without GnRHa.[128] The protocol for ovulation induction in low responders follows.

Protocol: CC + HMG + HCG + IUI

1. Baseline TVUS on cycle day 1 to 3.
2. CC 100 mg on days 3 through 7.
3. Start HMG 300 to 450 IU IM daily on cycle day 5.
4. Start monitoring on the 4th day of HMG stimulation with serial serum E2, LH, and TVUS and repeat every 2 to 3 days.
5. Adjust dose of HMG to maintain progressive follicular growth and doubling of E2 every other day.
6. When at least 4 leading follicles reach a mean diameter of > 12 mm, decrease the dose of HMG by 75 to 150 IU.
7. Administer HCG 5000 to 10000 IU IM when at least 4 leading follicles reach a mean diameter of 18 mm, 34 hours prior to oocyte retrieval.

IX. LUTEAL PHASE SUPPORT

Luteal phase defect (LPD) is diagnosed with a finding of endometrial histological dating more than 2 days out of phase and has long been associated with infertility.[129]

LPD is thought to result from inadequate quantity and/or duration of progesterone secretion by the corpus luteum. Interestingly, LPD has been shown to coexist with normal serum levels of progesterone,[130] indicating that progesterone levels alone do not reflect endometrial histology.[131] Relative to this discrepancy, researchers suggest that LPD and implantation failure may result from abnormal serum P:E2 ratio[132,133] or abnormal P:E2 receptor ratios.[134] Others have suggested specific deficiencies of cytosol E2 receptors at midluteal phase.[135] Therapy for LPD has included ovulation induction.[136–140] However, abnormalities of the luteal phase may also stem from ovarian stimulation,[141,142] particularly with induction of high estradiol levels.[143,144] Goldstein et al. evaluated different P:E2 relationships and how they influenced endometrial development and pregnancy rates.[145] They demonstrated that the most normal endometrium and best pregnancy rates were associated with high E2 levels balanced by high progesterone levels. While progesterone supplementation may mitigate the deleterious effects of hyperestrogenism on endometrial development,[146] the benefits of routine progesterone supplementation in cycles stimulated without GnRHa down regulation have not been confirmed by randomized controlled trials.

On the other hand, we know that cycles stimulated after down regulation with GnRHa result in luteal insufficiency.[147] The GnRHa induced block of LH secretion during the luteal phase results in suppression of progesterone pulsatility.[148] Decreased luteal E2 and P levels may also impair endometrial maturation and morphology.[149–151] The benefit of luteal phase support in down regulated cycles has been proven in prospective randomized trials.[152–156] Luteal phase support with both HCG and P appears to be effective.[154–156] However, some controversy remains regarding the best approach to supplementation. In choosing the best approach, one should consider the advantages and disadvantages of both. HCG requires less frequent dosing intervals of every 3 days. Progesterone, on the other hand requires daily administration. The disadvantages of HCG are serious. HCG supplementation increases the incidence of OHSS.[157,158] HCG may also increase luteal E2 to undesirable levels, inducing an unfavorable P:E2 ratio which may hinder implantation[159] and ongoing pregnancy rates.[133] Progesterone may neutralize the negative effect of hyperestrogenism on endometrial development[146] and have an immunosuppressive effect[160] which may facilitate implantation. While comparative randomized trials suggest equal efficacy of progesterone and HCG luteal support,[155,156] the increased risk of OHSS makes HCG a less safe alternative.

No consensus exists as to when progesterone supplementation should be initiated and how long it should be administered in ART cycles.[161] Some advocate beginning supplementation the day before oocyte retrieval[162] or on the day of embryo transfer.[155] Treatment duration has been recommended to be as short as 14 days[155,156] or as long as up to the 12th week of gestation.[162] Progesterone levels may fall on two occasions. The first is during the midluteal phase just prior to corpus luteum rescue by the HCG of a newly implanted blastocyst.[161] The second is at the time of luteoplacental shift, which may not be completed before the 7th to 9th week of gestation.[163] In the absence of definitive evidence to the contrary, this author recommends that P supplementation commence the day before oocyte retrieval for day 3 transfers and the day after retrieval for day 5 transfers. In either case, transfer occurs on the 5th day of progesterone supplementation, which is in agreement with others.[164] Furthermore, we recommend that it should be continued through the 12th gestational week.

For some researchers, vaginal progesterone appears as efficacious as IM progesterone.[156,162] This is in spite of lower serum levels of P found in women after vaginal P treatment.[165] Higher uterine tissue levels of progesterone have been found after vaginal administration[165] because of a 'first uterine pass effect.'[166] In spite of these findings, others have been unable to confirm that vaginal progesterone is equal to IM progesterone.[167]

At University of Nebraska Medical Center, we have used both IM and vaginal progesterone for supplementation of stimulated ART cycles. We do not use vaginal progesterone prior to embryo transfer because of lack of data regarding any embryo toxic effects of the currently available vaginal gel if transfer is done while the substance is in the vagina. As such, we use IM progesterone on the days prior to transfer and switch to vaginal progesterone after the transfer has been completed. This approach markedly improves patient comfort. Three protocols will be described, progesterone supplementation after ovulation induction and IUI, serial IM to vaginal progesterone for day 3 transfers, and serial IM to vaginal progesterone for day 5 transfers.

Progesterone Supplementation Protocol #1: Vaginal Progesterone Only for Ovulation Induction / IUI Cycles

1. On day 4 after HCG, start progesterone vaginal gel (Crinone 8%; Serono Laboratories, MA) one premeasured applicatorful daily per vagina and continue daily until the end of the 12th gestational week.

Progesterone Supplementation Protocol #2: Serial IM to Vaginal Progesterone for IVF / Day 3 Embryo Transfers

1. On the day prior to oocyte retrieval (day R-1), start progesterone-in-oil 50 mg IM in the morning.
2. On the morning of oocyte retrieval (day R), increase dose to 100 mg daily and repeat on days 1, 2, and 3 after retrieval (R+1, R+2, R+3).
3. Embyro transfer on day R+3.
4. Start progesterone vaginal gel one premeasured applicatorful on the morning after embryo transfer and continue daily through the 12th gestational week.

Progesterone Supplementation Protocol #3: Serial IM to Vaginal Progesterone for IVF / Day 5 Transfers

1. On the day after oocyte retrieval (R+1), start progesterone-in-oil 100 mg IM in the morning and repeat on days R+2, R+3, R+4, R+5.
2. Embryo transfer on day R+5.
3. Start progesterone vaginal gel one premeasured applicatorful on the morning after embryo transfer and continue daily through the 12th gestational week.

REFERENCES

1. Guzick, D. S., Carson, S. A., Coutifaris, C. et al., Efficacy of supraovulation and intrauterine insemination in the treatment of infertility, *N. Engl. J. Med.*, 340, 177, 1999.
2. Guzick, D. S., Sullivan, M. W., Adamson, G. D. et al., Efficacy of treatment for unexplained infertility, *Fertil. Steril.*, 70, 207, 1998.
3. Tummon, I. S., Asher, J. L., Martin, J. S. B., and Tulandi, T., Randomized control of trial of supraovulation and insemination and infertility associated with minimal or mild endometriosis, *Fertil. Steril.*, 68, 8, 1997.
4. Fedele, L., Bianchi, S., Marchini, M., Villa, L., Brioschi, D., and Parazzini, F., Superovulation with human menopausal gonadotropins in the treatment of infertility associated with minimal or mild endometriosis: a controlled randomized study, *Fertil. Steril.*, 58, 28–31, 1992.
5. Soto-Albors, C., Dailey, D. C., and Ying, Y.-K., Efficacy of human menopausal gonadotropins as therapy for abnormal cervical mucus, *Fertil. Steril.*, 51, 58, 1989.
6. Glazener, C. M. A., Coulson, C., Lambert, P. A., Watt, E. M., Hinton, R. A., Kelly, N. G., and Hull, M. G. R., Clomiphene treatment for women with unexplained infertility: placebo controlled study of hormonal responses and conception rates, *Gynecol. Endocrinol.*, 4, 75–83, 1990.
7. Wellner, S., DeCherney, A. H., and Polan, M. L., Human menopausal gonadotropins: a justifiable therapy in ovulatory women with longstanding idiopathic infertility, *Am. J. Obstet. Gynecol.*, 58, 111–17, 1988.
8. Melis, G. B., Paoletti, A. M., Strigini, F., Fabrais, F. M., Canale, D., and Fioretti, P., Pharmacologic induction of multiple follicular development improves the success rate of artificial insemination with husband's semen in couples with male related or unexplained infertility, *Fertil. Steril.*, 47, 441–45, 1987.
9. Serafini, P., Stone, B., Kerin, J., Batzofin, J., Queen, P., and Marrs, R. P., An alternate approach to controlled ovarian hyperstimulation in "poor responders": pretreatment with a gonadotropin releasing hormone analog, *Fertil. Steril.*, 49, 90–95, 1988.
10. Tummon, I. S., Maclin, V. M., Radwanska, E., Binor, Z., and Dmowski, W. P., Occult ovulatory dysfunction in women with minimal endometriosis or unexplained infertility, *Fertil. Steril.*, 50, 716–20, 1988.
11. Nulsen, J. C., Walsh, S., Dumez, S., and Metzger, D. A., A randomized and longitudinal study of human menopausal gonadotropin with intrauterine insemination and the treatment of infertility, *Obstet. Gynecol.*, 82, 780–6, 1993.
12. Jennings, J. C., Moreland, K., and Peterson, C. M., *In vitro* fertilisation: a review of drug therapy and clinical management, *Drugs*, 52, 331–43, 1996.
13. Fauser, B. C. J. M. and Van Heusden, A. M. V., Manipulation of human ovarian function: physiological concepts and clinical consequences, *Endocrine Reviews*, 18, 71–104, 1997.
14. Erickson, G. F., Physiologic basis of ovulation induction, *Semin. Reprod. Endocrinol.*, 14, 287–97, 1996.
15. Gougeon, A., Dynamics of follicular growth in the human: a model from preliminary results, *Hum. Reprod.*, 2, 81–87, 1986.
16. Hillier, S. G., Roles of follicle stimulating hormone and luteinizing hormone in controlled ovarian hyperstimulation, *Hum. Reprod.*, 11 Suppl 3, 113–21, 1996.
17. Speroff, L., Glass, R. H., and Kase, N. G., Regulation of the menstrual cycle, in *Clinical Gynecologic Endocrinology and Infertility*, 5th ed., Williams and Wilkins, Baltimore, MD, c. 1994, 183–230.

18. McNatty, K. P., Hunter, W. M., McNeilly, A. S. et al., Change in the concentration of pituitary and steroid hormones in the follicular fluid of human Graafian follicles throughout the menstrual cycle, *J. Endocrinol.*, 64, 555–71, 1975.

19. Brown, J. B., Pituitary control of ovarian function: concepts derived from gonadotropin therapy, *Aust. NZ J. Obstet. Gynaecol.*, 18, 47–54, 1978.

20. Van Weissenbruch, M. M., Schoemaker, H. C., Drexhage, H. A., and Schoemaker, J., Pharmaco-dynamics of human menopausal gonadotropin (HMG) and follicle-stimulating hormone (FSH). The importance of the FSH concentration in initiating follicular growth in polycystic ovary-like disease, *Hum. Reprod.*, 8, 813–21, 1993.

21. Van Der Meer, M., Hompes, P. G. A., Scheele, F., Schoute, E., Veersema, S., and Schoemaker, J., Follicle stimulating hormone (FSH) dynamics of low dose step-up ovulation induction with FSH in patients with polycystic ovary syndrome, *Hum. Reprod.*, 9, 1612–17, 1994.

22. Fauser, B. C., Donderwinkel, P., and Schoot, D. C., The step-down principle in gonadotropin treatment and the role of GnRh analogues, *Baillieres Clin. Obstet. Gynaecol.*, 7, 309–30, 1993.

23. Fathalla, M. F., Incessant ovulation-a factor in ovarian neoplasia?, *Lancet*, 2, 163, 1971.

24. Fishel, S. and Jackson, P., Follicular stimulation for high tech pregnancies: are we playing it safe?, *Br. Med. J.*, 299, 309–11, 1989.

25. Whittemore, A. S., Harris, R., and Itnyre, J., The Collaborative Ovarian Cancer Group. Characteristics related to ovarian cancer risk: collaborative analysis of twelve US case-control studies. II. Invasive epithelial cancer in white women, *Am. J. Epidemiol.*, 136, 1184–1203, 1992.

26. Harris, R., Whittemore, A. S., and Intyre, J., The Collaborative Ovarian Cancer Group. Characteristics related to ovarian cancer risk: collaborative analysis of twelve US case-control studies. III. Epithelial tumors of low malignant potential in white women, *Am. J. Epidemiol.*, 136, 1204–11, 1992.

27. Rossing, M. A., Daling, J. R., Weiss, N. S., Moore, D. E., and Self, S. G., Ovarian tumors in a cohort of infertile women, *N. Engl. J. Med.*, 331, 771–6, 1994.

28. Shushan, A. Paltiel, O., Iscovich, J., Elchalal, U., Peretz, T., and Schenker, J. G., Human menopausal gonadotropin and the risk of epithelial ovarian cancer, *Fertil. Steril.*, 65, 13–18, 1996.

29. Bristow, R. E. and Karlan, B. Y., Ovulation induction, infertility, and ovarian cancer risk, *Fertil. Steril.*, 66, 499–507, 1996.

30. Mosgaard, B. J., Lidegaard, O., Kruger-Kjaer, S., Schou, G., and Andersen, A. N., Infertility, fertility drugs, and invasive ovarian cancer: a case-control study, *Fertil. Steril.*, 67, 1005–1012, 1997.

31. Potashnik, G., Lerner-Geva, L., Genkin, L., Chetrit, A., Lunenfeld, G., and Porath, A., Fertility drugs and the risk of breast and ovarian cancers: results of a long term follow-up study, *Fertil. Steril.*, 71, 853–59, 1999.

32. Derman, S. G. and Adashi, E. Y., Adverse effects of fertility drugs, *Drug Saf.*, 11, 408–21, 1994.

33. Bonhoff, A. J., Naether, O. G., and Johannisson, E., Effects of clomiphene citrate stimulation on endometrial structure in infertile women, *Hum. Reprod.*, 11, 844–49, 1996.

34. Hock, D. L., Bohrer, M. K., Ananth, C. V., and Kemmann, G., Sonographic assessment of endometrial pattern and thickness inpatients treated with clomiphene citrate, human menopausal gonadotropins and intrauterine insemination, *Fertil. Steril.*, 68, 242, 1997.

35. *Physician's Desk Reference.* 53rd edition, Medical Economics Company, Inc., Montvale, NJ, c. 1999, 2995–97.
36. Bassil, S., Godin, P. A., Stallert, S., Nisolle, M., De Cooman, S., Donnez, J., and Gordts, S., Ovarian hyperstimulation syndrome: a review, *Assisted Reprod. Rev.*, 5, 90–96, 1995.
37. Navot, D., Margolioth, E. J., Laufer, N., Birkenfeld, A., Relon, A., Rosler, A., and Schenker, J. G., Direct correlation between plasma renin activity and severity of ovarian hyperstimulation syndrome, *Fertil. Steril.*, 48, 57–61, 1987.
38. Ong, A. C. M., Eisen, V., Rennie, D. P., Homburg, R., Lachelin, G. C. L., Jacobs, H. S., and Slater, J. D. H., The pathogenesis of the ovarian hyperstimulation syndrome (OHS): A possible role for ovarian renin, *Clin. Endocrinol.*, 34, 43–49, 1991.
39. Schenker, J. G. and Polishuk, W. Z., An experimental model of ovarian hyperstimulation syndrome, in *Proc. Int. Congress Animal Reprod.*, Vol 4, Tischner, M. and Pilc, J., Eds., Drukarnia Naukowa, Krakow, 1976, 635.
40. Knox, G. E., Dowd, A., Spiesel, S., and Hong, R., Antihistamine blockade of the ovarian hyperstimulation syndrome. II. Possible role of antigen-antibody complexes in the pathogenesis of the syndrome, *Fertil. Steril.*, 26, 418–21, 1975.
41. Balasch, J., Arroyo, V., Carmona, F., Llach, J., Jimenez, W., Pare, J. C., and Vanrell, J. A., Severe ovarian hyperstimulation syndrome: role of peripheral vasodilation, *Fertil. Steril.*, 56, 1077–83, 1991.
42. Erlik, Y., Naot, Y., Friedman, M., Ben-David, E., and Paldi, E., Histamine levels in ovarian hyperstimulation syndrome, *Obstet. Gynecol.*, 53, 580–82, 1979.
43. Haning, R. V., Strawn, E. Y., and Nolten, W. E., Pathophysiology of the ovarian hyperstimulation syndrome, *Obstet. Gynecol.*, 66, 220–24, 1985.
44. Doldi, N., Bassan, M., Messa, A., and Ferrari, A., Expression of vascular endothelial growth factor in human luteinizing granulosa cells and its correlation with the response to controlled ovarian hyperstimulation, *Gynecol. Endocrinol.*, 11, 263–7, 1997.
45. McClure, N., Healy, D. L., Rogers, P. A. W., Sullivan, J., Beaton, L., Haning, R. V. et al., Vascular endothelial growth factor as a capillary permeability agent in ovarian hyperstimulation syndrome, *Lancet*, 344, 235–6, 1994.
46. Neulen, J., Yan, Z., Raczek, S., Weindel, K., Keck, C., Weich, H. A. et al., Human chorionic gonadotropin-dependent expression of vascular endothelial growth factor/vascular permeability factor in human granulosa cells: importance in ovarian hyperstimulation syndrome, *J. Clin. Endocrinol. Metab.*, 80, 1967–71, 1995.
47. Christenson, L. K. and Stouffer, R. L., Follicle stimulating hormone and luteinizing hormone/chorionic gonadotropin stimulation of vascular endothelial growth factor production by macaque granulosa cells and from pre- and periovulatory follicles, *J. Clin. Endocrinol. Metab.*, 82, 2135–40, 1997.
48. Tanbo, T., Dale, P. O., Kjekshus, E., Haug, E., and Abyholm, T., Stimulation with human menopausal gonadotropin versus follicle stimulating hormone after pituitary suppression in polycystic ovarian syndrome, *Fertil. Steril.*, 53, 798–803, 1990.
49. Larsen, T., Larsen, J. F., Schioler, V., Bostofte, E., and Felding, C., Comparison of urinary follicle stimulating hormone and human menopausal gonadotropin for ovarian stimulation in polycystic ovarian syndrome, *Fertil. Steril.*, 53, 426–31, 1990.
50. *Physician's Desk Reference.* 53rd edition, Medical Economics Company, Inc., Montvale, NJ, c. 1999, 2988–89.
51. Howles, C. M., Genetic engineering of human FSH (Gonal-F), *Hum. Reprod. Update*, 2, 172–91, 1996.

52. Loumaye, E., Campbell, R., and Salat-Baroux, J., Human follicle stimulating hormone produced by recombinant DNA technology: a review for clinicians, *Hum. Reprod. Update*, 1, 188–99, 1995.

53. Bergh, C., Howles, C. M., Borg, K., Hamberger, L., Josefsson, B., Nilsson, L., and Wikland, M., Recombinant human follicle stimulating hormone (r-hFSH; Gonal F) versus highly purified urinary FSH (Metrodin HP): results of a randomized comparative study in women undergoing assisted reproductive techniques, *Hum. Reprod.*, 12, 2133–2139, 1997.

54. *Physician's Desk Reference*. 53rd edition, Medical Economics Company, Inc., Montvale, NJ, c. 1999, 2997–98.

55. Hugues, J. N. and Durnerin, C., Revisiting gonadotropin-releasing hormone agonist protocols and management of poor ovarian responses to gonadotropins, *Hum. Reprod Update*, 4, 83–101, 1998.

56. Racowsky, C., Prather, A. L., Johnson, M. K., Olvera, S. P., and Gelety, T. J., Prematurely condensed chromosomes and meiotic abnormalities in unfertilized human oocytes after ovarian stimulation with and without gonadotropin-releasing hormone agonist, *Fertil. Steril.*, 67, 932–8, 1997.

57. Plachot, M., Veiga, A., Montagut, J., de Grouchy, J., Calderon, G., Lepretre, S. et al., Are clinical and biological IVF parameters correlated with chromosomal disorders in early life?, *Hum. Reprod.*, 3, 627–35, 1988.

58. *Physician's Desk Reference*. 53rd edition, Medical Economics Company, Inc., Montvale, NJ, c. 1999, 3136–37.

59. Scott, R. T. and Hofmann, G. E., Prognostic assessment of ovarian reserve, *Fertil. Steril.*, 63, 1–11, 1995.

60. Scott, R. T., Toner, J. P., Muasher, S. J., Oehninger, S., Robinson, S., and Rosenwaks, Z., Follicle-stimulating hormone levels on cycle day 3 are predictive of *in vitro* fertilization outcome, *Fertil. Steril.*, 651–654, 1989.

61. Ramey, J. W., Seltman, H. J., and Toner, J. P., Superior analytic characteristics of an immunometric assay for gonadotropins also provides useful clinical prediction of *in vitro* fertilization outcomes, *Fertil. Steril.*, 65, 661–3, 1996.

62. Seifer, D. B., Lambert-Messerlian, G., Hogan, J. W., Gardiner, A. C., Blazer, A. S., and Berk, C. A., Day 3 serum inhibin-B is predictive of assisted reproductive technologies outcome, *Fertil. Steril.*, 67, 110–4, 1997.

63. Hofmann, G. E., Danforth, D. R., and Seifer, D. B., Inhibin-B: the physiologic basis of the clomiphene citrate challenge test for ovarian reserve screening, *Fertil. Steril.*, 69, 474–7, 1998.

64. Scott, R. T., Hofmann, G. E., Oehninger, S., and Muasher, S. J., Intercycle variability of day 3 follicle-stimulating hormone levels and its effect on stimulation quality in *in vitro* fertilization, *Fertil. Steril.*, 54, 297–302, 1990.

65. Smotrich, D. B., Widra, E. A., Gindoff, P. R., Levy, M. J., Hall, J. L., and Stillman, R. J., Prognostic value of day 3 estradiol on *in vitro* fertilization outcome, *Fertil. Steril.*, 64, 1136–40, 1995.

66. Buyalos, R. P., Daneshmand, S., and Brzechffa, P. R., Basal estradiol and follicle-stimulating hormone predict fecundity in women of advanced reproductive age undergoing ovulation induction therapy, *Fertil. Steril.*, 68, 272–7, 1997.

67. Evers, J. L. H., Slaats, P., Land, J. A., Dumoulin, J. C. M., and Dunselman, A. J., Elevated levels of basal estradiol-17 B predict poor response in patients with normal basal levels of follicle-stimulating hormone undergoing *in vitro* fertilization, *Fertil. Steril.*, 69, 1010–4, 1998.

68. Mukherjee, T., Copperman, A. B., Lapinski, R., Sandler, B., Bustillo, M., and Grunfeld, L., An elevated day 3 follicle-stimulating hormone:luteinizing hormone ratio (FSH:LH) in the presence of a normal day 3 FSH predicts a poor response to controlled ovarian hyperstimulation, *Fertil. Steril.*, 65, 588–93, 1996.

69. Padilla, S. L., Bayati, J., and Garcia, J. E., Prognostic value of the early serum estradiol response to leuprolide acetate in *in vitro* fertilization, *Fertil. Steril.*, 53, 288–294, 1990.

70. Winslow, K. L., Toner, J. P., Brzyski, R. G., Oehninger, S. C., Acosta, A. A., and Muasher, S. J., The gonadotropin-releasing hormone agonist stimulation test—a sensitive predictor of performance in the flare-up *in vitro* fertilization cycle, *Fertil. Steril.*, 56, 711–17, 1991.

71. Ranieri, D. M., Quinn, F., Maklouf, A., Khadum, I., Ghutmi, W., McGarrigle, H., Davies, M., and Serhal, P., Simultaneous evaluation of basal follicle-stimulating and 17 B-estradiol response to gonadotropin-releasing hormone analogue stimulation: an improved predictor of ovarian reserve, *Fertil. Steril.*, 70, 227–33, 1998.

72. Chang, M. Y., Chiang, C. H., Hsieh, T. T., Soong, Y. K., and Hsu, K. H., Use of the antral follicle count to predict the outcome of assisted reproductive technologies, *Fertil. Steril.*, 69, 505–10, 1998.

73. Tomas, C., Nuojua-Huttunen, S., and Martikainen, H., Pretreatment transvaginal ultrasound examination predicts ovarian responsiveness to gonadotropins in *in vitro* fertilization, *Hum. Reprod.*, 12, 220–3, 1997.

74. Chang, M. Y., Chiang, C. H., Chiu, T. H., Hsieh, T. T., and Soong, Y. K., The antral follicle count predicts the outcome of pregnancy in a controlled ovarian hyperstimulation/intrauterine insemination program, *J. Assist. Reprod. Genet.*, 15, 12–17, 1998.

75. Tanbo, T., Dale, P. O., Lunde, O., Norman, N., and Abyholm, T., Prediction of response to controlled ovarian hyperstimulation: a comparison of basal and clomiphene citrate-stimulated follicle-stimulating hormone levels, *Fertil. Steril.*, 57, 819–24, 1992.

76. Navot, D., Rosenwaks, Z., and Margolioth, E. J., Prognostic assessment of female fecundity, *Lancet*, 2, 645–47, 1987.

77. Loumaye, E., Billion, J. M., Mine, J. M., Psalti, I., Pensis, M., and Thomas, K., Prediction of individual response to controlled ovarian hyperstimulation by means of a clomiphene citrate challenge test, *Fertil. Steril.*, 53, 295–301, 1990.

78. Scott, R. T., Leonardi, M. R., Hofmann, G. E., Illions, E. H., Neal, G. S., and Navot, D., A prospective evaluation of clomiphene citrate challenge test screening of the general infertility population, *Obstet. Gynecol.*, 82, 539–44, 1993.

79. Hofmann, G. E., Sosnowski, J., Scott, R. T., and Thie, J., Efficacy of selection criteria for ovarian reserve screening using the clomiphene citrate challenge test in a tertiary fertility center population, *Fertil. Steril.*, 66, 49–53, 1996.

80. Scott, R. T., Opsahl, M. S., Leonardi, M. R., Neall, G. S., Illions, E. H., and Navot, D., Life table analysis of pregnancy rates in a general infertility population relative to ovarian reserve and patient age, *Hum. Reprod.*, 10, 1706–10, 1995.

81. Lim, A. S. T. and Tsakok, M. F. H., Age-related decline in fertility: a link to degenerative oocytes?, *Fertil. Steril.*, 68, 265–71, 1997.

82. Munne, S., Lee, A., Rosenwaks, Z., Grifo, J., and Cohen, J., Diagnosis of major chromosome aneuploidies in human preimplantation embryos, *Hum. Reprod.*, 8, 2185–91, 1993.

83. Benadiva, C. A., Kligman, I., Munne, S., Aneuploidy 16 in human embryos increases significantly with maternal age, *Fertil. Steril.*, 66, 248–55, 1996.

84. Battaglia, D. E., Goodwin, P., Klein, N. A., and Soules, M. R., Influence of maternal age on meiotic spindle assembly in oocytes from naturally cycling women, *Hum. Reprod.*, 11, 2217–22, 1996.

85. Hanoch, J., Lavy, Y., Holzer, H., Hurwitz, A., Simon, A., Revel, A., and Laufer, N., Young low responders protected from untoward effects of reduced ovarian response, *Fertil. Steril.*, 69, 1001–04, 1998.

86. Kettel, L. M. and Hummel, W. P., Ovulation induction in the estrogenized anovulatory patient, *Semin. Reprod. Endocrinol.*, 14, 309–15, 1996.

87. Ergur, A. R., Yergok, Y. Z., Ertekin, A., Kucuk, T., Mungen, E., and Tutuncu, L., Clomiphene citrate-resistant polycystic ovary syndrome: preventing multifollicular development, *J. Reprod. Med.*, 43, 185–90, 1998.

88. Van Voorhis, B. J., Sparks, A. E. T., Allen, B. D., Stovall, D. W., Syrop, C. H., and Chapler, F. K., Cost-effectiveness of infertility treatments: a cohort study, *Fertil. Steril.*, 67, 830–6, 1997.

89. Tummon, I. S., Maclin, V. M., Radwanska, E., Binor, Z., and Dmowski, W. P., Occult ovulatory dysfunction in women with minimal endometriosis or unexplained infertility, *Fertil. Steril.*, 50, 716–20, 1988.

90. Bohrer, M. K., Hock, D. L., Rhoads, G. G., and Kemmann, E., Sonographic assessment of endometrial pattern and thickness in patients treated with human menopausal gonadotropins, *Fertil. Steril.*, 66, 244–47, 1996.

91. Ransom, M. X., Doughman, N. C., and Garcia, A. J., Menotropins alone are superior to a clomiphene citrate and menotropin combination for superovulation induction among clomiphene citrate failures, *Fertil. Steril.*, 65, 1169–74, 1996.

92. Gentry, W. L., Thomas, S., and Critser, E. S., Use of endometrial measurement as an exclusion criterion for *in vitro* fertilization using clomiphene citrate, *J. Reprod. Med.*, 41, 545–47, 1996.

93. Tohma, H., Hasegawa, I., Sekizuka, N., and Tanaka, K., Uterine blood flow. Assessment in an intrauterine insemination program for unexplained infertility, *J. Reprod. Med.*, 42, 463–66, 1997.

94. Lu, P. Y., Chen, A. L. J., Atkinson, E. J., Lee, S. H., Erickson, L. D., and Ory, S. J., Minimal stimulation achieves pregnancy rates comparable to human menopausal gonadotropins in the treatment of infertility, *Fertil. Steril.*, 65, 583–87, 1996.

95. Balasch, J., Fabregues, F., Creus, M., Moreno, V., Puerto, B., Penarrubia, J., Carmona, F., and Vanrell, J. A., Pure and highly purified follicle-stimulating hormone alone or in combination with human menopausal gonadotropin for ovarian stimulation after pituitary suppression in *in vitro* fertilization, *Hum. Reprod.*, 11, 2400-04, 1996.

96. Balasch, J., Fabregues, F., Penarrubia, J., Creus, M., Vidal, R., Casamitjana, R., Manau, D., and Vanrell, J. A., Follicular development and hormonal levels following highly purified or recombinant follicle-stimulating hormone administration in ovulatory women and WHO group II anovulatory infertile patients, *J. Assist. Reprod. Genet.*, 15, 552–59, 1998.

97. Bennink, H. J. T. C., Fauser, B. C. J. M., and Out, H. J., Recombinant follicle-stimulation hormone (FSH; Puregon) is more efficient than urinary FSH (Metrodin) in women with clomiphene citrate-resistant, normogonadotropic, chronic anovulation: a prospective, multicenter, assessor-blind, randomized, clinical trial, *Fertil. Steril.*, 69, 19–25, 1998.

98. Homburg, R., Levy, T., Berkovitz, D., Farchi, J., Feldberg, D., Ashkenazi, J. et al., Gonadotropin-releasing hormone agonist reduces the miscarriage rate for pregnancies achieved in women with polycystic ovarian syndrome, *Fertil. Steril.*, 59, 527–31, 1993.

99. Sagle, M., Bishop, K., Ridley, N., Alexander, F. M., Michel, M., Bonney, R. C. et al., Recurrent early miscarriage and polycystic ovaries, *Br. Med. J.*, 297, 1027–8, 1988.

100. Homburg, R., Armar, N. A., Eshel, A., Adams, J., and Jacobs, H. S., Influence of serum luteinizing hormone concentrations on ovulation, conception, and early pregnancy loss in polycystic ovary syndrome, *Br. Med. J.*, 297, 1024–6, 1988.

101. Romeu, A., Monzo, A., Peiro, T., Diez, E., Peinado, J. A., and Quintero, L. A., Endogenous LH surge versus hCG as ovulation trigger after low-dose highly purified FSH in IUI: a comparison of 761 cycles, *J. Assist. Reprod. Genet.*, 14, 518–24, 1997.

102. Lewit, N., Kol, S., Manor, D., and Itskovitz-Eldor, J., Comparison of gonadotropin-releasing hormone analogues and human chorionic gonadotropin for the induction of ovulation and prevention of ovarian hyperstimulation syndrome: a case-control study, *Hum. Reprod.*, 11, 1399–1402, 1996.

103. Di Donato, P., Nola, V. F., Pittman, T. V., Marr, V., Stubbs, C., and Meldrum, D. R., Leuprolide acetate for inducing ovulation in women undergoing ovarian stimulation, *J. Reprod. Med.*, 40, 715–16, 1995.

104. Scott, R. T., Evaluation and treatment of low responders, *Semin. Reprod. Endocrinol.*, 14, 317–37, 1996.

105. Hofmann, G. E., Toner, J. P., Muasher, S. J., and Jones, G. S., High-dose follicle stimulating hormone (FSH) ovarian stimulation in low responder patients for *in vitro* fertilization, *J. In Vitro Fert. Embryo Transfer*, 6, 285–89, 1993.

106. Sungurtekin, U. and Jansen, R. P. S., Profound luteinizing hormone suppression after stopping the gonadotropin-releasing hormone-agonist leuprolide acetate, *Fertil. Steril.*, 63, 663–5, 1995.

107. Surrey, E. S., Bower, J., Hill, D. M., Ramsey, J., and Surrey, M. W., Clinical and endocrine effects of a microdose GnRH agonist flare regimen administered to poor responders who are undergoing *in vitro* fertilization, *Fertil. Steril.*, 69, 419–24, 1998.

108. Greenblatt, E. M., Meriano, J. S., and Casper, R. F., Type of stimulation protocol affects oocyte maturity, fertilization rate, and cleavage rate after intracytoplasmic sperm injection, *Fertil. Steril.*, 64, 557–63, 1995.

109. Scott, R. T. and Navot, D., Enhancement of ovarian responsiveness with microdoses of gonadotropin-releasing hormone agonist during ovulation induction for *in vitro* fertilization, *Fertil. Steril.*, 61, 880–5, 1994.

110. Schoolcraft, W., Schlenker, T., Gee, M., Stevens, J., and Wagley, L., Improved controlled ovarian hyperstimulation in poor responder *in vitro* fertilization patients with a microdose follicle-stimulating hormone flare, growth hormone protocol, *Fertil. Steril.*, 67, 93–7, 1997.

111. Suikara, A. M., Maclachlan, V., Koistinen, R., Seppala, M., and Healy, D. L., Double-blind placebo controlled study: human biosynthetic growth hormone for assisted reproductive technology, *Fertil. Steril.*, 65, 800–5, 1996.

112. Smitz, J., Devroey, P., Braekmans, P., Camus, M., Khan, I., Staessen, C. et al., Management of failed cycles in an IVF/GIFT programme with the combination of a GnRH analogue and hMG, *Hum. Reprod.*, 2, 309–14, 1987.

113. Ron-El, R., Herman, A., Golan, A. et al., The comparison of early follicular and midluteal administration of long-acting gonadotropin-releasing hormone agonist, *Fertil. Steril.*, 54, 233–37, 1990.

114. Urbancsek J. and Witthaus, E., Midluteaal buserelin is superior to early follicular phase buserelin in combined gonadotropin-releasing hormone analog and gonadotropin stimulation in *in vitro* fertilization, *Fertil. Steril.*, 65, 966–71, 1996.

115. Knodaveeti-Gordon, U., Harrison, R. F., Barry-Kinsella, C., Gordon, A. C., Drudy, L., and Cottell, E., A randomized prospective study of early follicular or midluteal initiation of long protocol gonadotropin-releasing hormone in an *in vitro* fertilization program, *Fertil. Steril.*, 66, 582–6, 1996.

116. Devreker, F., Govaerts, I., Bertrand, E., Van den Bergh, M., Gervey, C., and Englert, Y., The long-acting gonadotropin-releasing hormone analogues impaired the implantation rate, *Fertil. Steril.*, 65, 122–6, 1996.

117. Fabregues, F., Balasch, J., Creus, M., Civico, S., Carmona, F., Puerto, B., and Vanrell, J. A., Long term down-regulation does not improve pregnancy rates in an *in vitro* fertilization program, *Fertil. Steril.*, 70, 46–51, 1998.

118. Simon, C., Velasco, J. J. G., Valbuena, D., Peinado, J. A., Moreno, C., Remohi, J., and Pellicer, A., Increasing uterine receptivity by decreasing estradiol levels during the preimplantation period in high responders with the use of a follicle-stimulating hormone step-down regimen, *Fertil. Steril.*, 70, 234–9, 1998.

119. Tortoriello, D. V., McGovern, P. G., Colon, J. M., Skurnick, J. H., Lipetz, K., and Santoro, N., "Coasting" does not adversely affect cycle outcome in a subset of highly responsive *in vitro* fertilization patients, *Fertil. Steril.*, 69, 454–60, 1998.

120. Tiitinen, A., Husa, L. M., Tulppala, M., Simberg, N., and Seppala, M., The effect of cryopreservation in prevention of ovarian hyperstimulation syndrome, *Br. J. Obstet. Gynaecol.*, 102, 326–9, 1995.

121. Dahl Lyons, C. A., Wheeler, C. A., Frishman, G. N., Hackett, R. J., Seifer, D. B., and Haning, R. V., Early and late presentation of ovarian hyperstimulation syndrome: two distinct entities with different risk factors, *Hum. Reprod.*, 9, 792–9, 1994.

122. Paulson, R. J., Sauer, M. V., and Lobo, R. A., Embryo implantation after human *in vitro* fertilization: importance of endometrial receptivity, *Fertil. Steril.*, 53, 870–4, 1990.

123. Kowalik, A., Barmat, L., Damario, M., Liu, H.-C., Davis, O., and Rosenwaks, Z., Ovarian estradiol production *in vivo*: inhibitory effect of leuprolide acetate, *J. Reprod. Med.*, 43, 413–17, 1998.

124. Corson, S. L., Batzer, F. R., Gocial, B., Eisenberg, E., Hupert, L. C., and Nelson, J. R., Leuprolide acetate-prepared *in vitro* fertilization-gamete intrafallopian transfer cycles: efficacy versus controls and cost analysis, *Fertil. Steril.*, 57, 601–5, 1992.

125. Pantos, K., Meimeth-Damianaki, T., Vaxevanoglou, T., and Kapetanakis, E., Prospective study of a modified gonadotropin-releasing hormone agonist long protocol in an *in vitro* fertilization program, *Fertil. Steril.*, 61, 709–13, 1994.

126. Fujii, S., Sagara, M., Kudo, H., Kagiya, A., Sato, S., and Saito, Y., A prospective randomized comparison between long and discontinuous-long protocols of gonadotropin-releasing hormone agonist for *in vitro* fertilization, *Fertil. Steril.*, 67, 1166–6, 1997.

127. Faber, B. M., Mayer, J., Cox, B., Jones, D., Toner, J. P., Oehninger, S., and Muasher, S. J., Cessation of gonadotropin-releasing hormone agonist therapy combined with high-dose gonadotropin stimulation yields favorable pregnancy results in low responders, *Fertil. Steril.*, 69, 826–30, 1998.

128. Benadiva, C. A., Davis, O., Kligman, I., Liu, H. C., and Rosenwaks, Z., Clomiphene citrate and HMG: an alternative stimulation protocol for selected failed *in vitro* fertilization patients, *J. Assist. Reprod. Genet.*, 12, 8–12, 1995.

129. Noyes, R. W., The underdeveloped secretory endometrium, *Am. J. Obstet. Gynecol.*, 77, 929–44, 1959.

130. Zorn, J. R., Cedard, L., Nessmann, C., and Savale, M., Delayed endometrial maturation in women with normal progesterone levels: the dysharmonic luteal phase syndrome, *Gynecol. Obstet. Invest.*, 17, 157–62, 1984.
131. Batista, M. C., Cartledge, T. P., Merino, M. J., Axiotis, C., Platia, M. P., Merriam, G. R. et al., Midluteal phase endometrial biopsy does not accurately predict luteal function, *Fertil. Steril.*, 59, 294–300, 1993.
132. Gidley-Baird, A. A., O'Neill, C., Sinosich, M. J., Proter, R. N., Pike, I. L., and Saunders, D. M., Failure of implantation in human *in vitro* fertilization and embryo transfer patients: the effects of altered progesterone/estrogen ratios in humans and mice, *Fertil. Steril.*, 45, 69–74, 1986.
133. Maclin, V. M., Radwanska, E., Binor, Z., and Dmowski, W. P., Progesterone:estradiol ratios at implantation in ongoing pregnancies, abortions and nonconception cycles resulting from ovulation induction, *Fertil. Steril.*, 54, 238–44, 1990.
134. Abd-el-Maeboud, K. H., Eissa, S., and Kamel, A. S., Altered endometrial progesterone/oestrogen receptor ratio in luteal phase defect, *Dis. Markers*, 13, 107–16, 1997.
135. Hirama, Y. and Ochiai, K., Estrogen and progesterone receptors of the out-of-phase endometrium in female infertile patients, *Fertil. Steril.*, 63, 984–8, 1995.
136. DiZerega, G. S. and Hodgen, G. D., Follicular phase treatment of luteal phase dysfunction, *Fertil. Steril.*, 35, 428, 1981.
137. Huang, K., Muechler, E. K., and Bonfiglio, T. A., Follicular phase treatment of luteal phase defect with follicle-stimulating hormone in infertile women, *Obstet. Gynecol.*, 64, 32, 1984.
138. Minassian, S. S., Wu, C. H., Groll, M., Gocial, B., and Goldfarb, A. F., Urinary follicle stimulating hormone treatment of luteal phase defect, *J. Reprod. Med.*, 33, 11, 1988.
139. Muechler, E. K., Huang, K.-E., and Zongrone, J., Superovulation of habitual aborters with subtle luteal phase deficiency, *Int. J. Fertil.*, 32, 359, 1987.
140. Shapiro, A. G., New treatment for the inadequate luteal phase, *Obstet. Gynecol.*, 40, 826, 1972.
141. Olson, J. L., Rebar, R. W., Schreiber, J. F., and Vaitukaitis, J. L., Shortened luteal phase after ovulation induction with human menopausal gonadotropin and human chorionic gonadotropin, *Fertil. Steril.*, 39, 284, 1983.
142. Laatikkainen, T., Kurunmaki, H., and Koshimies, A., A short luteal phase in cycles stimulated with clomiphene and human menopausal gonadotropin for *in vitro* fertilization, *J. In Vitro Fert. Embryo Transfer*, 5, 14, 1988.
143. Howles, C. M., Macnamee, M. C., and Edwards, R. G., Follicular development and early luteal function of conception and nonconception cycles after human *in vitro* fertilization: endocrine correlates, *Hum. Reprod.*, 2, 17, 1987.
144. Berquist, C., Nillius, S. J., and Wide, L., Human gonadotropin therapy. II. Serum estradiol and progesterone patterns during nonconceptual cycles, *Fertil. Steril.*, 39, 766, 1983.
145. Goldstein, D., Zuckerman, H., Harpaz, S., Barkai, J., Gera, A., Gordon, S., Shalev, E., and Schwartz, M., Correlation between estradiol and progesterone in cycles with luteal phase deficiency, *Fertil. Steril.*, 37, 348, 1982.
146. Garcia, J., Jones, C., Agosta, A., and Wright, G., Corpus luteum function after follicle aspiration for oocyte retrieval, *Fertil. Steril.*, 46, 903, 1981.
147. Smitz, J., Devroey, P., Camus, M., Deshacht, J., Khan, I., Staessen, C. et al., The luteal phase and early pregnancy after combined GnRH agonist/HMG treatment for superovulation in IVF or GIFT, *Hum. Reprod.*, 3, 585, 1988.
148. Kubic, C. J., Luteal phase dysfunction following ovulation induction, *Semin. Reprod. Endocrinol.*, 4, 293, 1986.

149. Van Steirteghem, A. C., Smitz, J., Camus, M., Van Waesberghe, L., Deschacht, J. et al., The luteal phase after *in vitro* fertilization and related procedures, *Hum. Reprod.*, 3, 161, 1988.

150. Macnamee, M. C., Edwards, R. G., and Howles, C. M., The influence of stimulation regimens and luteal phase support on the outcome of IVF, *Hum. Reprod.*, 3, 43, 1988.

151. Dehou, M. F., Lejeune, B., Arijs, C., and Leroy, F., Endometrial morphology in stimulated *in vitro* fertilization cycles and after steroid replacement therapy in cases of primary ovarian failure, *Fertil. Steril.*, 48, 995, 1987.

152. Smith, E. M., Anthony, F. W., Gadd, S. C., and Masson, G. M., Trial of support treatment with human chorionic gonadotropin in the luteal phase after treatment with buserelin and human menopausal gonadotropin in women taking part in an *in vitro* fertilisation programme, *Br. Med. J.*, 298, 1483, 1989.

153. Belaisch Allart, J., DeMouzon, J., Lapousterie, C., and Mayer, M., The effect of HCG supplementation after combined GnRH agonist/HMG treatment in an IVF programme, *Hum. Reprod.*, 5, 163, 1990.

154. Claman, P., Domingo, M., and Leader, A., Luteal phase support in *in vitro* fertilization using gonadotropin releasing hormone analogue before ovarian stimulation: a prospective randomized study of human chorionic gonadotropin versus intramuscular progesterone, *Hum. Reprod.*, 7, 487–9, 1992.

155. Araujo, E., Bernardini, J., Frederick, J. L., Asch, R. H., and Balmaceda, J. P., Prospective randomized comparison of human chorionic gonadotropin versus intramuscular progesterone for luteal-phase support in assisted reproduction, *J. Assist. Reprod. Genet.*, 11, 74–78, 1994.

156. Artini, P. G., Volpe, A., Angioni, S., Galassi, M. C., Battaglia, C., and Genazzani, A. R., A comparative, randomized study of three different progesterone support of the luteal phase following IVF/ET program, *J. Endocrinol. Invest.*, 18, 51–6, 1995.

157. Buvat, J., Marcoiln, G., Herbaut, J. C., Dehaene, J. L., Verbeck, P., and Fourlinnie, J. C., A randomized trial human chorionic gonadotropin support following *in vitro* fertilization and embryo transfer, *Fertil. Steril.*, 49, 458, 1988.

158. Navot, D., Bergh, P. A., and Laufer, N., Ovarian hyperstimulation syndrome in novel reproductive technologies: prevention and treatment, *Fertil. Steril.*, 58, 249–61, 1992.

159. Mochtar, M. H., Hogerzeil, H. V., and Mol, B. W., Progesterone alone versus progesterone combined with HCG as luteal support in GnRHa/HMG induced IVF cycles: a randomized clinical trial, *Hum. Reprod.*, 11, 1602–1605, 1996.

160. Kinel, F. A. and Ciaccio, L. A., Suppression of immune response by progesterone, *Endocrinol. Exp.*, 14, 27, 1980.

161. Akande, A. V., Mathur, R. S., Keay, S. D., and Jenkins, J. M., The choice of luteal support following pituitary down regulation, controlled ovarian hyperstimulation and *in vitro* fertilisation, *Br. J. Obstet. Gynecol.*, 103, 963–66, 1996.

162. Smitz, J., Devroey, P., Faguer, B., Bourgain, C., Camus, M., and Van Steirteghem, A. C., A prospective randomized comparison of intramuscular or intravaginal natural progesterone as luteal phase and early pregnancy supplement, *Hum. Reprod.*, 7, 168–75, 1992.

163. Csapo, A. I., Pulkkinen, M. O., Ruttner, B., Sauvage, J. P., and Wiest, W. G., The significance of human corpus luteum in pregnancy maintenance, *Am. J. Obstet. Gynecol.*, 112, 1061, 1972.

164. Lelaidier, C., de Ziegler, D., Freitas, S., Oliveness, F., Hazout, A., and Frydman, R., Endometrium preparation with exogenous estradiol and progesterone for the transfer of cryopreserved blastocysts, *Fertil. Steril.*, 63, 919–21, 1995.

165. Miles, R. A., Paulson, R. J., Lobo, R. A., Press, M. F., Dahmoush, L., and Sauer, M. V., Pharmacokinetics and endometrial tissue levels of progesterone after administration by intramuscular and vaginal routes: a comparative study, *Fertil. Steril.*, 5, 276–81, 1990.
166. de Ziegler, D., Hormonal control of endometrial receptivity, *Hum. Reprod.*, 10, 4–7, 1995.
167. Perino, M., Brigandi, A., Abate, F. G., Costabile, L., Balzano, E., and Abate, A., Intramuscular versus vaginal progesterone in assisted reproduction: a comparative study, *Clin. Exp. Obstet. Gynecol.*, 24, 228–31, 1997.

7 Oocyte and Pre-Embryo Classification

Kathy L. Sharpe-Timms and Randall L. Zimmer

CONTENTS

I. INTRODUCTION

A variety of factors may affect oocyte and pre-embryo characteristics and subsequent outcome of assisted reproductive technologies (ART). These factors include patient demographics, ovarian stimulation protocols, oocyte retrieval methods, oocyte processing, fertilization procedure, and pre-embryo processing and transfer (Table 7.1). Oocyte maturity and quality at the time of retrieval reflect the individual's response to controlled ovarian hyperstimulation (COH) and can provide diagnostic and prognostic information based on gamete status. Human oocytes produced by various ovarian stimulation protocols may vary widely in maturity, quality, and rate of development *in vitro*. In the laboratory, rapid evaluation enables the oocyte to be maintained under optimal culture conditions of temperature, osmolarity, and pH, as an alteration of any of these parameters may be detrimental to the continuing oocyte development. Accurate assessment of oocyte maturity is critical to the timing and success of insemination, whereas errors in assessment may lead to abnormal fertilization and/or poor development potential.[1,2] Additionally, patient response to COH protocols and male factor infertility may be difficult to interpret based on fertilization results when insemination is improperly timed.[2] Correct assessment of oocyte quality may identify gamete anomalies, indicate reduced opportunity for success, and elucidate the need for oocyte donation.[3] Assessment of pre-embryo viability is of paramount importance when determining the number and selection of pre-embryos for intrauterine transfer. Although other factors such as maternal age and uterine receptivity undoubtedly affect the outcome of pre-embryo transfer, pre-embryo viability will determine the success of such procedures. Further, improved knowledge of characteristics influencing pre-embryo quality and an accurate system for viability assessment could reduce the number of pre-embryos transferred per patient, reduce the potential for high risk, multiple gestation, and provide some prediction of implantation success.[4] Thus, a rapid and accurate assessment of oocyte maturity at retrieval and a pre-embryo grading system that enables some prediction of implantation after IVF-ET are important components of any ART program. A standardized, universal scoring system may facilitate communication among embryologists, serve as an adjunct in patient counseling, and most importantly, improve the quality and outcome of ART procedures.

II. OOCYTE CLASSIFICATION

A. OOCYTE MATURATIONAL STATUS

To date, no reliable biochemical test of follicular fluid has been developed that can accurately and rapidly assess oocyte maturational status. Therefore, most oocyte classification systems rely on direct visualization of maturational status, morphology of the oocyte, and appearance of companion cumulus oophorus and corona radiata cells. Classification by maturational status is based on biological time points during oogenesis. For a review of meiosis and oogenesis see Alberts et al.[5] Here, oogenesis will be discussed in relation to oocyte classification. Germ cells in the fetal ovary multiply mitotically, but at approximately 11 to 12 weeks of pregnancy they enter meiosis and become arrested at the diplotene stage of prophase of the first meiotic division. Thus, the primordial follicle contains a germinal vesicle stage oocyte that is surrounded initially by a single layer of follicular cells. In response to appropriate gonadotropin stimulation at puberty, follicles are recruited and two processes ensue: follicular development accompanied by oocyte growth. In developing follicles, the primary or "immature" oocyte remains arrested in first meiotic prophase, but it grows, synthesizes cortical granules, and begins to synthesize the zona pellucida. Meanwhile, follicular cells proliferate to form multiple layers. Thus, immature oocytes are in prophase I of meiosis I and characterized by the germinal vesicle, prominent nucleolus, no polar body (Figures 7.1 and 7.2), and tightly packed or condensed cumulus and corona cells that give the appearance of a bull's-eye target (Table 7.2). Dissolution of the nuclear membrane or germinal vesicle breakdown indicates that the oocyte has resumed meiosis.

As meiosis resumes, the oocyte enters into metaphase I of meiosis I. This "intermediate" oocyte has not extruded the first polar body (Figures 7.1 and 7.2), and though the cumulus may be expanded, the corona is compact or displays varying degrees of expansion (Table 7.2). This stage is accompanied by continued follicular

TABLE 7.1
Factors That May Affect Oocyte and Embryo Quality and ART Outcomes

Patient demographics	Female age
	Diagnosis: male factor, tubal factor, endometriosis, ovulatory dysfunction,
	uterine factor (polyps, fibroids, septum, DES exposure, unexplained, other)
	Geographic factors
	Parity
	Genetic disorders
Stimulation protocols	GnRH protocol: flare vs. down regulation
	Follicle stimulating hormone
	Luteinizing hormone
	Clomiphene citrate
	Human menopausal gonadotropin
	Other
Oocyte retrieval	Anesthesia
	Laparoscopic vs. vaginal
	Manual vs. mechanical
	Number of oocytes retrieved
Oocyte processing	Time from retrieval to incubator
	Cumulus removal: mechanical/chemical
	Media and protein supplementation
	Incubator environment
	CO_2, O_2, humidity, temperature, recovery times
	Laboratory environment
	Light, temperature, air filtration/flow
	Culture volume
	Oil overlay
	Co-culture
	Cell type
	Human vs. nonhuman
Fertilization procedure	IVF, ICSI, SUZI
	Zona thickness
	Number of sperm used for insemination
	Mature vs. immature sperm
	Mature at retrieval vs. *in vitro* matured oocytes
Embryo processing	Culture conditions as stated for oocytes
	Duration of culture prior to transfer
	Cryopreservation

growth, expansion of the fluid-filled antrum, further development of the zona pellucida, and migration of cortical granules to the cortex.

Meiotic cleavage is uneven in oocytes. Each primary oocyte gives rise to one large secondary oocyte and one small polar body. The polar body, which is present within the zona pellucida of the ovulated oocyte, is destined to degenerate. Extrusion of the polar body marks the transition from intermediate metaphase I to "mature" metaphase II (Figures 7.1 and 7.2). Mature ovulated oocytes are arrested at metaphase II of meiosis II and remain so until fertilization. They have no germinal vesicle; the first meiotic division is completed with the extrusion of the first polar body; and, both the cumulus and corona radiata are optimally expanded (Table 7.2).

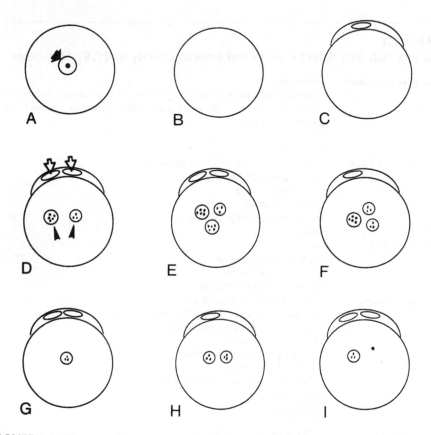

FIGURE 7.1 Diagram of oocyte maturational classification and assessment of fertilization. (A) Meiosis I, Prophase I oocyte, germinal vesicle (arrow) present in cytoplasm; (B) Meiosis I, Metaphase I, germinal vesicle absent, no polar body present; (C) Meiosis II, Metaphase II, germinal vesicle present, polar body in perivitelline space; (D) Normal fertilization: one male pronucleus and one female pronucleus (arrowheads) in the ooplasm, two polar bodies (open arrows) in perivitelline space; (E) Polyspermic fertilization: more than one male pronuclei plus one female pronucleus, two polar bodies; (F) Polygynic fertilization: more than one female pronuclei and one male pronucleus, one polar body; (G) Oocyte activation: one female pronucleus, two polar bodies; (H) Oocyte activation: one female pronucleus, one polar body; (I) Suspected failure of sperm to decondense: one refractile body, one female pronucleus, two polar bodies. (Zona pellucida, corona radiata, and granulosa cells not shown.) Photomicrograph examples shown in Figure 7.2.

Fertilization triggers the completion of the meiotic division with the extrusion of another small polar body. Technically, the oocyte does not become fully mature until fertilization triggers meiosis completion; however, oocytes are considered mature when they are capable of fertilization and embryonic development.

Normal maturation and growth of oocytes depends on adequate support from ovarian thecal and granulosa cells of the follicle. Folliculogenesis is influenced by hormones, primarily follicle stimulating hormone, and estrogens. Other growth promoting factors, such as epidermal growth factor, fibroblast growth factor, and

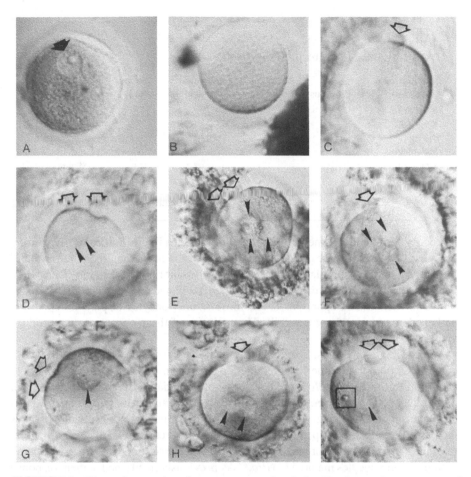

FIGURE 7.2 Photomicrographs of oocyte maturational classification and assessment of fertilization. [solid arrow = germinal vesicle; open arrow = polar body; arrowhead = pronucleus; box = refractile body] (A) Meiosis I, Prophase I oocyte, germinal vesicle present in cytoplasm; (B) Meiosis I, Metaphase I, germinal vesicle absent, no polar body present; (C) Meiosis II, Metaphase II, germinal vesicle present, polar body in perivitelline space; (D) Normal fertilization: one male pronucleus and one female pronucleus in the ooplasm, two polar bodies in perivitelline space; (E) Polyspermic fertilization: more than one male pronuclei, one female pronucleus, two polar bodies; (F) Polygynic fertilization: more than one female pronuclei and one male pronucleus, one polar body; (G) Oocyte activation: one female pronucleus, two polar bodies; (H) Oocyte activation: one female pronucleus, one polar body; (I) Suspected failure of sperm to decondense: one refractile body, one female pronucleus, two polar bodies.

insulin-like growth factors, also influence follicle growth by binding to the specific cell surface receptors on granulosa cells. COH protocols override this system leading to development of a cohort of follicles. COH can be induced therapeutically with clomiphene citrate, follicle-stimulating hormone (FSH), gonadotropin-releasing hormone agonists (GnRHa), or human menopausal gonadotropins (hMG). With these

TABLE 7.2
Maturational Status of the Oocyte

Maturational Status	Cumulus	Corona	Germinal Vesicle	Polar Body	Classification
Meiosis I, Prophase I	C	C	+	−	Immature (IM)
Meiosis I, Metaphase I	E	V	−	−	Intermediate (INT)
Meiosis II, Metaphase II,	E	E	−	+	Mature (M)

Note: C = condensed; V = variable; E = expanded; + = present; − = absent.

protocols, follicle recruitment may not be uniform, leading to follicular asynchrony that yields oocytes that are developmentally asynchronous at the time of retrieval.[6–10] Further, COH may stimulate an oocyte beyond its normal maturation point when performed in the presence of drugs designed to block endogenous gonadotropin secretion (i.e., GnRH agonists). These "postmature" oocytes display clumped and darkened cumulus and coronal cells. The majority of these oocytes do not produce viable pre-embryos.

Accordingly, one must assess maturational status of each oocyte at retrieval to determine appropriate time for insemination. Errors in the assessment may lead to abnormal fertilization and/or poor development potential.[1,2] Sperm can penetrate an immature oocyte; however, early insemination can result in failure of sperm head decondensation and oocyte activation failure.[1,11] Insemination of postmature oocytes increases the risk of polyspermy and parthenogenetic activation. Higher fertilization rates have been reported for mature meiosis II, metaphase II oocytes when compared with immature oocytes matured *in vitro*.[2,7] As previously mentioned, patient response to COH protocols and male factor infertility may be difficult to interpret based on fertilization results when insemination is timed improperly.[2]

B. Oocyte Morphological Quality

Morphology assessment reveals oocyte quality (Table 7.3). Morphology of human oocytes has been described extensively in the past.[2,11–13] The overall appearance of the cytoplasm, zona pellucida, and polar body, as well as the granulosa, cumulus, and corona companion somatic cells are considered. In the mature oocyte, the cytoplasm should be clear, shiny, uniform in color and granularity, and occupy most of the space within the zona pellucida. The zona pellucida should be intact, even in thickness, and symmetrical. Granulosa and cumulus oophorus cells associated with high quality oocytes are clear, shiny, and uniformly spread out, with a stringiness and propensity to attach to the culture dish. Coronal expansion should be optimal and radiant. Oocytes are downgraded for any of the following characteristics: dark, granular, or shrunken cytoplasm, vacuoles, refractile bodies, a thick or cracked zona pellucida or a dark, clumpy, free-floating, or absent cumulus-coronal complex.

TABLE 7.3
Assessment of Oocyte Morphology

Feature	Positive Characteristics	Negative Characteristics
Cytoplasm	Clear, shiny, homogeneous	Dark, granular, pitted
	Occupies most space within zona	Shrunken
	Uniform color and granularity	Refractile body
		Vacuoles
Zona pellucida	Appropriate thickness for	Cracked
	developmental stage	Too thick for developmental stage
Granulosa cells	Clear, shiny	Dark
(at retrieval and	Stringinous	Clumpy
in vitro)	Attachment to culture dish	Free-floating
Cumulus cells	Clear, shiny	Dark
(at retrieval and	Stringiness	Clumpy
in vitro)	Attachment to culture dish	Free-floating
Coronal cells	Optimal, radiant	Incomplete, uneven expansion
(maturational or		Condensed
morphological?)		

Postmature oocytes display a clumping and darkening of the cumulus-coronal morphology, may have a larger than normal perivitelline space, and show a slightly degenerative first polar body. Degenerating or atretic oocytes display a much wider perivitelline space, irregular shape, and very dark, granular cytoplasm, and may or may not exhibit a polar body.

As with maturity, oocyte quality may affect fertilization, cleavage, pre-embryo quality, and pregnancy rate. As the quality of oocytes obtained from patients undergoing COH will vary, a scoring system becomes an important tool in selecting those oocytes most conducive to successful outcomes.

C. Techniques Used for Oocyte Evaluation

Initial evaluation of oocyte maturity historically is based on direct visualization of the appearance of the cumulus-coronal complex. Oocytes with an expanded, elastic cumulus oophorus and a radiant sunburst corona radiata are considered mature meiosis II, metaphase II oocytes. Those oocytes exhibiting an expanded cumulus, but only varying degrees of coronal expansion (slight or uneven), indicate less mature or meiosis I, metaphase I intermediate oocytes. The absence of cumulus expansion typifies immature or meiosis I, prophase I oocytes. These initial observations can be made quickly while searching through follicular aspirates. However, cumulus-coronal expansion is correlated only indirectly with oocyte maturity, and as stated above, asynchrony has been reported between cumulus-coronal morphology and nuclear maturity.[6-10] In order to assess the true nuclear status, one must visualize the oocyte directly, either with or without the cumulus-coronal mass.

Several techniques allow direct assessment of oocyte nuclear maturity, ranging from a thinning or spreading of the cumulus-coronal complex, to various degrees of somatic cell removal. The Veeck spreading technique involves placing the cumulus-coronal complex in a small droplet of culture medium or follicular fluid on the flat surface of a Petri dish, jarring the dish and/or slowly removing the fluid in order to use the resulting surface tension to flatten or spread out the cumulus for better visualization of the ooplasm and perivitelline space.[11] Care must be taken to avoid temperature, pH, and osmolarity changes due to evaporation of medium. If, after employing the surface tension spreading technique, the granulosa cell density obscures the cumulus complex or the oocyte, the additional step of removing overlaying cell layers may provide an unobstructed view of the ooplasm. Granulosa and cumulus cells may be removed manually using the beveled edge of fine gauge needles in a slicing manner or by drawing the oocyte in and out of a fine bore denuding pipette. Take care not to damage the oocyte with the needles or with the excessive pressure of an undersized pipette. Alternatively, one can remove all of the cumulus-coronal cells enzymatically by exposing the oocyte-cumulus complex briefly to hyaluronidase and subsequently stripping the cells with a denuding pipette.[6,14] Following removal of granulosa cells, the unobscured oocyte can be evaluated for maturational status and graded in regard to quality. In attempts to visualize nuclear status, one must avoid overmanipulation of the oocytes which could negatively affect fertilization, pre-embryo quality, and subsequent outcome.

A direct relationship between proliferative capacity of cumulus oophorus and corona radiata cells *in vitro* and ART outcome has been determined.[15] While cell proliferation does not correlate with etiology of infertility, COH protocol, patient age, ovarian response and quality of oocytes, fertilization, or pre-embryo morphology, a direct relationship occurs between cell proliferation and the incidence of clinical pregnancy. Further, progesterone production of the oocyte-cumulus complex correlates with the cleavage potential of pre-embryos in an IVF system.[16]

D. Oocyte Classification Systems

A comprehensive scoring or grading system should include evaluation of oocyte maturational status, morphological quality, and fertilization capacity. Most classification systems divide maturational status of the oocyte into three to five stages and may include classes of immature, intermediate, and mature, or prophase I, metaphase I, and metaphase II, respectively. Metaphase II oocytes may be subdivided to include postmature and atretic classes. Other classification systems distinguish between early and late metaphase I in which the divisive point is approximately 15 hours to attain meiotic competence, or morphologically, the cumulus is expanded greatly, but the corona radiata is less expanded.[2] Some classify the oocyte-cumulus cell complex by assigning a grade on a scale of 1 to 5 with grade 1 = immature, grade 2 = intermediate, grade 3 = mature, grade 4 = postmature, and grade 5 = atretic.[14] This system creates confusion with other oocyte and pre-embryo grading systems that use a similar grading format to represent morphological grading (described below) rather than maturational status.

Oocyte morphology is graded according to characteristics that may correlate to reduced fertilization success. Variation between morphology grading scales exists in the field, and oocyte morphology grades may range from 1 to 4 or 1 to 5 with either 1 or 4/5 representing the best grade. Anomalies of oocyte morphology are listed in Table 7.3. Generally, oocyte grade is altered one point for each morphological anomaly.

At retrieval, many embryologists will classify each oocyte as to both its maturational and morphological status. Examples include an oocyte that exhibits an expanded cumulus, an expanded corona, clear cytoplasm, and one polar body, and second oocyte that displays an expanded cumulus, a condensed corona, slightly darkened cytoplasm, and no polar body. Using a maturational scale of immature (IM also called PI), intermediate (INT also called MI), mature (M also called MII), and postmature (PM) and using a morphology grade (G) of excellent (4), good (3), fair (2), and poor (1), the first oocyte would be graded M (or MII), G4 and the second would be graded INT (or MI), G3. This system provides valuable information relating to the subsequent time of insemination, offers some insight into the efficacy of the COH protocol on oocyte maturity and quality, and provides diagnostic and prognostic information based on gamete status.

Others have designed a point system for describing oocyte morphology at retrieval.[7] In this system, a maximum of four points each for cumulus expansion, cumulus appearance, amount of cumulus, corona expansion, corona appearance, and oocyte appearance may be assigned. The first oocyte in the example above would score a maximum of 24 points, the second would score in the 19 to 20 range. An atretic or very immature oocyte would score a minimum of 6, receiving one point for each category. In both classification systems, a higher grade or score correlates significantly with the percentage of high-quality oocytes in meiosis II, metaphase II and with better fertilization rates. The oocyte maturity and morphology, as reflected by the oocyte score, affect the subsequent outcome of both fertilization and pre-embryo quality.

E. OTHER METHODS FOR EVALUATING OOCYTES

Hormone and growth factor content of follicular fluid have been evaluated for predictive value of oocyte maturity and fecundability. Although concentrations of some parameters vary with oocyte maturational status, no difference in estradiol, progesterone, testosterone, prolactin, insulin-like growth factor, and growth hormone have been found in follicular fluid between fertilized and unfertilized oocytes.[17,18]

III. DOCUMENTATION OF FERTILIZATION

Fertilization checks of oocytes inseminated *in vitro* are performed 16 to 18 h post-insemination. Fertilization checks performed prior to pronuclear formation (< 16 h) or after pronuclear dissolution (>20 h) may conceal nuclear status of resultant pre-embryos or cause oocytes to be classified as unfertilized. Fertilization assessment should be performed rapidly, yet efficiently. If present, the cumulus-coronal complex should be removed sufficiently to visualize nuclear status. Fine gauge needles or finely drawn pipets may remove these cells mechanically. Needles cost less, but may pierce the zona. A pipet works faster, but may cause zona compression rupture and fail to remove sufficient cells. Alternatively, hyaluronidase may be used to remove the cells chemically.[6,14] To visualize nuclear status, observe the oocytes from different angles using inverted phase contrast microscopy to ensure that two, and only two, pronuclei are present. Photo or video micrography, when used, should be simple and rapid, minimizing oocyte exposure to harmful changes in temperature, light, and pH.

Normal fertilization is characterized by the presence of one male and one female pronuclei in the ooplasm and two polar bodies in perivitelline space (Figures 7.1 and 7.2). Abnormal fertilization may include polypronuclear fertilization or more than two pronuclei in the ooplasm. Polypronuclear fertilization can be polyspermic (penetration by more than one sperm) or polygynic (formation of more than one female pronuclei) in nature (Figures 7.1 and 7.2). An increased risk of polyspermic fertilization is associated with early or late inseminations, rupture of the zona pellucida, insemination with high numbers of motile sperm, and micro-operative procedures including partial zona dissection and subzonal insertion of spermatozoa. Avoid transfer of polypronuclear oocytes because of potential genetic anomalies, formation of hydatidiform moles, or even triploid infants. Visualization of the pronuclear status is essential as abnormally fertilized oocytes may cleave normally and are then morphologically indistinguishable from normally fertilized oocytes. Oocyte activation or failure of the sperm head to decondense can result in observation of one female pronuclei and one or two polar bodies when checking fertilization status. Failed fertilization also is characterized by the absence of pronuclei and the persistence of one or two degenerating polar bodies. Fertilization failure may result from a variety of causes including poor quality oocytes, poor quality sperm, bad culture medium, or technical failure. Incorrect evaluation of fertilization status may occur from use of low-powered microscopes, insufficient denuding of oocytes, incorrect classification of oocytes, visualization of polar bodies (rather than nuclear status) to determine fertilization, and classification of cytoplasmic vacuoles as pronuclei.

IV. PRE-EMBRYO ASSESSMENT AND CLASSIFICATION

A. BACKGROUND

Correlations exist among morphological appearance of a pre-embryo, assessments of cleavage rates, and IVF pregnancy success rates.[4,19–21] Pre-embryo morphology may be affected by intrinsic factors such as developmental and genetic errors and/or extrinsic factors such as the stimulation protocol or suboptimal culture conditions. Abnormalities also may arise from anomalies in oocyte maturation and the events of fertilization *in vitro*. A number of grading systems assist in the evaluation of pre-embryos for viability and implantation success based on morphological appearance under low-light microscopy and/or the developmental rate of cleavage stage pre-embryos in culture. Accurate pre-embryo assessment could reduce the number of pre-embryos transferred per patient and thereby reduce the potential for high risk, multiple gestation.[4] Noninvasive methods of assessing pre-embryo metabolism and nutrient uptake also are being developed.

B. Methods of Assessing Pre-Embryo Viability

1. Assessment of Morphology

Morphology of human pre-embryos has been described extensively in the past.[2,12,13] Reports comparing pre-embryo morphological appearance and IVF pregnancy success rates traditionally associate blastomere size and regularity, granularity, and the presence or absence of cytoplasmic fragments with the capacity for continued development after transfer.[20] Accurate scoring of pre-embryo appearance to quantify pre-embryo development is, however, subjective, difficult, and notoriously inaccurate.[8,22] Pre-embryos that appear microscopically normal may be multinucleate or possess intracellular abnormalities. Moreover, some morphological anomalies do not correspond necessarily to decreased viability. Further, as each blastomere of a pre-embryo is believed to retain totipotency for several of the early cell divisions, cleavage stage pre-embryos can rid themselves of defective cells destined for degeneration and still produce a viable pre-embryo.

Examples of morphological characteristics used to establish the score of human pre-embryos in culture appear in Table 7.4 and Figure 7.3. Each blastomere must possess a single nucleus, have equal size and shape, maintain uniform color and granularity, and occupy most of the space within the zona pellucida. Multinucleation, unequal size, irregular shape, and dark or granular cytoplasm are undesirable characteristics of blastomeres. The presence and degree of cytoplasmic fragmentation is considered particularly inferior if ≥20% of the surface area. Pre-embryos in the blastocyst stage must have a single cavity, visible inner cell mass, regular trophoblast cells, and adequate expansion with appropriate cell numbers. Human blastocysts grown *in vitro* may have visible morphological abnormalities including more than one cavity, necrotic areas, no visible inner cell mass, irregular trophoblast cells, severe contraction, and variable cell numbers.

Thickness of the zona pellucida, the glycoprotein membrane that surrounds the pre-embryo, appears to predict pre-embryo potential.[23] Cleaved pre-embryos with thinned patches in their zonae, as compared to pre-embryos with zonae of regular thickness, appear to implant more frequently. Zona pellucida thinning normally occurs during blastocyst expansion. Thickening of the zona pellucida or failure of zonae rupture may result from *in vitro* culture conditions, cryopreservation, or a phenomenon inherent to many human pre-embryos, irrespective of their *in vivo* or *in vitro* conception.[23,24] Implantation rates of pre-embryos with zona thickness ≥15 μm may improve with assisted hatching; however, patients whose pre-embryos have thin zonae (≤13 μm) may suffer from these procedures.[23] Assisted hatching not only facilitates pre-embryo hatching mechanically, but also allows earlier embryo-endometrium contact thereby enhancing synchrony between the endometrium and pre-embryo and thus potentially implantation.

As with oocyte assessment, pre-embryo assessment systems using morphological criteria generally categorize pre-embryos into one of four or five grades. Pre-embryos can be classified using terms such as excellent, good, fair, or poor or by using numbers on a scale of 1 to 4 or 1 to 5. As mentioned above for oocyte grading, one must take care when reviewing pre-embryo scores between ART programs as

TABLE 7.4
Assessment of Pre-Embryo Morphology

Feature	Positive Characteristics	Negative Characteristics
Blastomeres	Equal size and shape	Fragments
	Occupy most of the space within the zona	Blebs
	Uniform in color and granularity	Vacuoles
	Single nucleus	Refractile bodies
Nuclei	Zygote with two pronuclei	Multinucleate blastomeres
Zona pellucida	Appropriate thickness for developmental stage	Thickness ≥15 µ may be enhanced by assisted hatching.
	Varying evenness of thickness	Thin zonae ≥13 µ may be jeopardized by these procedures.[23]
		Zona pellucida hardening
Blastocyst	Single cavity	More than one cavity
	Distinct inner cell mass	Necrotic areas
	Regular trophoblast cells	No visible inner cell mass
	Adequate expansion	Irregular trophoblast cells
	Appropriate cell numbers	Severe contraction
		Variable cell numbers

some grading systems will designate 1 as the best category while others will use 4 or 5 to indicate the best pre-embryo score. Pre-embryo grades usually are adjusted one grade for each undesirable morphological characteristic.

Grading scales using only blastomere conformation and degree of fragmentation show significant correlations to implantation success.[25–27] A grade 1 pre-embryo, representing perfect morphology, would have equal size blastomeres with no cytoplasmic fragments. A grade 2 pre-embryo would have blastomeres of equal size and minor fragmentation. Pre-embryos with distinctly unequal blastomeres are grade 3, and those with moderate to heavy fragmentation would be grade 4. Grade 5 pre-embryos resemble amorphous masses with few blastomeres of any size and with major or complete fragmentation.

Several studies indicate that neither day 2 nor day 3 morphology nor cell number predicts embryo ability to form a blastocyst.[28–30] However, blastocyst morphology combined with hatching, adherence, growth, and amount of human chorionic gonadotropin (hCG) secretion have successfully predicted embryo viability.[28] Viable blastocysts had better morphology, produced more hCG, and showed larger nuclei counts than poorer quality, nonviable blastocysts. Interestingly, hCG secretion was similar in hatched blastocysts and blastocysts that remained within the zona pellucida, yet, hatched blastocysts showed adherence that significantly increased hCG secretion.[31]

2. Assessment of Cleavage Rates

Human pre-embryos rely on maternal messenger ribonucleic acid processed during oogenesis for the first two cleavage divisions. Embryonic transcripts seem to be activated and expressed during the 4- to 8-cell stages of preimplantation development. As human pre-embryos may be transferred before or at the 8-cell stage, the

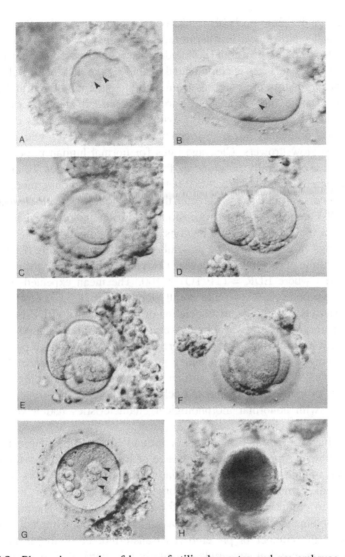

FIGURE 7.3 Photomicrographs of human fertilized oocytes and pre-embryos. (A and B) Normal fertilization (one male pronucleus and one female pronucleus in the ooplasm, arrowheads). Fertilized oocyte A is of excellent quality whereas fertilized oocyte B may be downgraded for morphological features such as irregular shape, cytoplasm shrunken and does not fill zona pellucida, and uneven cytoplasmic granularity. (C and D) Two-cell pre-embryos. Preembryo C is of near perfect morphology whereas pre-embryo D may be downgraded for features including uneven blastomeres, uneven cytoplasmic granularity, and cytoplasmic fragments. (E and F) Four-cell pre-embryos. Pre-embryo E is of near perfect morphology whereas pre-embryo F may be downgraded for features including uneven blastomeres, uneven cytoplasmic granularity, and cytoplasmic fragments. (G) Abnormally fertilized human oocyte. This oocyte displays three pronuclei (arrowheads) which are distinguishable from cytoplasmic vacuoles as the pronuclei possess nucleoli while the vacuoles are empty. (H) Atretic oocyte 16 hours post-insemination. This oocyte was postmature at retrieval (note clumped cumulus cells in background) and deteriorated rapidly.

initial cleavage divisions probably reflect oocyte maturation rather than pre-embryo developmental competence. Furthermore, human oocytes can be parthenogenetically activated or polyspermic and still undergo apparently normal cleavage. Quality evaluation by cleavage rate is complicated further by the fact that development rate variation occurs within pre-embryos from a single patient cultured under identical conditions. Despite this intrapatient variation, retarded cleavage rates seem to indicate reduced pre-embryo viability while faster cleavage rates correspond to higher clinical pregnancy rates.[13,32] Pregnancies occur, however, with concepti considered to be slow growers. Cleavage rates for normal human pre-embryos post-insemination are generally observed as follows: 2-cell between 22 and 44 hours, 4-cell between 36 and 50 hours, 8-cell between 48 and 72 hours, morulae between 72 and 96 hours, and blastocyst greater than 120 hours. Uneven cleavage (i.e., 3, 5, or 7 cells) may be observed occasionally during meiotic division; however, persistent uneven cleavage would be considered an anomaly.

Cummings et al.[33] developed a pre-embryo development rating (EDR) based on the observed time of pre-embryo cleavage (TO) and the expected time of pre-embryo cleavage (TE) where EDR = (TE/TO) × 100. The mean expected times for the pronuclear pre-embryo, 2-, 4-, and 8-cell stages were 24.7, 33.6, 45.5, and 56.4 hours, respectively. A significant association of pregnancy with EDR in multiple and single pre-embryo transfers was found. Average EDRs fell between 90 and 109. Pre-embryos with an EDR of 110 to 130 were more likely to produce pregnancy than slower cleaving pre-embryos. Pregnancy prediction improved further by adding a pre-embryo quality rating based on pre-embryo morphology including symmetry of blastomeres, proportion of fragmented cells, and clarity of blastomere cytoplasm. Pre-embryos with abnormal morphological characteristics had lowered viability irrespective of their cleavage rates.

Others have proposed that the main influences on implantation rate include cleavage, achieving the 4-cell stage, absence of irregular blastomeres, and absence of anucleate fragments.[4, 34–36] The Cumulative Embryo Score (CES), as developed by Steer et al.,[37] multiplies the pre-embryo grade at transfer by the number of blastomeres to produce a quality score for each pre-embryo. The scores are then summed to obtain the CES, which is used as an index to predict implantation success, regardless of the number of pre-embryos transferred. Pre-embryos fall into four grades based on morphology: grade 4, equally symmetrical blastomeres; grade 3, uneven blastomeres with 10% or less fragmentation; grade 2, 10 to 50% fragmentation; and grade 1, greater than 50% fragmentation, or those not exhibiting cleavage. Pregnancy rates increased as CES increased to a maximum of 42, but multiple gestations rose with scores above 42.

Giorgetti et al.[35] devised a 4-point scale in which pre-embryos received 1 point for each of the following attributes: cleavage, 4-cell stage, absence of irregular blastomeres, and fragmentation of less than 20% of the embryonic surface. Higher pregnancy rates not only resulted from those pre-embryos of perfect morphology, but 4-cell pre-embryos implanted twice as often as those with 2, 3, or 5 plus cells. Pre-embryos that did not cleave received no score and produced no pregnancies.

3. Assessment of Pre-Embryo Metabolism

Rapid advances in technology produce noninvasive techniques for studies of pre-embryo nutrient uptake and metabolism. For example, a microfluorometric technique has been used to show that mouse and human preimplantation pre-embryos consume pyruvate before glucose which becomes the predominate substrate for the blastocyst.[38] Other procedures including fluorometric assays, enzymatic cycling, and bioluminescence assays assess metabolism in human pre-embryos. Detailed descriptions of these procedures for monitoring nutrient uptake are available elsewhere.[38] Studies of pre-embryo metabolism enhance our understanding of pre-embryo physiology, facilitate the development of more suitable culture conditions, and ultimately lead to the development of quantitative tests of pre-embryo viability.

Dye exclusion (trypan blue, eosin Y) tests, dye affinity tests (DAPI), and dye retention tests (fluorescein diacetate, FDA) help test the viability of a variety of cells including mammalian pre-embryos. Results of such dye tests reflect basic cell functions rather than developmental potential. Abnormal pre-embryos may retain basic cell functions. Furthermore, dye use necessitates pre-embryo exposure to nonphysiological compounds and should be restricted to human pre-embryos not destined for replacement. However, this data may be useful in improving culture methods.[38]

Pre-embryo production of platelet activating factor (PAF) correlates strongly with human pre-embryo viability. Pre-embryo-derived PAF capable of inducing transient maternal thrombocytopenia has been proposed as both an *in vitro* and *in vivo* marker of pre-embryo viability.[13]

Assessment of glycolytic activity determines viability in murine embryos. Blastocysts with low glycolytic activity had significantly higher viability than those with abnormally elevated levels of glycolysis.[39] At present, researchers require more specific assays to confirm the utility of this assay for evaluating pre-embryo viability.[38]

4. Pre-Embryo Biopsy for Preimplantation Assessment

Pre-embryo biopsy techniques have been developed for diagnosis of genetically transmitted diseases. One or more pre-embryo blastomeres are removed by microoperative techniques and the pre-embryo is cryopreserved while genetic analysis ensues. A variety of biopsy methods, each with inherent problems, have been reported including blastomere aspiration, blastomere extrusion, mechanical distortion, and trophectoderm herniation.[40] The proposed limit of cellular mass that may be removed by biopsy from human pre-embryos without affecting subsequent pre-embryo development may be around one quarter of the total cellular mass.[40] Accurate assessment of biopsied blastomeres relies on successful amplification of the genetic material via such techniques as polymerase chain reaction and subsequent DNA analysis.

V. SUMMARY

Oocyte and pre-embryo classification traditionally are based on morphological characteristics. Evaluation and classification by morphology alone, however, can be subjective, can vary among embryologists, does not distinguish between intrinsic or extrinsic causes of anomalies, and may not predict success. In the past decade, systems have evolved that, in addition to morphological criteria, incorporate cleavage rate to predict pre-embryo viability and subsequent implantation. More recently, components of follicular fluid and culture media are being evaluated for their prognostic value, and microsurgical techniques are being used for preimplantation diagnosis. Correct identification of oocyte maturational status maximizes fertilization and embryonic development. To date, however, a standardized oocyte and pre-embryo classification system has not been adopted by the profession. Further, classification systems currently in place differ greatly between clinics. An accurate, standardized oocyte and pre-embryo classification system could improve communication among embryologists, serve as an adjunct in patient counseling, and improve the quality and outcome of ART procedures by improving our knowledge of characteristics influencing pre-embryo quality. An accurate system for assessment of viability could reduce the number of pre-embryos transferred per patient, reduce the potential for high risk, multiple gestation, and provide for some prediction of implantation success.

REFERENCES

1. Sathananthan, A. H. and Trounson, A. O., *Atlas of Fine Structure of Human Sperm Penetration, Eggs and Embryos Cultured In Vitro*, Praeger, New York, 1986, 2.
2. Veeck, L. L., The morphological assessment of human oocytes and early concepti, *Handbook of the Laboratory Diagnosis and Treatment of Infertility*, Keel, B. A. and Webster, B. W., Eds., CRC Press, Boca Raton, FL, 1990, 353–69.
3. Ezra, Y., Simon, A., and Laufer, N., Defective oocytes: a new subgroup of unexplained infertility, *Fertil. Steril.*, 58, 24–7, 1992.
4. Staessen, C., Camus, M., Bollen, N., Devroey, P., and Van Steirteghem, A., The relationship between embryo quality and the occurrence of multiple pregnancies, *Fertil. Steril.*, 57, 626–630, 1992.
5. Alberts, B., Bray, D., Lewis, J., Raff, M., Roberts, K., and Watson, J., *Molecular Biology of the Cell*, 2nd ed., Garland Publishing, Inc., New York, NY, 1989, 845–867.
6. Laufer, N., Tarlatzis, B. C., DeCherney, A. H., Masters, J. T., Haseltine, F. F. P., MacLusky, N., and Naftolin, F., Asynchrony between human cumulus-corona cell complex and oocyte maturation after human menopausal gonadotropin treatment for *in vitro* fertilization, *Fertil. Steril.*, 42, 366–72, 1984.
7. Mahadevan, M. M. and Fleetham, J., Relationship of a human oocyte scoring system to oocyte maturity and fertilizing capacity, *Int. J. Fertil.*, 35, 240–244, 1990.
8. Hammitt, D. G., Syrop, C. H., Van Voorhis, B. J., Walker, D. L., Miller, T. M., Barud, K. M., and Hood, C. C., Prediction of nuclear maturity from cumulus-coronal morphology: influence of embryologist experience, *J. Assist. Reprod. Genet.*, 9, 439–446, 1992.
9. Hammitt, D. G., Syrop, C. H., Van Voorhis, B. J., Walker, D. L., Miller, T. M., and Barud, K. M., Maturational asynchrony between oocyte cumulus-coronal morphology and nuclear maturity in gonadotropin-releasing hormone agonist stimulations, *Fertil. Steril.*, 59, 375–381, 1993.

10. Greenblatt, E. M., Meriano, J. S., and Casper, R. F., Type of stimulation protocol affects oocyte maturity, fertilization rate and cleavage after intracytoplasmic sperm injection, *Fertil. Steril.*, 64, 557–63, 1995.
11. Veeck, L. L., Oocyte assessment and biological performance, *Ann. NY Acad. Sci.*, 541, 259–74, 1988.
12. Veeck, L. L., Preembryo grading, *Atlas of the Human Oocyte and Early Conceptus*, Vol. 2, Williams and Wilkins, Baltimore, MD, 1991, 121–150.
13. Wolf, D. P., Analysis of embryonic development, in *In Vitro Fertilization and Embryo Transfer*, Plenum Press, New York, NY, 1988, 137–145.
14. Osborn, J., Oocyte retrieval and maturation, in *Handbook of In Vitro Fertilization*, Trounson, A. O. and Gardner, D. K., Eds., CRC Press, Boca Raton, FL, 1993, 17–32.
15. Gregory, L., Booth, A. D., Wells, C., and Walker, S. M., A study of the cumulus-corona cell complex in in vitro fertilization and embryo transfer; a prognostic indicator of the failure of implantation, *Hum. Reprod.*, 9, 1308–17, 1994.
16. Wiswedel, K., Granulosa cell metabolism and the assessment of oocyte quality in IVF, *Hum. Reprod.*, 2, 589–91, 1987.
17. Rosenbusch, D., Djalai, M., and Sterzik, K., Is there any correlation between follicular fluid concentrations, fertilizability and cytogenetic constitution of human oocytes recovered for in vitro fertilization?, *Fertil. Steril.*, 57, 1358–60, 1992.
18. Artini, P. G., Battaglia, C., D-Ambrogio, G., Barreca, A., Droghini, F., Volpe, A., and Genazzani, A. R., Relationship between human oocyte maturity, fertilization and follicular fluid growth factors, *Hum. Reprod.*, 9, 902–6, 1994.
19. Shulman, A., Kaneti, H., Ben-Nun, I., Shilon, M., Ghetler, Y., and Beyth, Y., Relationship between embryo morphology and implantation rate after in vitro fertilization treatment in conception cycles, *Fertil. Steril.*, 123–6, 1993.
20. Trounson, A. and Osborn, J., In vitro fertilization and embryo development, in *Handbook of In Vitro Fertilization*, Trounson, A. and Gardner, D. K., Eds., CRC Press, Boca Raton, FL, 1993, 63–84.
21. Cooperman, A. B., Sandler, B., Selick, C. E., Bustillo, M., and Grunfeld, L., Cumulative number and morphological score of embryos resulting in success: realistic expectations from in vitro fertilization-embryo transfer, *Fertil. Steril.*, 64, 88–92, 1995.
22. May, J. T. and Sharpe-Timms, K. L., Lack of consensus in human oocyte grading among ART laboratory personnel, *J. Assist. Reprod. Genet.*, 14 (5S), OC-19–168, 1997.
23. Cohen, J., Zona pellucida micromanipulation and consequences for embryonic development and implantation, in *Micromanipulation of Human Gametes and Embryos*, Raven Press, New York, NY, 1992, 211–212.
24. Tucker, M. J., Cohen, J., Massey, J. B., Mayer, M. P., Wiker, S. R., and Wright, G., Partial dissection of the zona pellicuda of frozen-thawed human embryos may enhance blastocyst hatching, implantation and pregnancy rates, *Am. J. Obstet. Gynecol.*, 165, 341–4, 1991.
25. Scott, R. T., Hofmann, G. E., Veeck, L. L., Jones, H. W., and Muasher, S. J., Embryo quality and pregnancy rates in patients attempting pregnancy though in vitro fertilization, *Fertil. Steril.*, 55, 426–428, 1991.
26. Erenus, M., Zouves, C., Rajamahendran, P., Leung, S., Fluker, M., and Gomel, V., The effect of embryo quality on subsequent pregnancy rates after in vitro fertilization, *Fertil. Steril.*, 56, 707–710, 1991.
27. Puissant, F., Van Rysselberge, M., Barlow, P., Deweze, J., and Leroy, F., Embryo scoring as a prognostic tool in IVF treatment, *Hum. Reprod.*, 2, 705–708, 1987.

28. Dokras, A., Sargent, I. L., and Barlow, D. H., Human blastocyst grading: an indicator of developmental potential?, *Hum. Reprod.*, 8, 2119–27, 1993.
29. Gardner, D. K., Vella, P., Lane, M., Wagley, L., Schlenker, T., and Schoolcraft, W. B., Culture and transfer of human blastocysts increases implantation rates and reduces the need for multiple embryo transfers, *Fertil. Steril.*, 69, 84–8, 1998.
30. Rijnders, P. M. and Jansen, C. A., The predictive value of day 3 embryo morphology regarding blastocyst formation, pregnancy and implantation rate after day 5 transfer following *in vitro* fertilization or intracytoplasmic sperm injection, *Hum. Reprod.*, 13, 2869–73, 1998.
31. Dokras, A., Sargent, I. L., Ross, C., Gardner, R. L., and Barlow, D. H., The human blastocyst: morphology and human chorionic gonadotropin secretion *in vitro*, *Hum. Reprod.*, 6, 1143–51, 1991.
32. Shoukir, Y., Chardonnens, D., Campana, A., Bischof, P., and Sakkas, D., The rate of development and time of transfer play difference roles in influencing the viability of human blastocysts, *Hum. Reprod.*, 13, 676–81, 1998.
33. Cummins, J. M., Breen, T. M., Harrison, K. L., Shaw, J. M., Wilson, L. M., and Hennessey, J. F., A formula for scoring human embryo growth rates in *in vitro* fertilization: its value in predicting pregnancy and in comparison with visual estimates of embryo quality, *J. In Vitro Fertil. and Embryo Transfer*, 3, 284–295, 1986.
34. Hill, G. A., Freeman, M., Bastias, M. C., Rogers, B. J., Herbert III, C. M., Osteen, K. G., and Wentz, A. C., The influence of oocyte maturity and embryo quality on pregnancy rate in a program for *in vitro* fertilization-embryo transfer, *Fertil. Steril.*, 52, 801–806, 1989.
35. Giorgetti, C., Terriou, P., Auquier, P., Hans, E., Spach, J.-L., Salzmann, J., and Roulier, R., Embryo score to predict implantation after *in vitro* fertilization: based on 957 single embryo transfers, *Hum. Reprod.*, 10, 2427–2431, 1995.
36. Hoover, L., Baker, A., Check, J. H., Lurie, D., and O'Shaughnessy, A., Evaluation of a new embryo-grading system to predict pregnancy rates following *in vitro* fertilization, *Gynecol. Obstet. Invest.*, 40, 151–157, 1995.
37. Steer, C. V., Mills, C. L., Tan, S. L., Campbell, S., and Edwards, R. G., The cumulative embryo score: a predictive embryo scoring technique to select the optimal number of embryos to transfer in an *in vitro* fertilization and embryo transfer program, *Hum. Reprod.*, 7, 117–119, 1992.
38. Gardner, D. K. and Leese, H. J., Assessment of embryo metabolism and viability, in *Handbook of In Vitro Fertilization*, Trounson, A. O. and Gardner, D. K., Eds., CRC Press, Boca Raton, FL, 1993, 195–211.
39. Lane, M. and Gardner, D. K., Selection of viable mouse blastocysts prior to transfer using a metabolic criterion, *Hum. Reprod.*, 11, 1975–8, 1996.
40. Tarin, J. J. and Trounson, A. O., Embryo biopsy for preimplantation diagnosis, in *Handbook of In Vitro Fertilization*, Trounson, A. O. and Gardner, D. K., Eds., CRC Press, Boca Raton, FL, 1993, 115–127.

8 Oocyte and Embryo Culture

Lynette A. Scott

CONTENTS

I. INTRODUCTION

Most forms of assisted reproduction require that either or both the male and female gametes and the resulting embryos be maintained *in vitro*. This has been accomplished, with varying degrees of success, in many species for a number of years. Most of the early success in human assisted reproduction technologies (ART) came as a direct consequence of the work in laboratory animals, such as mice, rats, and hamsters, and domestic animals such as cows and sheep. These species are still used as models for the development and refinement of many of the systems used in human ART procedures. In most species studied, researchers observed that the embryos arrested at specific stages of preimplantation development *in vitro*. The developmental blocks and retardation seen in animal modes have also appeared in human embryos between the 4- and 16-cell stages,[26] which is the point at which embryonic products of transcription and translation become functional,[55] and reach the morula stage.[69,78] This led to the practice of using early cleavage stage embryos for embryo transfer in human IVF.[45] Embryos are not blocked in development if they have proceeded to the blastocyst stage. The use of co-culture systems (bovine uterine fibroblasts,[140] vero cells,[69,78] and granulosa cells,[57] resulted in more advanced human embryos and blastocysts for embryo transfer in certain instances. Recently, investigators have a renewed interest in developing culture media specifically for extended culture to avoid the use of a co-culture system. Further, in all systems studied to date, the embryos become growth retarded and asynchronous compared with those developing *in vitro*, which is probably due to suboptimal culture conditions.[15,18,95] This retardation is considered when using animal models where embryo transfers occur with the recipients timed to be synchronous or slightly behind the developmental stage of the embryos grown *in vitro*. In human IVF, the cycle from which the embryos are derived is usually the transfer cycle, thus this timing is not a feasible option.

A variety of culture systems have been used for human *in vitro* fertilization and embryo culture with approximately equivalent pregnancy and delivery rates. Many of the culture media are based on an acellular culture system consisting of simple balanced salt solutions based on either Earle's Balanced salt solution or on Tyrode's medium. These media typically contain between 1 and 10% human serum as a protein additive, at least 2.78 mM glucose with some containing as much as 5.0 mM glucose, and pyruvate. Some contain lactate, EDTA, and glutamine as additives at varying concentrations. These media provide adequate development to at least the 8-cell stage[36] and some to the blastocyst stage.[107]

Over the last few years, advances in oocyte and embryo culture from a wide variety of species, including the human, provide successful *in vitro* maturation and fertilization of oocytes and the alleviation of the *in vitro* developmental blocks. In many instances, such advances allow complete *in vitro* development to the expanded blastocyst stage and subsequent fetal development.

Oocyte and embryo development *in vitro* is a study, either directly or indirectly, of metabolism since it is through metabolism that oocytes and embryos grow and differentiate. Mammalian oocytes and preimplantation embryos rely on exogenous substances to fuel metabolism. Metabolism is a coordinated and complex series of events in which multi-enzyme systems regulate the acquisition and exchange of energy substrates and co-factors between the oocyte or embryo and its environment. Exogenous nutrients transform into the precursors of macromolecules required for growth such as nucleic acids, proteins, and lipids. The embryo takes up nutrients in response to its energy requirements rather than the concentration of available nutrients, which are then used in metabolism. Metabolism regulation includes the regulation of the rate of enzymatic reactions that can be affected by pH, intracellular concentrations of substrates, the products of the reactions, and the availability of co-factors required for these reactions. Metabolism control occurs through regulatory enzymes that function by a feedback mechanism in which the regulatory enzyme is inhibited by the end product of the sequence of reactions it regulates. Finally, the availability or actual production (transcription and translation) of the enzymes necessary for the metabolic process can act as a regulating mechanism.

Oocytes initially develop in the ovary in a highly specialized environment that changes dramatically through the growth and maturation phases of the oocyte. The ovulated oocyte and subsequent embryo develop in the oviduct *in vivo*. The oviduct environment is dynamic and different from the conditions found *in vitro*. An understanding of the *in vivo* events, metabolism, and controls of metabolism occurring in oocytes and embryos is an essential part of developing systems for the *in vitro* culture of both oocytes and embryos.

II. *IN VIVO* DEVELOPMENT

Mammalian oogenesis begins in the fetus with the deposition of the primordial germ cells in the developing gonads.[129] The germ cells migrate into the sex cords, begin to divide, change their morphology, and become known as oogonia. During fetal development some of the oogonia enter the first meiotic division through the pre-leptotene phase[49] and replicate their DNA for entry into meiosis thus transforming the oogonia into oocytes. During this transition a large attrition of oogonia occurs.[5] The signal for this transformation is unknown. By birth all the oogonia have progressed to various stages of the first meiotic prophase.[49,129] Once the first meiotic division begins, no endocrine, or even gonadal-location, requirement for its continuation occurs.[37] By birth all of the oogonia that have survived have entered at least the diplotene and most the dictyate stage of the first meiotic division, and soon after birth all arrest at the dictyate stage. These small oocytes are the only source of oocytes available to the adult for recruitment into the growing and ovulation cycle.

During this phase the somatic cells in the gonad enclose individual oocytes forming "primordial follicles" that contain the oocyte without a zona pellucida enveloped in a complete basement membrane[5] and surrounded by a flattened layer of somatic cells (pre-granulosa cells). These follicles appear in the neonate and either degenerate over the lifetime of the female or enter the growing phase and may form Graafian follicles and potentially ovulate. We do not know the specific signals that initiate the growth of a primordial follicle. However, when the signals occur, growth resumes, the flattened somatic (squamous granulosa) cells proliferate, and the mass and volume of the oocyte increase dramatically.[49,100] This corresponds to an increased protein content.[123] During this phase of growth the follicle is known as a pre-antral follicle. The granulosa cells form three layers of cuboidal cells with the recruitment of mesechymal-derived cells.[5,129] During this phase of oocyte growth, the zona pellucida is laid down and the oocyte increases in size by about 300 times, the granulosa cells proliferate, and an antrum forms in the follicle which contains the oocyte surrounded by two or more layers of granulosa cells. The layers closest to the oocyte become columnar in shape and are known as the corona radiata. This structure is the Graafian follicle or antral follicle. The ovary contains pools of these fully grown and growing or nongrowing oocytes all arrested in prophase of the first meiotic cell division. Only the fully grown oocytes can resume meiosis.

As the oocyte grows, its metabolism changes. The germinal vesicle increases in size, altering the nuclear to cytoplasmic ration. The few nucleoli that are present also increase in size, indicative of ribosomal-RNA synthesis.[8] Dramatic changes in the ultrastructure of the mitochondria occur. Oocyte growth is characterized by a change from elongated mitochondria with many transverse cisternae and a single vacuole to round and oval-shaped mitochondria with columnar-shaped cisterna and containing vacuoles.[8,9] The golgi change in activity and structure and the cortical granules, small membrane-bound vesicles involved in fertilization, move to the subcorticle region of the growing oocyte.[10] The number of ribosomes also increases dramatically as the oocyte grows.[21]

During follicle growth, a network of capillaries appears connected with the follicle and the thecal cells differentiate into distinct layers: the theca interna which are steroidogenic cells, and the theca externa which are connective tissues. Thus, the granulosa and thecal cells of the fully formed follicle are specialized with specific functions that include acting as receptors for follicle stimulating hormone (FSH), luteinizing hormone (LH), and the steroidogenic enzymes necessary for the synthesis of progesterone, androgens, and estradiol.[5,143]

Oocytes in primordial and pre-antral follicles cannot resume meiosis.[126] However, during the growing phase the molecules required for the initiation of meiosis are synthesized. Once the oocyte is fully grown (in the antral follicle) it can undergo meiotic maturation which involves nuclear progression from the dictyate stage of the first meiotic prophase to metaphase II of the second meiotic division (first meiotic reduction) forming an unfertilized egg. Only these oocytes can be fertilized and develop normally. The granulosa cells adjacent to the oocyte (cumulus cells) secrete hyaluronic acid in a process known as cumulus expansion or mucification. The granulosa cells in the follicle wall transform to produce the corpus luteum after the oocyte has been ovulated. *In vivo*, these events are stimulated by FSH and the LH surge. The gap junctions between the follicle wall, cumulus cells, and the oocyte are essential for oocyte maturation.[48] Oocyte maturation with germinal vesicle breakdown occurs when the flow of meiosis arresting substances to the oocyte via the gap junctions decreases. Researchers postulate that the granulosa cells produce a substance that overcomes the meiosis arresting action of cAMP[48] which is stimulated by either FSH or epidermal growth factor. Research also indicates that the gap junctions do not entirely disappear as the oocyte matures. During the growth phase of the oocyte both nuclear and cytoplasmic maturation must proceed in a coordinated manner for the successful development of the mature oocyte and subsequent fertilization. Either can proceed without the other, but the resulting oocytes, even if they are fertilized and embryonic development ensues, generally are not viable.[49,51,126] Nuclear maturation includes the resumption of the first meiotic division and progression to metaphase II. Cytoplasmic maturation encompasses all the events that prepare an oocyte for successful fertilization such as zona pellucida acquisition, ability to release calcium and cortical granules, mitochondrial changes, protein synthesis during the growing phase, and cytoskeletal changes.[8-10,49]

After ovulation, surrounded by the cumulus cells which have been its source of nutrition, growth stimulators (cAMP), and hormones, the oocyte enters the oviduct. As the ovulated oocyte completes maturation, the microvilli that extend from the cumulus cells in order to "feed" the oocyte are withdrawn. These cells remain around the oocyte until after fertilization and in the mouse can still be found associated with the embryo until near the end of the first cleavage division. The cumulus cells metabolize glucose and produce pyruvate[41] which the early embryo uses in an obligatory manner.[23] The cumulus cells also produce progesterone and estrogen, and they can act as both a buffer to the oviduct environment and as a specialized culture environment for the developing embryo.[68] Sperm that have traveled up from the cervix penetrate the cumulus layer, attach to the oocyte, and proceed with fertilization.

The oviduct provides a dynamic and complex environment for the gametes and resulting embryos.[91] The composition of the oviduct fluid is different from plasma and varies with the stage of the reproductive cycle and the region of the oviduct.[24,25,92] For example, at the time of ovulation only 0.3 to 0.5 mM glucose appears in the oviduct[61] in contrast with serum (5.5 mM) and other parts of the reproductive tract such as the uterus (3.5 to 5.0 mM).[91] The oviduct contains a preponderance of ciliated epithelial cells at the ampulla with a gradation to more nonciliated forms in the isthmus.[93,110] The cilia move the oocytes and embryos continually, functioning as a mixing system and moving metabolites, proteins, byproducts, growth factors, and hormones.[95] The embryo is separated from the rest of its environment by the zona pellucida and it is not in direct contact with any other cells in the oviduct.

The embryo begins to divide as it moves down the oviduct towards the uterus. In humans the embryo enters the uterus at the morula stage which is approximately 3 days after fertilization (72 hours or 96 hours after ovulation). At the morula stage the embryo begins to differentiate, forming tight junctions and two cell lines, innermost cells that will form the innercell mass, and outer cells that will form the trophectoderm. The embryo movement into the uterus also coincides with new protein formation, with an increase in embryo size, and with the initiation of glycolysis. As the embryo begins to cavitate it interacts more with the environment, actively taking up water and expanding. After 2 additional days (at 110 hours after fertilization) the zona pellucida disappears and implantation begins, providing a receptive endometrium exists for the blastocyst.

The endometrium changes through the cycle in response to endocrine factors, characterized by numerous biochemical, cellular, and molecular events.[114,128] The blastocyst stimulates site specific changes[114] making a part of the endometrium receptive to the implanting blastocyst.[101] The time during which a blastocyst can stimulate changes in the endometrium is referred to as the "implantation window." The endometrium remains unresponsive to the blastocyst before and after this implantation window. Human embryos implant in a manner similar to that seen in rhesus monkeys utilizing "intrusion penetration,"[47] characterized by the syncytiotrophoblast cells penetrating the surface epithelial cells, the gap junctions breaking down, and the gap junctions reforming with the surface epithelial cells. The trophoblast cells interpose themselves between the epithelial cells without the apoptosis or sloughing off of the epithelium[101] seen in other species such as the mouse and rat.[128]

Thus, from primordial follicle to implanting blastocyst many systems, located in different parts of the reproductive system with different growth patterns, requirements, and cellular interactions are involved. *In vitro* culture for any of the oocyte and embryo stages should reflect systems specifically designed to accomplish the growth or maturational events occurring during that particular sequence of events. An understanding of the metabolism of the oocyte and embryo also could aid in developing systems for these media refinements.

III. OOCYTE AND EMBRYO METABOLISM, METABOLIC CONTROLS, AND *IN VITRO* CULTURE

A. OOCYTES: METABOLISM

We know little about the metabolism of the primordial and early growing follicle although researchers assume that these follicles use oxidative phosphorylation or the pentose phosphate shunt for metabolic needs. Because the oocyte is surrounded by the ovarian tissue and follicle cells *in vivo*, the metabolism of the oocyte cannot be measured directly or separated from that of the follicle cells. Further, once isolated from the ovary, the surrounding cells' metabolic requirements must be met in order to keep the oocyte viable. In the early stages of development the follicle utilizes oxidative phosphorylation to generate energy for growth. The ultrastructure of the mitochondria in the oocyte changes through development, as described above, transforming from an elongated organelle containing transverse cisternae and a single vacuole to a round and oval-shaped structure with columnar-shaped cisterna and containing vacuoles.[8,9] Investigators assume that the oocyte also utilizes oxidative phosphorylation during the early growing phases.

As the follicle reaches the pre-antral and antral stages of development, the blood supply, and therefore oxygen supply, become vital for normal development. Indirect evidence for this is the fact that oocytes derived from follicles with aberrant capillary development are nonviable.[67,71] A hypoxic environment in the developing follicle also has been associated with decreased fertilization and implantation rates and increased spindle defects and chromosomal anomalies in human oocytes.[133] Further, mature metaphase II oocytes with disorganized cytoplasm appear to have a lower cystolic pH and ATP content than oocytes with normal appearing cytoplasm.[134,135] This is associated with a state of hypoxia in the follicle.[133] The levels of vascular endothelial growth factor, which will stimulate angiogenesis and therefore blood and oxygen supply to the follicle, appear lower in underoxgenated follicles. Dissolved oxygen concentrations below 2% were inconsistent with oocyte normality, and concentrations ranging from 3 to 5% correspond to high incidence of normality. Van Blerkom et al.[134] also have shown that oocytes with low ATP levels (<0.2 pmol) fail to develop normally and establish successful pregnancies. Low ATP levels presumably reflect a lowered or compromised metabolism specifically at the level of oxidative phosphorylation. Taken together these data suggest that the developing oocyte and follicle rely on oxidative phosphorylation, and disruption or depressions in metabolism adversely affect the subsequent embryo.

The first major regulatory enzyme in glycolysis is hexokinase (see below). Human[130] and mouse[27,38] oocytes have low levels of hexokinase activity which further suggests preovulatory oocytes do not use glycolysis for metabolism, but rely on oxidative phosphorylation for energy generation. Glucose 6-phosphate dehydrogenase activity, the first enzyme in the pentose phosphate shunt, is high in mouse oocytes,[39] but the activity of 6-phosphogluconate dehydrogenase, the next metabolic enzyme, was very low[38] indicating that the pentose phosphate shunt is probably not a means of energy generation in oocytes. Further, isolated oocytes from both the mouse and the rhesus monkey preferentially use pyruvate,[23,96] again suggesting they rely on oxidative phosphorylation for energy needs.

B. Oocytes: *In Vitro* Maturation and Culture

The recovery, maturation, and fertilization of immature oocytes with resultant embryo development and implantation has been achieved in a number of species. Currently the starting point, whether it be primordial/pre-antral or antral stage oocytes, dictates procedural success. The ideal situation would be to harvest and mature primordial follicles *in vitro* since they make up the majority of the oocytes in the ovary at any one time. This stage of oocyte produces minimal success and so far is limited to the mouse,[50] Pre-antral and antral stage oocytes/follicles yielded better success with live young in the bovine, mouse, and human models. The disadvantage of using these larger oocytes and follicles in humans is the limited number at any point in the ovary due to follicular atresia.

In a human, a primordial follicle takes approximately 85 days to grow into the antral stage. During this time the changes in the cell types, described above, take place. A culture system that will take a primordial follicle to the stage where the oocyte acquires both nuclear and cytoplasmic competence is inherently complex. Development of systems that can mature oocytes *in vitro* is still experimental with many of the basic physical and metabolic problems unresolved.[71,120]

The isolation of follicles containing immature oocytes from the ovary generally is performed using enzyme digestion with some mechanical separation. The isolated follicles can be grown in suspension to ensure a spherical development, or on a base with attachment. It is still unclear which method will give the best results. Many media systems test for follicle cultures with all having gonadotropin supplementation to aid in maturational events.

The *in vitro* maturation and culture of pre-antral and antral stage human oocytes has been accomplished successfully in a number of laboratories. The oocytes produced have been fertilized, grown to cleavage stages, and subsequently transferred with resulting pregnancies. Oocytes have been obtained from both stimulated and nonstimulated ovaries. Oocytes retrieved from unstimulated ovaries generally are recovered between days 9 and 11 of the menstral cycle. Follicles that have begun the growth phase and attained the size of approximately 2 mm are thus visible on ultrasound and aspirated. Clinicians separate oocyte-cumulus complexes from the other ovarian tissue and culture them in a tissue culture medium such as Medium 199 or alpha essential medium containing fetal calf or human serum.[13,76] Typically these media will be supplemented with FSH, hCG, pyruvate, and antibiotics. Oocytes that proceed to the metaphase II stage can then be inseminated conventionally or fertilized more efficiently using intracytoplasmic sperm injection.

Due to the paucity of follicles in a human ovary compared to experimental animal models, *in vitro* maturation and culture of oocytes provides an inefficient method of assisting patients in achieving a pregnancy. Until a system can be developed that cultures and matures many follicles *in vitro* with correct cytoplasmic and nuclear maturation this technique will not be offered on a broad clinical scale.

Only a well-defined and dynamic system can meet the needs of the complex, developing follicle.

C. EMBRYOS: METABOLISM AND CULTURE

Recent developments in embryo culture indicate that, among other factors, glucose, inorganic phosphate, glutamine, EDTA, and amino acids play vital and connected roles in both the developmental blocks and retardation *in vitro* when an acellular culture system is used.[15,33,61,72,82,86,87,95,115,124,127] Understanding how these alterations affect embryo development *in vitro* could lead to the design of improved culture systems.

1. Glucose and Inorganic Phosphate

Recent evidence demonstrates that certain combinations of energy substrates and/or ions in embryo culture media contribute to the *in vitro* blocks and developmental retardation. Glucose and inorganic phosphate have been implicated in the developmental blocks of mouse,[31,33,87,124] hamster,[16,121,122,125] rat,[82,106] and human[54,115,116] embryos.

The concentration of glucose used in most embryo culture media was originally 5.0 to 5.5 mM, which is equivalent to that reported for the female reproductive tract.[24,25,91] More recent studies[59,61] show that the concentration of glucose in the oviduct at the time of ovulation is between 0.3 and 0.5 mM. Merely removing glucose from medium for the early stages of culture in a number of strains of mouse embryos overcame the 2-cell block.[31,33,124]

The concentration of inorganic phosphate in various regions of the oviduct falls between 3.90 mM (ampulla) and 8.46 mM (isthmus) in the mouse[119] and between 5.84 mM and 11.07 mM in human tubal fluid.[24] This concentration is considerably higher than that found in any culture media used for embryos and may be more in line with that found in serum (0.4 mM). The removal of inorganic phosphate from culture medium containing glucose overcomes the developmental blocks of mouse embryos.[87,124] These results contradict the concentrations of inorganic phosphate present in the oviduct to which the embryo would be subject. However, the possibility exists that high inorganic phosphate concentrations coupled with the high glucose concentrations generally found in media cause an imbalance between glycolysis and oxidative phosphorylation. Lowering the concentration of inorganic phosphate to that found in serum (0.4 mM) rather than the oviduct (3 to 10 mM) conveyed benefit on mouse embryos from a wide variety of strains, with or without glucose (Scott and Whittingham, unpublished).

Quinn et al.[115] demonstrated an increased rate of development of mouse and human embryos in a medium based on original Tyrode's[139] in which only 0.37 mM inorganic phosphate and 2.78 mM glucose (HTF medium) occurred. This inorganic phosphate concentration was one fourth of that found in most other media in use at that time (0.8 to 1.4 mM). Utilizing the system described by Chatot et al. (glucose free for the first 2 days of culture),[33] FitzGerald and DiMattina achieved increased human blastocyst formation.[54] More recently, increased blastocyst development, increased implantation, and increased delivery rates have been reported using a medium devoid of both glucose and inorganic phosphate for the complete *in vitro* fertilization and culture of human embryos.[116] A sequential, serum-free medium system, with a step from 0.3 mM to 3.15 mM glucose and 0.5 mM inorganic phosphate also increased blastocyst development, implantation rates, and delivery rates.[60]

The effects of glucose and inorganic phosphate on early embryo development most likely result from imbalance and/or deregulation of certain metabolic functions when embryos are placed in the artificial environment *in vitro*.

Ovulated oocytes arrest at metaphase II of the second meiotic division. Downs et al.[42] demonstrated that glucose is necessary for the resumption of meiosis in cumulus-enclosed mouse oocytes *in vitro*. Summers et al.[127] showed that *in vitro* fertilization and mouse embryo development benefited from a medium (KSOM) containing 5.5 mM glucose and 0.35 mM inorganic phosphate. Research also shows that glucose facilitates fertilization in the mouse and that nonmetabolized analogs of glucose could not substitute.[131] The action of glucose on this process occurred as hyperactivity ensued in the sperm, allowing them to penetrate the zona pellucida.[132] In a limited study, human fertilization was not affected by the lack of glucose in a tyrodes-based medium; however, researchers noted that the sperm velocity fell requiring an increased density of sperm for insemination.[115] Granulosa cells use glucose, converting it to pyruvate, which in turn can be used by the embryo.[41] Although there is a trend away from the use of glucose in human embryo culture media,[115,116] it is prudent, based on the above data, to include at least 0.3 to 0.5 mM glucose[60,61] in oocyte culture and insemination media to help cumulus cells and sperm in the process of fertilization.

Embryos primarily utilize pyruvate in early development, via oxidative phosphorylation.[35,66,70,96] The first cleavage division relies absolutely on pyruvate.[23] Glucose use begins at approximately the 8-cell/morula stage in human embryos.[66,97] Embryos use oxidative phosphorylation rather than glycolysis for energy production for two reasons. First, the complete reduction of glucose in anaerobic glycolysis generates a net of 2 molecules of ATP, whereas the use of one pyruvate molecule in the TCA cycle, with oxidative phosphorylation, generates 15 molecules of ATP. Thus, anaerobic glycolysis is an inefficient means of energy generation. The second limitation on the use of glycolysis by oocytes and embryos is that key allosteric regulatory enzymes of glycolysis are either nonfunctional (phosphofructokinase) or are inhibited and thus switch off glycolysis in the early stages of development (hexokinase).

The rate limiting steps in glycolysis are the feedback mechanism of glucose-6-phosphate on hexokinase,[75,142] the inhibition of phosphofructokinase by citrate (from the TCA cycle), and the inhibition of pyruvate kinase by fructose biphosphate and ATP.[104] Regulatory inhibition or lack of enzyme expression could explain some of the observed effects of glucose and inorganic phosphate on embryo development. This has been shown in mouse embryos where an excessive production of lactate, indicating a loss of glycolytic control, was associated with nonviability.[63] When the lactate production of human blastocysts was measured, those with normal glycolytic activity had a fourfold increase in implantation rate compared to those selected at random.[60]

The first point of glucose regulation by an embryo is uptake, which occurs either through passive transport down concentration gradients or through facilitative uptake using specific transporter molecules.[96] Facilitative glucose uptake is mediated by a family of glucose transporters that are highly homologous, membrane-associated proteins.[20,80] Fetal tissue relies predominantly on GLUT-1 for all its glucose uptake. Research shows that mouse embryos contain at least one type of facilitative glucose transporter which is operational from the 1-cell stage onward.[62] Research also indicates, at both the gene expression[73] and protein level,[2] that mouse oocytes and all the preimplantation embryonic states do contain the glucose transporter GLUT-1. We can assume that human oocytes and embryos also express GLUT-1. Facilitative glucose uptake can be blocked utilizing the compound phloretin.[62] The use of phloretin in medium containing 2.78 mM glucose overcame the glucose-inorganic phosphate mediated 2-cell block in certain strains of mouse embryos,[124] indicating that at least some of the reported effects of glucose and inorganic phosphate on embryo development could result from uncontrolled uptake when they are placed in unphysiologic concentrations of glucose (5 mM compared with 0.3 to 0.5 mM in the oviduct). The reduction or removal of either or both glucose and inorganic phosphate from culture media for the early stages of development in human IVF may afford the embryos the same benefit reported for mouse, hamster, and rat embryos.

Once glucose has entered the cell it is rapidly and irreversibly phosphorylated to form glucose-6-phosphate (G6P) by the enzyme hexokinase, the first site of glycolytic control. Of the four isozymes of hexokinase (Types I–IV) three (Types I–III) are under allosteric regulation by their product, G6P.[142] Type I hexokinase is found in most tissue, is primarily responsible for introducing glucose into metabolism and into the TCA cycle for energy production, and is the isotype predominantly found in embryos.[75] The inhibition of hexokinase by G6P halts in the presence of inorganic phosphate since both products bind at the same site on the enzyme.[46] However, at concentrations greater than 3 mM, as found in the oviduct (3.9 to 11.07 mM), inorganic phosphate inhibits hexokinase Type I.[142] Thus, the concentration of inorganic phosphate most often found in culture media (1 to 1.8 mM) could be removing the allosteric inhibition of hexokinase by G6P. Concentrations of phosphate greater than 2 mM, as found in some media (B2 medium, 2.27 mM) may be beneficial. However, in a mouse system, with or without glucose, increasing inorganic phosphate concentrations (up to 2 mM) resulted in a decrease of blastocyst formation even in an F2 strain, normally not experiencing developmental blocks (Scott and Whittingham, unpublished). Reduced inorganic phosphate concentrations (0.5 mM), coupled with a low glucose concentration for the early stages of development, resulted in increased development of human embryos.[60]

Inorganic phosphate (Pi) is usually taken up in the form of HPO_4. We know that cells differ in their permeability to inorganic phosphate in vitro,[77] that this uptake reacts to the presence or concentrations of other substances,[84,113] and that phosphate levels can affect the uptake of other substances.[29] Embryos in vitro may lack a mechanism to regulate Pi uptake or cytosolic Pi concentrations leading to internal concentrations that remove the allosteric inhibition of hexokinase. Although the embryo cannot proceed with glycolysis until phosphofructokinase is functional, the imbalance caused by hexokinase activity could lead to developmental blocks and retardation of development.

Embryos rely on hexokinase Type I.[75] The activity level of hexokinase increases progressively from the oocyte stage to the blastocyst stage with activity increasing dramatically at the morula stage,[74] at which point glucose uptake and utilization increases in both mouse and human embryos. This dramatic increase of hexokinase activity lags by approximately 12 hours in embryos cultured *in vitro*, presumably due to culture-related retardation of development.

The most important point of glycolysis regulation is the second allosteric enzyme, 6-phosphofructokinase which is inhibited by high concentrations of ATP, citrate, and isocitrate, end products of the TCA cycle. As oxidative phosphorylation leads to a high ATP/ADP ratio, phosphofructokinase will be inhibited when a cell uses oxidative phosphorylation under aerobic conditions to produce energy. This in itself is a control mechanism since the overproduction of these products in the TCA cycle will inhibit glycolysis and therefore reduce the amount of pyruvate resulting from glucose in glycolysis for entry into the TCA cycle. However, phosphofructokinase activity does not begin in embryos until the morula stage of development,[11,12,95,137] thus glycolysis cannot proceed beyond this point, regardless of metabolic controls. If glucose uptake is not regulated and sufficient inorganic phosphate occurs in the system to inhibit the allosteric inhibition of hexokinase by G6P, the embryo could be compromised, having an unphysiological build-up of fructose-6-phosphate, which cannot be further metabolized until the morula stage.

This glucose and inorganic phosphate could interact at the level of glucose uptake and deregulation of hexokinase inhibition, causing an imbalance in the embryo leading to developmental retardation and arrest. After the morula stage, when phosphofructokinase is active, a surge in glycolytic activity would occur, utilizing the fructose-6-phosphate. Increased glycolytic activity in early blastocysts has been associated with low implantation rates in human embryos.[60]

Embryos primarily use pyruvate in the TCA cycle and oxidative phosphorylation for energy requirements. Pyruvate dehydrogenase is a complex of three enzymes: pyruvate dehydrogenase, dihydrolipoamide acetyltransferase, and dihydrolipoamide reductase attached to the inner mitochondrial wall.[109] In addition, two other regulatory enzymes occur within the complex, pyruvate dehydrogenase kinase and pyruvate dehydrogenase phosphase. The reaction is unidirectional and driven by pyruvate. The reaction slows with high levels of ATP through the phosphorylation of the enzyme complex by one of the regulatory enzymes, pyruvate dehydrogenase kinase, which inhibits the production of Acetyl CoA thus depressing the TCA cycle. The pyruvate dehydrogenase moiety is phosphorylated to form the inactive "b" form, turning off the entire complex. When the ADP concentration is high, the pyruvate dehydrogenase complex activates by dephosphorylation of the "b" form to the "a" form by pyruvate dehydrogenase phosphatase. Physiologic levels of inorganic phosphate can protect pyruvate dehydrogenase from the inactivation by ATP.[34] However, the activity of pyruvate dehydrogenase decreases proportionally with phosphate concentration from 0 to 10 mM.[83,111] Thus, a reduction or absence of inorganic phosphate ions in culture media in the initial stages of development could improve pyruvate utilization. The inhibition of pyruvate dehydrogenase also depends on the presence of potassium ions, the absence of which negates the inhibitory effects of high phosphate concentration. In a commonly used medium for IVF (HTF),[115] increased K+ ion concentration occurs, but reduced inorganic phosphate and glucose concentrations accompany them. The authors attributed the increased development to the increased K+ concentration. However, this is inconsistent with the explanation of the K+/inorganic phosphate inhibition of the pyruvate dehydrogenase complex. The benefits of HTF medium probably result from its reduced inorganic phosphate and glucose concentrations compared to other media.

The bicarbonate concentration in cells also influences the regulation of pyruvate dehydrogenase activity.[118] The effect is indirect in that bicarbonate compels citrate to exit the mitochondria which increases citrate synthase activity, lowering the concentration of Acetyl CoA which in turn stimulates pyruvate dehydrogenase activity to form more Acetyl CoA. Intracellular pH changes can occur with different concentrations of bicarbonate buffer which have been shown to affect embryo development.[7,30] Further, mouse embryos cultured without bicarbonate-CO_2 have poor to no developmental potential[117,139] and hamster embryos suffer from significant reduction in developmental competence when exposed to HEPES buffer, because of the lack of bicarbonate-CO_2[52] which could be inhibiting the pyruvate dehydrogenase activity. One should therefore limit the use of HEPES buffered media in human IVF since human embryos use pyruvate preferentially in the first cleavage divisions.[94,97,137]

Changing the culture environment in accordance with the embryo's developmental requirements[64,103] or providing energy substrates[28] overcomes the 2-cell block and increases development *in vitro* of mouse embryos. Recent evidence shows that this system can be used effectively for the development of human blastocysts with resultant high implantation and pregnancy rates.[60] This is a logical course considering the dynamic nature of the *in vitro* environment complex character of the embryo as it develops.

In conclusion, oocyte preincubation and insemination media should contain both glucose and inorganic phosphate, but in lower concentrations than found in most conventional culture media. Concentrations of 0.5 mM glucose and 0.3 mM inorganic phosphate have proven effective in mouse embryo culture (Scott and Whittingham, unpublished)[64] and in humans (G1/G2 culture media).[60] This same formulation should be used for the early developmental stages. Once the embryo begins to compact and phosphofructokinase is active, an increase in glucose concentration to a physiological concentration of approximately 3 mM should provide the embryo with sufficient glucose for glycolysis initiation.

2. EDTA and Glutamine

EDTA use in human embryo culture media came from the reports of its benefit in overcoming the 2-cell block of various strains of mouse embryos. Abramczuk et al.[1] first reported that the addition of 0.11 mM EDTA to Whitten's medium (5.56 mM glucose, 1.19 mM inorganic phosphate)[138] overcame the 2-cell block in random bred mouse embryos. The extent of blastocyst formation depended on both embryo age at collection and EDTA concentration, with approximately 0.1 mM giving maximum development. Nasr-Esfahani et al.[108] also reported increased development of random bred mouse embryos through the 2-cell block in a medium that had 5.55 mM glucose, 0.39 mM inorganic phosphate, and a number of cation chelating agents. Other reports indicate that amino acids can perform a similar function to EDTA.[53,105]

EDTA action stems from its ability to chelate cations that may appear in the culture system. These cations, such as iron, are thought to function as co-factors in the conversion of reactive oxygen species into free radicals. Mouse embryos that suffer *in vitro* developmental blocks have transient rises in reactive oxygen species at the 2-cell stage[98,108] that are though to be converted into the toxic free radicals, causing loss of cell function, damage to cell membranes, and prevention of cell division.[3] Fissore et al.[53] showed that EDTA or proteins could act equally as well as protectants in an Earl's Balanced Salt solution. The addition of EDTA and selected amino acids to medium increased implantation and fetal development after *in vitro* fertilization of mouse embryos.[105] EDTA use (0.01 mM) in human embryo culture media has been widely adopted, has had no detrimental effects on fertilization or implantation rates, and is recommended while serum continues as a fixed nitrogen source in IVF.

Glutamine is becoming a common component of human embryo culture media in general and is an additive in certain complex media used for human IVF (Hams F10, Hams F12, B2 media). Researchers added glutamine to mouse embryo culture media as an alternative energy source in glucose-free media.[33] Investigations show that mouse embryos grown without glutamine have reduced abilities to grow to the blastocyst stage and have a significantly reduced internal store of glutamine.[136] Further, when culture medium is supplemented with essential amino acids, glutamine enhances mouse blastocyst formation *in vitro*.[85] The nonessential amino acids (alanine, asparagine, aspartate, glycine, proline, serine, and glutamine) are the most beneficial to embryos *in vitro*.[85]

Glutamine can counteract the inhibitory effects of glucose on mouse embryos in the presence of inorganic phosphate,[4] and the negative effects that high sodium ion concentrations have on embryos by acting as an organic osmolyte.[88] It is an important ingredient in the culture media used for a number of cell systems including mouse[32,124] and hamster[121,122] embryos. Researchers speculate that glutamine could be used by the embryos as a more accessible energy substrate, thus allowing the embryo sufficient metabolic activity for continued growth through the early developmental blocks.

No negative effects of these media additives appear, but many positive effects occur on embryo development, especially in the post-implantation phase. A limited study showed increased human embryo development, blastocyst formation, and implantation rates using a Tyrode's-based medium supplement with both EDTA and glutamine. Further, when this supplemented medium had the glucose and inorganic phosphate removed, further increases in pregnancy rates occurred.[115] Coupled with a decrease in glucose concentration for the early stages of development, the addition of EDTA and glutamine to media could benefit the embryos.

3. Other Ingredients

Certain media marketed for human embryo development contain taurine. Taurine has been shown to overcome the 2-cell block in mouse embryos grown in a Tyrode's-based medium, but this beneficial effect was limited to the first cleavage division.[43,44] Hamster embryos grown *in vitro* have an absolute requirement for hypotaurine, which is a precursor for taurine.[14] Both taurine and hypotaurine inhibit Na+/K+-ATPases. The Na+/K+-ATPases are only active at low levels in the early stages of embryo development, but increase to high levels at the morula to blastocyst stage.[58] At the blastocyst stage, its activity can be linked to the active uptake of water into the blastocoel[22,141] and amino acid transport into the blastocyst.[40] Throughout development, the prime function of ATPase is to regulate the intracellular concentrations of electrolytes. When embryos are taken out of the oviduct environment, this enzyme system deregulates, resulting in an electrolyte imbalance. This imbalance leads to a block or retardation in development. If the activity of the Na+/K+-ATPases is inhibited[6] these imbalances may not occur resulting in alleviation of the developmental blocks.[43,44] However, once the embryo requires water uptake, inhibition of the ATPase is detrimental. This problem is taken into account in a 2-step culture system which results in both increased blastocyst development and implantation rates in a human IVF program.[60] Investigators recommend that the addition of taurine to culture media remain limited to the first 48 h of culture, at a concentration of approximately 0.1 mM.[60]

Water transport into the embryo occurs passively through water channels and also down ion gradients. The water channels provide a source of passive entry for metabolites such as glucose and ions. Both Na+ and Cl– are important in maintaining and driving the osmotic gradient and facilitating water entry into the embryos. At the blastocyst stage the embryo accumulates water in a manner that is driven by the Na+ generated ion gradient.[102] Both Na+ and K+ ions have been implicated in the 2-cell block of mouse embryos.[86–88] *In vivo* embryos exist in a colloidal suspension of macromolecules, metabolites, salts, etc. The water is bound up and is thus not available to the embryo.[56] Water also can be accumulated by the blastocyst in an attempt to take up protein.[112] Embryos actively take up protein by pinocytosis.[8] When embryos are cultured without protein, they take up water more quickly which could upset the balance of ions and other constituents of the blastocoelic fluid. One must design a culture medium to meet this stage specific requirement of embryos, adding amino acids or protein to the system at the time the embryos would normally take it up for *de novo* synthesis of new protein. Researchers also suggest that amino acids can serve as regulators of the internal pH of embryos.[18,19]

Additionally, the embryo is subjected to, and in contact with, different hormones and growth factors within the oviduct and uterine environment. Adding insulin to culture media containing BSA increased embryo development and cell numbers,[72] indicating that without certain factors embryos could be compromised. The blastocyst stage embryo differentiates and grows dramatically, and *in vitro* embryos in this stage appear dramatically different from those isolated from *in vivo*. Investigators speculate that the addition of growth factors to culture media will benefit this stage of development, increasing the inner cell mass and increasing implantation and post-implantation development.[99]

During development embryos change in their *in vitro* requirements. One-cell and early cleavage stage embryos can develop adequately in simple media without any fixed nitrogen source and with only pyruvate as an energy substrate. However, the morula and blastocyst stages require a more complex environment which could reflect their more complex structure, metabolism, and stage of differentiation. This would indicate that the embryo changes in its needs, its form, and its rate of metabolism as it grows. Based on a knowledge of the mechanisms, regulations, and inhibition of metabolism and the empirical data gathered thus far, the possibility exists for a series of media that can meet the needs of all stages of embryo development.

4. Co-Culture

Co-culture as a means of increasing implantation and pregnancy rates and for human embryo development to the blastocyst stage receives much attention. However, a monolayer of feeder cells is not the equivalent of the complex and changing environment of the oviduct.[17,91] Many problems occur in the use of cell lines for co-culture. The cell lines may introduce harmful byproducts of metabolism into the medium; the medium and substrate requirements for the feeder cells could be different from those of embryos; cell lines must be maintained in long term cultures which can lead to contamination and the need for high concentrations and complex mixtures of antibiotics. Further, these cell lines may have widely different requirements from those of embryos. The results of embryo transfers in many species show that embryos derived from culture in systems devoid of feeder cells and their "factors" are viable and develop into viable offspring. Many of the cell lines that have provided the most benefit to embryos are derived from cattle or sheep sources, are not well characterized for viruses or other infectious agents, and are not standardized. Vero cells, which are a source of feeder cells that are well defined, immortal, and pathogen free, specifically derived for the production of human vaccines, have not proved as beneficial. When the rate of blastocyst formation and delivery rates per oocyte retrieval are compared between co-culture and standard culture systems utilizing day 1, 2, 3, 5, or 6 embryo transfers, no differences in pregnancy or delivery rates appear. The most benefit afforded to embryos is the development of a system specifically designed to meet their metabolic needs at each developmental stage, as shown by Gardner et al.,[60] in which both the rate of blastocyst formation and implantation can be increased with the use of a step culture system.

IV. CONCLUSIONS

The development of human oocytes and embryos *in vitro* requires a complex and changing series of culture media designed to meet the requirements of each developmental stage, primarily from a metabolic standpoint. Because *in vitro* aqueous systems are so different from the *in vivo* environment, understanding how controls in the metabolic pathways function can help in the design of media. Research interest increases in blastocyst development *in vitro* for increasing pregnancy rates, aiding in our ability to select more viable embryos and to reduce higher order multiple pregnancies without compromising pregnancy rates. This requires the development of media systems finely tuned to human embryo development. Blastocysts formed *in vitro* are very different from those formed *in vivo*[65] which may be due to a lack of growth factors or certain amino acids.[79] More work needs to be done on the requirements of the compacting embryo, specific growth factors required for optimum development, a more natural suspension phase for the embryos as they are not actually in an aqueous environment *in vivo*, and better systems for selecting embryos that are viable. The culture and maturation of immature oocytes *in vitro* is an area that holds much promise for the future.

REFERENCES

1. Abramczuk, J., Solter, D., and Koprowski, H., The beneficial effect of EDTA on development of mouse one-cell embryos in chemically defined medium, *Dev. Biol.*, 618, 378–38, 1977.

2. Aghayan, M., Rao, L. V., Smith, R. M., Jarrett, L., Charron, M. J., Thorens, B., and Heyner, S., Developmental expression and cellular localization of glucose transporter molecules during mouse preimplantation development, *Development*, 115, 305–312, 1992.

3. Aitken, R. J., Clarkson, J. S., and Fishel, S., Generation of reactive oxygen species, lipid peroxidation and human sperm function, *Biol. Reprod.*, 41, 183–197, 1989.

4. Ali, J., Whitten, W. K., and Shelton, J. N., Effect of culture systems on mouse early embryo development, *Hum. Reprod.*, 8, 1110–1114, 1993.

5. Anderson, L. D. and Hirshfield, A. N., An overview of follicular development in the ovary: from embryo to the fertilized ovum *in vitro*, *Maryland Med. J.*, 41, 614–620, 1992.

6. Anner, B. M., The receptor function of the Na+, K+,-activated adenosine triphosphate system, *J. Biochem.*, 227, 1–11, 1985.

7. Bagger, P., Byskov, A., and Christiansen, M. D., Maturation of mouse oocytes *in vitro* is influenced by alkalisation during their isolation, *J. Reprod. Fertil.*, 80, 251–55, 1987.

8. Baker, T. and Franchi, L., The structure of the chromosomes in human primordial oocytes, *Chromasoma*, 22, 358–377, 1967.

9. Balakier, H., Induction of maturation in small oocytes from sexually immature mice by fusion with mitotic cells, *Exp. Cell Res.*, 112, 137–141, 1978.

10. Balakier, H. and Czolowska, R., Cytoplasmic control of nuclear maturation in mouse oocytes, *Exp. Cell Res.*, 110, 466–469, 1977.

11. Barbehenn, E. K., Wales, R. G., and Lowry, O. H., The explanation for the blockade of glycolysis in early mouse embryos, *Proc. Nat. Acad. Sci. USA*, 71, 1056–1060, 1974.

12. Barbehenn, E. K., Wales, R. G., and Lowry, O. H., Measurement of metabolites in single preimplantation embryos: a new means to study metabolic control in early embryos, *J. Embryol. Exp. Morphol.*, 43, 29–46, 1978.

13. Barnes, F., Kausche, A., Tiglias, J., Wood, C., Wilton, L., and Trounson, A. O., Production of embryos from *in vitro* matured primary human oocytes, *Fertil. Steril.*, 65, 1151–1156, 1996.

14. Barnett, D. K. and Bavister, B. D., Hypotaurine requirement for *in vitro* development of golden hamster one-cell embryos into morulae and blastocysts, and production of term offspring from *in vitro*-fertilized ova, *Biol. Reprod.*, 47, 297–304, 1992.

15. Barnett, D. K. and Bavister, B. D., What is the relationship between the metabolism of preimplantation embryos and their developmental competence?, *Mol. Reprod. Developmental.*, 43, 105–133, 1996a.

16. Barnett, D. K. and Bavister, B. D., What is the relationship between the metabolism of preimplantation embryos and their developmental competence?, *Mol. Reprod. Developmental.*, 43, 105–133, 1996b.

17. Bavister, B. D., Co-culture for embryo development: is it really necessary?, *Hum. Reprod.*, 7, 1339–1341, 1992.

18. Bavister, B. D., Culture of preimplantation embryos: facts and artifacts, *Hum. Reprod. Update*, 1, 91–148, 1995.

19. Bavister, B. D. and McKieran, S. H., Regulation of hamster embryo development *in vitro* by amino acids, in *Preimplantation Embryo Development*, Bavister, B. D., Ed., Springer-Verlag, New York, 57–72, 1993.

20. Bell, G. I., Kayano, J. B., Buse, C. F., Burant, J., Takeda, D., Lin, H., Fukumoto, S., and Seino, S. D. C., Molecular biology of mammalian glucose transporters, *Diabetes Care*, 13, 198, 1990.

21. Biggers, J. D., New observations on the nutrition of the mammalian oocyte and the preimplantation embryo, in *Biology of the Blastocyst*, University of Chicago Press, Chicago, IL, 1971, pp. 319–325.

22. Biggers, J. D., Bell, J. E., and Benbos, D. J., Mammalian blastocysts: transport functions in a developing epithelium, *Am. J. Physiol.*, 255, C419–C432, 1988.

23. Biggers, J. D., Whittingham, D. G., and Donahue, R. P., The pattern of energy metabolism in the mouse oocyte and zygote, *Proc. Nat. Acad. Sci. USA*, 58, 506–567, 1967.

24. Borland, R. M., Biggers, J. D., and Taymor, M. L., Elemental composition of fluid in the human fallopian tube, *J. Reprod. Fertil.*, 58, 479–482, 1980.

25. Borland, R. M., Hazra, S., Biggers, J. D., and Lechene, C. P., The elemental composition of the environment of the gametes and preimplantation embryo during the initiation of pregnancy, *Biol. Reprod.*, 16, 147–157, 1977.

26. Braude, P., Bolton, V., and Moore, S., Human gene expression first occurs between the four and eight-cell stages of preimplantation development, *Nature*, 332, 459–461, 1988.

27. Brinster, R. L., Hexokinase activity in the preimplantation mouse embryo, *Enzymologia*, 34, 304–308, 1968.

28. Brown, J. J. G. and Whittingham, D. G., The dynamic provision of different energy substrates improves development of one-cell random bred mouse embryos *in vitro*, *J. Reprod. Fertil.*, 95, 503–511, 1992.

29. Cardelli, P., Fcori, A., Santulli, M. C., Ceci, F., Salerno, C., Savi, M. R., Peresempio, V., and Strom, R., Effect of inorganic phosphate on hypoxanthine transport in isolated brain microvessels, *Biochem. Int.*, 28, 823–834, 1992.

30. Carney, E. W. and Bavister, B. D., Stimulatory and inhibitory effects of amino acids on development of hamster eight cell embryos *in vitro*, *J. In Vitro Fertil. Embryo Transfer*, 4, 162–167, 1987.

31. Chatot, C. L., Lewis, J. L., Torres, I., and Ziomek, C. A., Development of 1-cell embryos from different strains of mice in CZB medium, *Biol. Reprod.*, 42, 432–440, 1990.

32. Chatot, C. L., Tasca, R. J., and Ziomek, C. A., Glutamine uptake and utilization by preimplantation mouse embryos in CZB medium, *Biol. Reprod.*, 89, 335–346, 1990.
33. Chatot, C. L., Ziomek, C. A., Bavister, B. D., Lewis, J. L., and Torres, I., An improved culture medium supports the development of random-bred 1-cell mouse embryos *in vitro*, *J. Reprod. Fertil.*, 86, 679–688, 1989.
34. Chiang, P. K. and Sackor, B., Control of pyruvate dehydrogenase activity in intact cardiac mitochondria. Regulation of the inactivation and activation of the dehydrogenase, *J. Biological Chem.*, 250, 3399–3408, 1975.
35. Conaghan, J., Handyside, A. H., Winston, R. M. L., and Leese, H. J., Effects of pyruvate and glucose on the development of human preimplantation embryos *in vitro*, *J. Reprod. Fertil.*, 99, 87–95, 1993.
36. Dawson, K. J., Conaghan, J., Ostera, G. R., Winston, R. M. L., and Hardy, K., Delaying transfer to the third day post-insemination, to select non-arrested embryos, increases development to the fetal heart stage, *Hum. Reprod.*, 10, 177–182, 1995.
37. De Felici, M. and McLaren, A., Isolation of mouse primordial germ cells, *Exp. Cell Res.*, 142, 476–482, 1982.
38. De Schepper, G. G., Van Noorden, C. J. F., and Koperdraad, F., A cytochemical method for measuring enzyme activity in individual preovulatory mouse oocytes, *J. Reprod. Fertil.*, 74, 709–716, 1985.
39. De Schepper, G. G., Vander Perk, C., Westerveld, A., Oosting, J., and Van Noorden, C. J. F., *In situ* glucose-6-phosphate dehydrogenase activity during development of pre-implantation mouse embryos, *Histochem. J.*, 25, 299–303, 1993.
40. Di Zio, S. M. and Tasca, R. J., Sodium-dependent amino acid transport in preimplantation mouse embryos, *Dev. Biol.*, 59, 198–205, 1977.
41. Donahue, R. P. and Stern, S., Follicular cell support of oocyte maturation: production of pyruvate *in vitro*, *J. Reprod. Fertil.*, 17, 395–398, 1968.
42. Downs, S. M., Coleman, D. L., and Eppig, J. J., Maintenance of murine oocyte meiotic arrest: uptake and metabolism of hypoxanthine and adenosine by cumulus cell-enclosed and denuded mouse oocytes, *Dev. Biol.*, 117, 174–183, 1986.
43. Dumoulin, J. C. M., Evers, J. L. H., Bakker, J. A., Bras, M., Pieters, M. H. E. C., and Geraedts, J. P. M., Temporal effects of taurine on mouse preimplantation development *in vitro*, *Hum. Reprod.*, 403–407, 1992.
44. Dumoulin, J. C. M., Evers, J. L. H., Bras, M., Pieters, M. H. E. C., and Geraedts, J. P. M., Positive effect of taurine on preimplantation development of mouse embryos *in vitro*, *J. Reprod. Fertil.*, 94, 373–380, 1992.
45. Edwards, R. G., Steptoe, P. C., and Purdy, J. M., Establishing full term human pregnancies using cleaving embryos grown *in vitro*, *Br. J. Obstet. Gynaecol.*, 87, 737–575, 1980.
46. Ellison, W. R., Lueck, J. D., and Fromme, H. J., Studies on the mechanism of orthophosphate regulation of bovine brain hexokinase, *J. Biol. Chem.*, 250, 1864–1871, 1975.
47. Enders, A. C., Implantation, *Encyclopedia of Human Biology*, 4, 423–430, 1991.
48. Eppig, J. J., Maintenance of meiotic arrest and the induction of oocyte maturation in mouse oocyte-granulosa cell complexes developed *in vitro* from preantral follicles, *Biol. Reprod.*, 45, 824–830, 1991.
49. Eppig, J. J., O'Brien, M., and Wigglesworth, K., Mammalian oocyte growth and development *in vitro*, *Mol. Reprod. Dev.*, 44, 260–273, 1996.
50. Eppig, J. J. and O'Brien, M. J., Development of mouse oocytes from primordial follicles, *Biol. Reprod.*, 54, 197–207, 1996.

51. Eppig, J. J., Schultz, R. M., O'Brien, M., Chesnal, F., and Smith, A., Relationship between the developmental programs controlling nuclear and cytoplasmic maturation of mouse oocytes, *Dev. Biol.*, 164, 1–9, 1994.

52. Farrel, P. S. and Bavister, B. D., Short-term exposure of two-cell hamster embryos to collection media is detrimental to viability, *Biol. Reprod.*, 31, 109–114, 1984.

53. Fissore, R. A., Jackson, K. V., and Kiessling, A. A., Mouse zygote development in culture medium without protein in the presence of ethylene-diaminetetraacetic acid, *Biol. Reprod.*, 41, 835–841, 1989.

54. FitzGerald, L. and DiMattina, M., An improved medium for the long term culture of human embryos overcomes the developmental block and increases blastocyst formation, *Fertil. Steril.*, 641–647, 1992.

55. Flach, G., Johnson, M. H., Braude, P. R., Taylor, R. A. S., and Bolton, V, N The transition from maternal to embryonic control in the 2-cell mouse embryo, *EMBO J.*, 1, 681–686, 1982.

56. Franks, F., Solvation and conformational effects in aqueous solutions of biopolymer analogues, *Philos. Trans. R. Soc. London*, 278, 33–57, 1977.

57. Freeman, M. R., Whitsworth, C. M., and Hill, G. A., Granulosa cell co-culture enhances human embryo development and pregnancy rate following *in vitro* fertilization, *Hum. Reprod.*, 10, 408–414, 1995.

58. Gardiner, C. S., Williams, J. S., and Menino, A. R., Sodium/Potassium adenosine triphosphate a- and °-submit and a-submit mRNA levels during mouse embryo development *in vitro*, *Biol. Reprod.*, 43, 788–794, 1990.

59. Gardner, D. K., Lane, M., Calderon, I., and Leeton, J., Metabolite concentrations in human oviduct and uterine fluids throughout the menstrual cycle, *Proc. AFS*, 78, 1994.

60. Gardner, D. K. and Lane, M., Culture and selection of viable blastocysts: a feasible proposition for human IVF?, *Hum. Reprod. Update*, 832, 367–382, 1997.

61. Gardner, D. K., Lane, M., Calderon, I., and Leeton, J., Environment of the preimplantation embryo *in vivo*: metabolite analysis and uterine fluids and metabolism of cumulus cells, *Fertil. Steril.*, 65, 349–353, 1996.

62. Gardner, D. K. and Leese, H. J., The role of glucose and pyruvate transport in regulating nutrient utilization by preimplantation mouse embryos, *Development*, 104, 423–429, 1988.

63. Gardner, D. K. and Leese, H. J., Concentrations of nutrients in mouse oviduct fluid and their effects on embryo development and metabolism *in vitro*, *J. Reprod. Fertil.*, 88, 361–368, 1990.

64. Gardner, D. K. and Sakkas, D., Mouse embryo cleavage, metabolism and viability: role of medium composition, *Hum. Reprod.*, 8, 288–295, 1993.

65. Gonzales, D. S. and Bavister, B. D., Zona pellucida escape by hamster blastocysts *in vitro* is delayed and morphologically different compared with zona escape *in vivo*, *Biol. Reprod.*, 52, 470–480, 1995.

66. Gott, A. L., Hardy, K., Winston, R. M. L., and Leese, H. J., The nutrition and environment of the early human embryo, *Proc. Nutr. Soc.*, 49, 2A, 1990.

67. Gregory, L., Booth, A., Wells, C., and Walker, S., A study of the cumulus-corona cell complex in *in vitro* fertilization and embryo transfer: a prognostic indicator of the failure of implantation, *Hum. Reprod.*, 9, 1308–1317, 1994.

68. Gregory, L. and Leese, H. J., Determinants of oocyte and preimplantation embryo quality: metabolic requirements and the potential role of cumulus cells, *J. Br. Fertil. Soc.*, 1, 96–102, 1996.

69. Guerin, J. F. and Nicollet, B., Interest in co-cultures for embryos obtained by *in vitro* fertilization: a French collaborative study, *Hum. Reprod.*, 12, 1043–1046, 1997.

70. Hardy, K., Hooper, M. A. K., Handyside, A. H., Rutherford, A. J., Winston, R. M. I., and Leese, H. J., Non invasive measurement of glucose and pyruvate uptake by the individual human ova and preimplantation embryo, *Hum. Reprod.*, 4, 188–191, 1989.

71. Hartshorne, G., Steroid production by the cummulus: relationship to fertilization *in vitro*, *Hum. Reprod.*, 7, 742–745, 1989.

72. Harvey, M. B. and Kaye, P. L., Insulin stimulates protein synthesis in compacted mouse embryos, *Endocrinology*, 122, 1182–1184, 1988.

73. Hogan, A., Heyner, S., Charron, M. J., Copeland, N. G., Gilbert, D. J., Jenkins, N. A., Thorens, B., and Schultz, G. A., Glucose transporter gene expression in early mouse embryos, *Development*, 113, 363–372, 1991.

74. Hooper, M. A. K. and Leese, H. J., Activity of hexokinase in mouse oocytes and preimplantation embryos, *Biochem. Soc. Trans.*, 546–547, 1988.

75. Houghton, F. D., Sheth, B., Moran, B., Leese, H. J., and Fleming, T. P., Expression and activity of hexokinase in the early mouse embryo, *Mol. Hum. Reprod.*, 1, 793–798, 1996.

76. Hovatta, O., Silye, R., Abir, R., Krausz, T., and Winston, R. M. L., Extracellular matrix improves survival of both stored and fresh primordial ovarian follicles in long-term culture, *Hum. Reprod.*, 12, 1032–1036, 1997.

77. Ibsen, K. H. and Fox, J. P., Substrate modification of the Crabtree effect in Ehrlich ascites tumor cells, *Arch. Biochem. Biophys.*, 112, 580–585, 1965.

78. Janney, L. and Menezo, Y., Maternal age effect on early human embryonic development and blastocyst formation, *Mol. Reprod. Dev.*, 45, 31–37, 1996.

79. Kane, M. T., Morgan, P. M., and Coonan, C., Peptide growth factors and preimplantation development, *Hum. Reprod. Update*, 3, 137–157, 1997.

80. Kasanicki, M. A. and Pilch, P. F., Regulation of glucose transporter function, *Diabetes Care*, 13, 219–223, 1990.

81. Pemble, L. B. and Kaye, P. O., Whole protein uptake and metabolism by mouse blastocysts, *J. Reprod. Fertil.*, 78, 149–157, 1986.

82. Kishi, J., Noda, Y., Narimoto, K., Umaoka, Y., and Mori, T., Block to development in cultured rat 1-cell embryos is overcome using medium HECM-1, *Hum. Reprod.*, 6, 1445–1448, 1991.

83. Koobs, D. H., Phosphate mediation of the Crabtree and Pasteur effects, *Science*, 13, 127–133, 1972.

84. Kotyk, A., Interaction of 2-deoxy-D-glucose and adenosine with phosphate anion in yeast, *Folia Microbiologica*, 37, 401–403, 1992.

85. Lane, M. and Gardner, D. K., Increase in postimplantation development of cultured mouse embryos by amino acids and induction of fetal retardation and exencephaly by ammonium ions, *J. Reprod. Fertil.*, 102, 305–312, 1994.

86. Lawitts, J. A. and Biggers, J. D., Optimization of mouse embryo culture media using simplex methods, *J. Reprod. Fertil.*, 91, 543–556, 1991.

87. Lawitts, J. A. and Biggers, J. D., Overcoming the 2-cell block by modifying standard components in a mouse embryo culture medium, *Biol. Reprod.*, 45, 245–251, 1991.

88. Lawitts, J. A. and Biggers, J. D., Joint effects of sodium chloride, glutamine and glucose in mouse preimplantation embryo culture medium, *Mol. Reprod. Dev.*, 31, 189–194, 1992.

89. Lawrence, C. J., Hiken, J. F., and James, D. E., Stimulation of glucose transport and glucose transporter phosphorylation by oxadaic acid in rat adipocytes, *J. Biol. Chem.*, 265, 19768–19776, 1990.

90. Lawrence, J. C., Hiken, J. F., and James, D. E., Phosphorylation of the glucose transporter in rat adipocytes, *J. Biol. Chem.*, 265, 2324–2332, 1990.

91. Leese, H. J., The formation and function of oviduct fluid, *J. Reprod. Fertil.*, 82, 843–856, 1988.

92. Leese, H. J., Energy metabolism of the blastocyst and uterus at implantation, in *Blastocyst Implantation*, Yoshinaga, K., Ed., Adams Publishing Group, Boston, MA, 39–44, 1989.

93. Leese, H. J., The environment of the preimplantation embryo, in *Establishing a Successful Human Pregnancy*, Vol. 66, Edwards, R. G., Ed., 143–154, 1990.

94. Leese, H. J., Metabolism of the preimplantation mammalian embryo, in *Oxford Reviews of Reproductive Biology*, Vol. 13, Mulligan, S. R., Ed., Oxford University Press, 35–72, 1991.

95. Leese, H. J., Metabolic control during preimplantation mammalian development, *Hum. Reprod. Update*, 1, 63–72, 1995.

96. Leese, H. J. and Barton, A. M., Pyruvate and glucose uptake by mouse ova and preimplantation embryos, *J. Reprod. Fertil.*, 72, 9–13, 1984.

97. Leese, H. J., Conaghan, J., Martin, K. L., and Hardy, K., Early human embryo metabolism, *Bioessays*, 15, 259–264, 1993.

98. Legge, M. and Sellens, M. H., Free radical scavengers ameliorate the 2-cell block in mouse embryo culture, *Hum. Reprod.*, 6, 867–871, 1991.

99. Lighten, A. D., Moore, G. E., Winston, R. M. L., and Hardy, K., Routine addition of human insulin-like growth factor-1 ligand could benefit clinical *in vitro* fertilization culture, *Hum. Reprod.*, 13, 3144–3150, 1998.

100. Lintern-Moore, A. and Moore, G. P., The initiation of follicle and oocyte growth in the mouse ovary, *Biol. Reprod.*, 20, 773–778, 1979.

101. Lopata, A., Blastocyst-endometrial interaction: an appraisal of some old and new ideas, *Mol. Hum. Reprod.*, 2, 519–525, 1996.

102. Manejewala, F. M., Cragoe, E. J., and Schultz, R. M., Blastocoel expansion in the preimplantation mouse embryo: role of extracellular sodium and chloride and possible apical routes of their entry, *Dev. Biol.*, 133, 210–220, 1989.

103. Martin, K. L. and Leese, H. J., Role of glucose in mouse preimplantation embryo development, *Mol. Reprod. Dev.*, 40, 436–443, 1995.

104. Masters, C. J., Metabolic regulation and the microenvironment, in *Metabolic Regulation*, Ochs, R. S., Hanson, R. W., and Hall, J., Eds., Elsevier Science Publishers, New York, 33–38, 1985.

105. Mehta, T. S. and Kiessling, A. A., Developmental potential of mouse embryos conceived *in vitro* and cultured in ethylenediaminetetraacetic acid with and without amino acids or serum, *Biol. Reprod.*, 43, 600–606, 1990.

106. Miyoshi, K., Okuda, K., and Niwa, K., Development of rat one-cell embryos in a chemically defined medium: effects of glucose, phosphate and osmolarity, *J. Reprod. Fertil.*, 100, 21–26, 1994.

107. Muggleton-Harris, A. L., Glazier, A. M., and Wall, M., A retrospective analysis of the *in vitro* development of "spare" human *in vitro* fertilization preimplantation embryos using "in-house" prepared medium and "Medi-Cult" commercial medium, *Hum. Reprod.*, 10, 2976–2984, 1995.

108. Nasr-Esfahani, M., Johnson, M., and Aitken, R. J., The effect of iron and iron chelators on the *in vitro* block to development of the mouse preimplantation embryo: BAT6 a new medium for the improved culture of mouse embryos *in vitro*, *Hum. Reprod.*, 5, 997–1003, 1990.

109. Newsholm, E. A. and Leech, D., *Biochemistry for the Medical Sciences*, John Wiley & Sons, London, 1989.

110. Nieder, G. L. and Macon, G. R., Uterine and oviductal protein secretion during early pregnancy in the mouse, *J. Reprod. Fertil.*, 81, 287–294, 1987.

111. Pawelczyk, T. and Olson, M. S., Regulation of pyruvate dehydrogenase kinase activity from pig kidney cortex, *Biochem. J.*, 288, 369–373, 1992.

112. Pembel, L. B. and Kaye, P. L., Whole protein uptake by mouse blastocysts, *J. Reprod. Fertil.*, 78, 149–157, 1986.

113. Polgreen, K. E., Kemp, G. J., Clarke, K., and Radda, G. K., Transsarcolemmal movement of inorganic phosphate in glucose-perfused rat heart: a 31P nuclear magnetic resonance spectroscopic study, *J. Mol. Cell. Cardiol.*, 26, 219–228, 1994.

114. Psychoyos, A., The implantation window: basic and clinical aspects, in *Perspectives in Assisted Reproduction*, Vol. 4, Mori, T., Aono, T., Tominaga, T., and Hiroi, M., Eds., Ares Serono Symposia, Rome, Italy, 57–62, 1993.

115. Quinn, P., Enhanced results in mouse and human embryo culture using a modified human tubal fluid medium lacking glucose and phosphate, *J. Assist. Reprod. Genet.*, 12, 97–105, 1995.

116. Quinn, P. and Margalt, R., Beneficial effects of coculture with cumulus cells on blastocyst formation in a prospective trial with supernumerary human embryos, *J. Assist. Reprod. Genet.*, 13, 9–14, 1996.

117. Quinn, P. and Wales, R. G., Growth and metabolism of preimplantation mouse embryos cultured in phosphate-buffered medium, *J. Reprod. Fertil.*, 35, 289–300, 1973.

118. Robinson, B. H., Oei, J., Cheema-Dhadli, S., and Halperin, M., Regulation of citrate transport and pyruvate dehydrogenase in rat kidney cortex mitochondria by bicarbonate, *J. Biol. Chem.*, 252, 5661–5665, 1977.

119. Roblero, L. S. and Riffo, M. D., High potassium concentration improves preimplantation development of mouse embryos *in vitro*, *Fertil. Steril.*, 45, 412–416, 1986.

120. Roy, S. K. and Greenwald, G. S., Methods for separation and *in vitro* culture of preantral follicles from mammalian ovaries, *Hum. Reprod. Update*, 2, 236–245, 1996.

121. Schini, S. A. and Bavister, B. D., Development of golden hamster embryos through the two-cell block in chemically defined medium, *J. Exp. Zool.*, 245, 111, 1988.

122. Schini, S. A. and Bavister, B. D., Two-cell block to development of cultured hamster embryos is caused by phosphate and glucose, *Biol. Reprod.*, 39, 1183–1192, 1988.

123. Schultz, R. M. and Wassarman, P. M., Biochemical studies of mammalian oogenesis: protein synthesis during oocyte growth and meiotic maturation in the mouse, *J. Cell Science*, 24, 167–194, 1977.

124. Scott, L. A. and Whittingham, D. G., The influence of genetic background and media components on the development of mouse embryos *in vitro*, *Mol. Reprod. Dev.*, 43, 336–346, 1996.

125. Seshagiri, P. B. and Bavister, B. D., Glucose and phosphate inhibit respiration and oxidative metabolism in cultured hamster eight-cell embryos: evidence for the "Crabtree effect", *Mol. Reprod. Dev.*, 30, 105–111, 1991.

126. Sorenson, R. A. and Wassarman, P. M., Relationship between growth and meiotic maturation of the mouse oocyte, *Dev. Biol.*, 50, 531–536, 1976.

127. Summers, M. C., Bhatnagar, P. R., Lawitts, J. A., and Biggers, J. D., Fertilization *in vitro* of mouse ova from inbred and outbred strains: complete preimplantation development in glucose-supplemented KSOM, *Biol. Reprod.*, 53, 431–437, 1995.

128. Tabibzadeh, S. and Babakina, A., The signals and molecular pathways involved in implantation, a symbiotic interaction between blastocyst and endometrium involving adhesion and tissue invasion, *Mol. Hum. Reprod.*, 1, 10, 1579–1602, 1995.

129. Tsafriri, A., Local nonsteroidal regulators of ovarian function, in *The Physiology of Reproduction*, Vol. 1, Knobil, E. and Neil, J. D., Eds., Raven Press, New York, 527–565, 1988.

130. Tsutsumi, O., Yano, T., Satoh, K., Mizuno, M., and Kato, T., Studies of hexokinase activity in human and mouse oocytes, *Am. J. Obstet. Gynecol.*, 162, 1301–1304, 1990.

131. Urner, F. and Sakkas, D., Glucose is not essential for the occurrence of sperm binding and zona pellucida-induced acrosome reaction in the mouse, *Int. J. Androl.*, 19, 91–96.

132. Urner, F. and Sakkas, D., Glucose participates in sperm-oocyte fusion in the mouse, *Biol. Reprod.*, 55, 917–922, 1996.

133. Van Blerkom, J., Antczak, M., and Schrader, R., The developmental potential of the human oocyte is related to the dissolved oxygen content of follicular fluid: association with vascular endothelial growth factor levels and perifollicular blood flow characteristic, *Hum. Reprod.*, 12, 1047–1055, 1997.

134. Van Blerkom, J., Davis, P. W., and Lee, J., ATP content of human oocytes and developmental potential and outcome after *in vitro* fertilization and embryo transfer, *Hum. Reprod.*, 10, 415–424, 1995.

135. Van Blerkom, J. and Henry, G., Oocyte dysmorphism and aneuploidy in meiotically-mature human oocytes after ovulation stimulation, *Hum. Reprod.*, 7, 379–390, 1992.

136. Van Winkel, L. J. and Dickinson, H. R., Differences in amino acid content of preimplantation mouse embryos that develop *in vitro* versus *in vivo*: *in vitro* effects of five amino acids that are abundant in oviductal secretions, *Biol. Reprod.*, 52, 96–104, 1995.

137. Wales, R. G., Whittingham, D. G., Hardy, K., and Craft, I. L., Metabolism of glucose by human embryos, *J. Reprod. Fertil.*, 79, 289–297, 1987.

138. Whitten, W. K., Nutrient requirements for the culture of preimplantation embryos *in vitro*, in *Schering Symposium on Intrinsic and Extrinsic Factors in Early Mammalian Development*, Vol. 6, Pergamon Press, Oxford, 129–141, 1971.

139. Whittingham, D. G., The culture of mouse ova, *J. Reprod. Fertil.* (Suppl.), 14, 7–21, 1971.

140. Wiemer, K. E., Cohen, J. C., Wiker, S. R., Metler, H. E., Wright, G., and Godke, R. A., Coculture of human zygotes on fetal bovine uterine fibroblasts: embryonic morphology and implantation, *Fertil. Steril.*, 52, 503–508, 1989.

141. Wiley, L. M., Cavitation in the mouse preimplantation embryo Na/K-ATPase and the origin of nascent blastocoele fluid, *Dev. Biol.*, 105, 330–342, 1984.

142. Wilson, J. E., Hexokinases: an introduction to the isozymes of mammalian hexokinase types I-III, *Biochem. Soc. Trans.*, 25, 103–106, 1997.

143. Zeleznik, A. J. and Hillier, S. G., The role of gonadotrophins in the selection of the preovulatory follicle, *Clin. Obstet. Gynaecol.*, 27, 927–940, 1981.

9 Micromanipulation of Human Gametes, Zygotes, and Embryos

Gianpiero D. Palermo and J. Michael Bedford

CONTENTS

I. INTRODUCTION

Since the first human birth following *in vitro* fertilization (IVF) in 1978 this procedure has been used extensively for alleviation of infertility. However, because spermatozoa cannot fertilize in many cases of male factor infertility, a number of supplementary techniques have been developed to overcome this inability, and these are referred to generally as *assisted fertilization, microsurgical fertilization,* or simply *micromanipulation.* The application of micromanipulation to human gametes has not only allowed fertilization in cases of severe oligozoospermia and even by defective spermatozoa, it has provided a powerful tool for understanding the basic elements of oocyte maturation, fertilization, and early development. Micromanipulation techniques also now permit the diagnosis and sometimes even the correction of genetic anomalies, as well as increases implantation rates in certain cases.

II. TECHNIQUES USED TO ACHIEVE FERTILIZATION

A. ZONA DRILLING, PARTIAL ZONA DISSECTION, SUBZONAL INSEMINATION

Where sperm density, motility, or morphology are inadequate, various techniques help to bypass the zona pellucida. The practical use of micromanipulation for this burst onto the scene in the mid 1980s with zona drilling and partial zona dissection. Since then, the field evolved so rapidly that these early approaches largely have been abandoned in favor of intracytoplasmic sperm injection (ICSI), with partial zona dissection confined to the 4 to 8-cell embryo stage (hatching) in an effort to promote implantation. Nevertheless, because several of the techniques used initially provide historical interest, these are discussed briefly to maintain some perspective in that regard.

Zona drilling (ZD) (Figure 9.1b) first reported by Gordon et al.[41] involves the creation of a circumscribed opening in the zona by acid Tyrode's solution (pH 2) applied through a fine glass micropipette. After insemination, more than one spermatozoon frequently enters such drilled zonas. Moreover, acid Tyrode's has a deleterious effect on the one-celled egg—an effect not seen to the same extent in 4-cell embryos using the "hatching" procedure, discussed later in this chapter. As ZD was being tested, mechanical *cutting* of a hole in the zona emerged as another technique, this for nuclear manipulation of fertilized eggs.[135] Alternative but similar procedures were zona *cracking* in which the zona was breached mechanically with two fine glass hooks controlled by a micromanipulator[99] and zona *softening* (Figure 9.1a) performed by a brief exposure to trypsin[40] or pronase. Partial zona dissection (PZD) (Figure 9.1c),[22] used extensively for a period in cases of fertilization failure, involved cutting the zona with glass pipettes just before exposure of the treated oocytes to spermatozoa.

For all these techniques, spermatozoa had to be progressively motile and to have undergone or to have the potential for an acrosome reaction. The techniques also carried a distinct risk of injury to the oocytes and the need to produce an opening in the zona of optimal size. Localized laser photoablation of the zona also has been

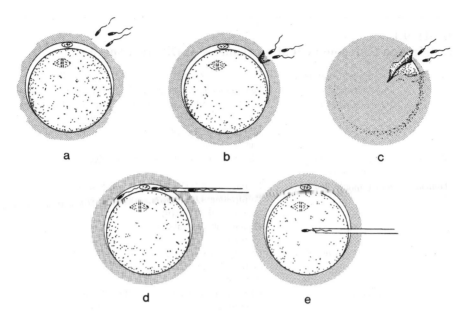

FIGURE 9.1 Different techniques of assisted fertilization: (a) zona softening; (b) zona drilling; (c) partial zona dissection; (d) subzonal insemination; (e) intracytoplasmic sperm injection.

used to produce a gap of precise dimensions in the zona, and this has resulted in a few healthy offspring.[32,2] However, not only did all these early procedures bring only a moderate fertilization rate, with PZD being the most useful in that regard, but they corresponded to a significant incidence of polyspermy.

Later, mechanical insertion of spermatozoa directly into the perivitelline space—subzonal sperm injection (SUZI)[69] (Figure 9.1d)—appeared as another way of overcoming inadequacies of sperm concentration and motility, and this proved to be more effective than ZD or PZD, particularly following prior induction of the acrosome reaction.[102,105] However, SUZI required that spermatozoa be normal, capacitated, and even hyperactivated or acrosome-reacted. Thus, this technique remained limited by an inability to overcome acrosomal abnormalities or dysfunction of the sperm-oolemma fusion process, and, ultimately, by unacceptably low fertilization rates.

B. INTRACYTOPLASMIC SPERM INJECTION

Because intracytoplasmic sperm injection (ICSI) involves insertion of a single selected spermatozoon directly into the oocyte (Figure 9.1e), this bypasses all the preliminary steps of fertilization. The technique was pioneered in animals (Table 9.1), initially by Hiramoto in the sea urchin,[53] then by Lin in mammalian (mouse) oocytes.[74] Later, Uehara and Yanagimachi observed relatively high rates of sperm nucleus decondensation after microinjection of human or golden hamster spermatozoa into hamster eggs,[138] and subsequently ICSI was used to study the determinants of male pronucleus formation.[96,112] This technique too may cause oocyte injury and lysis,[81] and in early

TABLE 9.1
Fertilization Outcome by ICSI on Gametes of Different Species

Gametes	Sperm Treatment	Results	Ref.
Rabbit	Intact, epididymal	Fertilization 60%; offspring 3%	Hosoi et al.;[55] Iritani[58]
Rabbit	Intact, epididymal	Fertilization 53%; cleavage 30%	Iritani;[58] Iritani and Hosoi[57]
Human	Intact	Fertilization 50% (6/12); ultrastructure	Lanzendorf et al.[67]
Rabbit	Intact, nuclei, 18 h preincubation	Cleavage 25%; fetal development	Keefer[60]
Human	Intact, motile, and immotile	Fertilization 8% (1/13)	Sathananthan et al.[116]
Human	Intact	Fertilization 32% (20/62); cleavage 58% (11/19) Eleven embryos transferred in 7 patients	Veeck et al.[141]
Bovine	Killed by freezing-thawing	Cleavage: 6-12 cells 15%; morula-blastocyst 10% A calf born	Goto et al.[42]
Bovine	Capacitated	Cleavage activated oocytes 28%; control 2%	Younis et al.;[152] Keefer et al.[61]
Human	Intact	Fertilization 15% (4/26) Four zygotes transferred by ZIFT in 2 patients	Ng et al.[98]
Rabbit	Testicular, and nuclei ("dead")	Fertilization 50%; cleavage 66% Twenty-five embryos transferred to 3 rabbits	Yanagida et al.[151]
Human	Intact, acrosome-reacted	Fertilization 66% (31/47); cleavage 58% (18/31) One twin and 3 singleton pregnancies, four babies born	Palermo et al.[103]

studies only about 30% of injected mouse eggs survived the procedure, even when fine micropipettes (4 to 6 mm diameter) were used under ideal conditions.[131]

Because the fusion step of fertilization is bypassed in ICSI, male pronucleus development generally requires oocyte activation in most species tested. This can be provoked by energetic suction of some cytoplasm immediately before or during sperm nucleus insertion.[113] In the hamster[54] and the bovine,[152] exposure to a calcium ionophore (e.g., A23187) appeared to increase the likelihood of oocyte activation.

The first live offspring using ICSI came from the rabbit following the transfer of sperm-injected eggs into the oviduct of a pseudopregnant female,[57] and soon after that the first ICSI live birth was reported in the bovine.[42] Although applied to human gametes some years earlier,[67] the first human pregnancies with ICSI occurred only in 1992,[103] since which time thousands of babies have been born after its use.[108]

1. Procedure

The pipettes are made from borosilicate glass capillary tubes (Drummond Scientific, Broomall, PA, U.S.) with a 0.97 mm external diameter, a 0.69 mm internal diameter, and a 78 mm length. Cleaning the capillary tubes involves (1) soaking overnight in

MilliQ water (Millipore Corporation, Bedford, MA, U.S.); (2) sonication; (3) rinsing at least 30 times in MilliQ water before drying in a hot air oven; and (4) heat sterilization. Pipettes are made by drawing the thin-walled glass capillary tubes using a horizontal microelectrode puller (Model 753, Campden Instruments Ltd., Loughborough, U.K.). The holding pipette is cut and fire-polished on a microforge (Narishige Co. Ltd., Tokyo, Japan) to a final outer diameter of 60 µm and an inner diameter of 20 µm. To prepare the injection pipette, the pulled capillary is opened and sharpened on a grinder (Narishige Co. Ltd.), with a bevel angle of 30°, an outer diameter of approximately 7 µm, and an inner diameter of approximately 5 µm. A spike is made on the injection pipette using a microforge, and both pipettes are bent to an angle of approximately 35° at a point positioned horizontally 1 mm from the edge, allowing injection with the tip in a plastic Petri dish (Model 1006, Falcon).

Immediately before injection, 1 ml of sperm suspension is diluted with 4 ml of a 10% polyvinyl pyrrolidone solution (PVP-K 90, MW 360,000, ICN Biochemicals, Cleveland, OH, U.S.) in HTF-Hepes medium placed in the middle of the Petri dish. The viscosity of PVP, which is used as it comes from the manufacturer, decelerates the aspiration and prevents the sperm cells from sticking to the injection pipette. Where less than 500,000 spermatozoa are available in an ejaculate, these are often concentrated in approximately 5 µl and transferred directly into the injection dish. A spermatozoon is then aspirated from the concentrated 5 µl sperm suspension and transferred into the central drop containing PVP solution, in order to remove debris and facilitate aspiration control.

After the spermatozoa are prepared, each oocyte is placed in a droplet of 5 µl medium surrounding the central drop containing the sperm suspension/PVP. With HTF-Hepes medium supplemented with 5 mg/ml BSA (A-3156, Sigma Chemical Co.) in the injection dish, the droplets are covered with lightweight paraffin oil (BDH Ltd., Poole, U.K.). No more than four oocytes go into the injection dish to avoid exposure to the Hepes buffered medium for any longer than 10 minutes. The droplets in each dish are used only once to avoid dilution of the buffered medium during oocyte transport.

The injection is performed at 400 X magnification using Hoffman Modulation Contrast optics on the heated stage (Easteach Laboratory, Centereach, NY, U.S.) of a Nikon Diaphot inverted microscope equipped with two motor-driven coarse control manipulators and two hydraulic micromanipulators (MM-188 and MO-109, Narishige Co., Ltd.). The micropipettes are fitted to a tool holder controlled by two IM-6 microinjectors (Narishige Co., Ltd.).

When the 1 µl of sperm suspension meets the drop containing PVP, motile spermatozoa progress into the viscous medium, whereas debris (other cells, bacteria, and immotile spermatozoa) floats in the PVP at its interface with the paraffin oil. We must emphasize that too many spermatozoa in the PVP-containing droplet may favor adherence of debris to the injection pipette and so contaminate the injection medium. In addition to decelerating the spermatozoon, the viscosity highlights its tridimensional motion patterns. This not only facilitates sperm aspiration into the pipette, but, while difficult with moving cells at ×400, it helps in the selection of normally-shaped spermatozoa from their form, light refraction, and motility pattern in this environment.

The spermatozoa preferred for aspiration are those that tend to stick to the bottom of the Petri dish by their heads and become immotile after displaying simple vibration patterns for a short period. Generally, these reside on the bottom of the dish at the edge of the droplet. Paradoxically, the ICSI technique works better with spermatozoa that are immotile rather than motile in the final stage. Thus, active spermatozoa must first be immobilized. This is accomplished by gently lowering the tip of the pipette so as to compress the mid region of the sperm flagellum against the bottom of the dish.

Once spermatozoa are immobilized, one must lift them from the bottom of the dish by gentle suction with a pipette. Once free, the sperm cell should be drawn into the injection pipette tail first. Then the injection needle is lifted slightly by turning the knob of the joystick clockwise to avoid damaging the needle spike on scratches in the dish. Note that as the needle is redirected by moving the microscope stage to the drop containing the oocyte, the difference in medium consistency (PVP vs. culture medium) may promote loss of the spermatozoon from the pipette at this point.

As the holding pipette is lowered, the oocyte is slowly rotated to locate the polar body and the associated area of cortical rarefaction (or polar granularity)—presumably the site from which the first polar body is extruded. While the polar body is not a wholly reliable reference point since it may move within the perivitelline space during the cumulus cell's removal, this area should be avoided during injection.

Subsequently, the depth of the holding pipette is adjusted such that its internal opening and the equator of the oocyte are both in focus. This allows for greater support of the holding pipette in a position opposite the injection point. The inferior pole of the oocyte should touch the bottom of the dish as this stabilizes the egg during the procedure. The injection pipette is then lowered and focused together with the outer right border of the oolemma on the equatorial plane at 3 o'clock. The spermatozoon within the injection pipette is then advanced slowly to lie close to the beveled opening, which is pushed against and through the zona, then further against the oolemma. A break in this membrane is signaled by a sudden quivering of its surface (at the site of invagination) above and below the needle. Penetration of the oolemma also brings an important flow of ooplasm up into the pipette, causing the spermatozoon to move back up with it, and this retrograde movement is encouraged to a point approximately 60 µm from the tip by active aspiration. To counteract the flow of ooplasm, which is important for oocyte activation, the spermatozoon is then ejected back with ooplasm, thereby avoiding a tendency to inject any significant volume of medium into the oocyte.

The physical character of the oolemma can vary and may be particularly soft or elastic according to the maturity of the oocyte or the time spent *in vitro*.[107] In such instances, one may need to withdraw the pipette slightly and to repeat the procedure slowly, hooking the upper or lower border of the invagination with the spike in order to penetrate the oocyte in a line parallel to its equatorial plane. Once entry is confirmed, the spermatozoon should then be ejected into the ooplasm well beyond the tip while withdrawing the pipette, at which point some surplus medium is reaspirated. This promotes association of the injected sperm with cytoplasmic organelles and final closure of the funnel-shaped opening at 3 o'clock. Where the surface of the oolemma becomes everted, the cytoplasmic organelles can leak and the oocyte may lyse. Thus, the penetration point is checked to ensure that the border of the opening maintains a funnel shape or vertex pointing into the egg. The average time required to inject a spermatozoon into an oocyte is up to one minute.[101,106]

2. Indications for ICSI

Despite agreement in some areas, no universal standards for patient selection exist and a lack of standardized criteria complicates attempts to quantify the therapeutic value of ICSI. The general consensus, however, is that it should be performed following failure in standard IVF with oocytes whose nuclear maturity was established properly and in initial failures where an appropriate sperm concentration was utilized even in microdrops—useful criteria for all male factor patients, even those who have not been treated before. The performance of the spermatozoon can improve further by adding kinetic stimulators such as pentoxifylline.

Although oocytes that failed to fertilize with standard IVF techniques can be reinseminated, this introduces a risk of fertilizing aged eggs.[95] In our own limited experience, six of eight pregnancies established by micromanipulation of such oocytes miscarried, and cytogenetic studies performed on the aborted fetuses provided evidence of chromosomal abnormalities. Thus, notwithstanding a recent report of normal pregnancies,[85] the reinsemination of unfertilized oocytes is currently performed only for research purposes.

In regard to sperm numbers, when the count is $<5 \times 10^6$/ml, the likelihood of fertilization with normal IVF procedures is reduced significantly, regardless of etiology.[153] A couple is considered unsuitable for standard IVF if the sperm concentration in the initial ejaculate is less than 500,000 progressively motile spermatozoa per ml, with $<4\%$ normal forms (strict criteria). Moreover, fertilization between apparently mature oocytes and motile spermatozoa may fail to occur.[12] One potential cause may be spontaneous hardening of the zona pellucida after *in vitro* culture[27] or an inherently impenetrable zona around oocytes that often reveal ooplasmic inclusions.[7,140] The rare sperm abnormality that prevents sperm fusion with the oolemma also justifies sperm injection.[65] In many instances, however, fertilization failure results from multiple sperm abnormalities seen in severe oligo-, astheno-, or teratozoospermia as defined by WHO.[150] A clear consensus now supports micromanipulation in such cases where IVF rates drop to less than 10%,[29] with ICSI being the only treatment option.[108] To give an idea of the performance of ICSI versus standard *in vitro* insemination, the overall fertilization and pregnancy rates with the two procedures appear in Table 9.2.

3. ICSI With Mature Spermatozoa

How effective is ICSI using ejaculated spermatozoa in cases judged, a priori, to be unsuitable for standard IVF? The ICSI procedure has been performed at Cornell in 2,143 such cases with 74.5% of oocytes being fertilized normally and 95.1% of patients receiving good quality embryos, this leading to a 44.2% clinical pregnancy rate, including 6 ectopic pregnancies and 81 miscarriages. The ongoing pregnancy and delivery rate was 39.7% per oocyte retrieval and 41.7% per replacement. These

TABLE 9.2
Outcome of ICSI and IVF Treatments in the Same Time Period

Number of	ICSI	(%)	IVF	(%)
Cycles	2,427		2,407	
Inseminated oocytes	20,899		25,365	
Fertilized oocytes	15,457	(73.9)*	16,924	(66.7)*
Embryo replacements	2,311	(95.2)	2,261	(93.9)
Mean embryos transferred	3.1		3.5	
Clinical pregnancies	1,105	(45.5)**	986	(41.0)**

* χ^2, 2×2, 1 df; Effect of insemination procedure on fertilization rate, $p = 0.0001$.
** χ^2, 2×2, 1 df; Effect of insemination procedure on pregnancy rate, $p = 0.001$.

results from ICSI were not related to the source of the spermatozoon (fresh or cryopreserved, or obtained by masturbation, electroejaculation, or bladder catheterization), but the concentration of normal motile spermatozoa in the ejaculate influenced the fertilization rate ($p = 0.0001$) and the actual pregnancy rate ($p < 0.01$) (Table 9.3). Thus the clinical outcome with ICSI is comparable to the best outcome of IVF in couples where no sperm abnormalities exist.

TABLE 9.3
ICSI Outcome According to Total Motile Spermatozoa

Groups	Cycles	Fertilization Rate (%)	Clinical Pregnancies (%)
0	92	511/864 (59.1)*	26 (28.3)**
1–500,000	328	2,165/3,125 (69.3)*	158 (48.2)**
>500,000	1,723	10,822/14,127 (76.6)*	764 (44.3)**
TOTAL	2,143	13,498/18,116 (74.3)	948 (44.2)

* χ^2, 2×3, 2 df; Effect of concentration of normal motile spermatozoa on fertilization rate, $p = 0.0001$.
** χ^2, 2×3, 2 df; Effect of concentration of normal motile spermatozoa on fertilization rate, $p < 0.01$.

4. ICSI With Immature or Abnormal Germ Cells

Early experience showed that isolated nuclei of testicular, caput, and cauda epididymal hamster spermatozoa decondensed soon after injection into mature hamster oocytes and were transformed into pronuclei in activated eggs.[137] Although conventional IVF of human oocytes has often been accomplished in man with functional epididymal spermatozoa,[124,129] only with the advent of ICSI has it been possible to obtain normal embryos with surgically retrieved *immature* epididymal spermatozoa.[106,123,134] Using ICSI a clinical pregnancy rate of 64.2% was achieved with spermatozoa collected microsurgically from the epididymis, and 44.2% of 104 couples became pregnant after ICSI using frozen epididymal sperm (Table 9.4). However, the therapeutic possibilities of ICSI go even further since testicular spermatozoa and even spermatids can be used in this way. Testicular biopsies have provided sperm cells from men who have a scarred epididymis and no possibility

TABLE 9.4
ICSI Outcome Using Immature Spermatozoa

	Epididymal Sperm	Cryopreserved Epididymal Sperm	Testicular Sperm	Cryopreserved Testicular Sperm
Cycles	123	104	53	4
Mean density (10^6/ml ± SD)	24.2 ± 37	18.4 ± 29	0.7 ± 2	0.2 ± 0.4
Mean motility (% ± SD)	19.0 ± 17	3.1 ± 7	6.7 ± 14	6.5 ± 12
Mean morphology (% ± SD)	2.2 ± 2	1.7 ± 2	0	0
Fertilization (%)	952/1318 (72.2)	674/925 (72.9)	306/503 (60.8)	27/37 (73.0)
Clinical pregnancies (%)	79 (64.2)	46 (44.2)	29 (54.71)	3 (75.0)

of sperm retrieval.[26,33,121] In 57 cycles where such testicular germ cells were used, the fertilization rate was 61.7%, and 32 (56.1%) pregnancies occurred with spermatozoa that were either totally immotile or slightly twitching.

A few men form only round-headed (acrosomeless) spermatozoa that can neither bind to nor penetrate zona-free hamster oocytes.[66] After ICSI with such acrosomeless spermatozoa, 15 of 45 oocytes were fertilized, 10 embryos were replaced in 4 cycles, and 3 pregnancies were established.[77]

5. Concerns About ICSI

Are the babies born in any way compromised by the use of ICSI per se? A recent report suggested a high incidence (33%) of sex chromosomal abnormalities in embryos created through ICSI,[56] but this is clearly incorrect. Liebaers et al.[73] reported only 1% of sex chromosomal anomalies after ICSI, and a large retrospective study of babies born in our own program after ICSI (n = 623) showed only a 1.6% incidence of congenital abnormalities compared to 3.5% in babies born as a result of standard IVF and 3.6% in the general population.[97] Thus, our data support the conclusions from many ICSI programs worldwide[8,9] that the incidence of fetal abnormalities is no higher than with standard IVF, despite the fact that its use often involves suboptimal spermatozoa.[110] On the other hand, meticulous follow-up of newborns throughout development seems to be prudent for obvious reasons. Researchers have a real reason to be concerned about the perpetuation of purely reproductive defects, i.e., that those particular problems that necessitated recourse to ICSI in some cases of astheno-, oligo-, and azoospermia could emerge at puberty in the male children so conceived.[28,111]

Finally, in considering the basis of some fetal anomalies, one must recognize that these can also arise from the oocyte, particularly those from the many women undergoing either standard IVF or ICSI who receive ovarian hyperstimulation. Although oocyte inclusions have been linked to a refractory state of the zona[7] and certain perturbations in cytoplasmic organization similarly to fertilization failure,[140] after ICSI morphological abnormalities of human oocytes appear to have little bearing on fertilization success or early cleavage at least.[1]

6. Future Developments

In principle, round spermatids can be used to create normal mammalian embryos.[100] Moreover, even secondary spermatocytes can "haploidize" themselves within the mouse egg at least and create normal offspring.[63] Nevertheless, to date only two term pregnancies have been reported using round spermatids recovered from ejaculates produced by azoospermic men,[130] and only one baby after using round spermatids retrieved from testicular tissue.[122]

An additional final step might be the cryopreservation of spermatogonia for their future transfer and maturation in a recipient testis. This type of transfer has been successful in the rat[4] and may have clinical applications in the future. For example, men likely to lose their germ cells (e.g., undergoing chemotherapy) may have spermatogonia cryopreserved for later recolonization of the irradiated testis. While one would hope that this would initiate normal spermatogenesis, if this is not so, one could at least harvest the haploid product for use in the ICSI procedure. On the other hand, selecting the round spermatids of man remains difficult, and, as noted above, their use has so far brought no more than modest results in the clinical setting.

III. THE CORRECTION OF FERTILIZATION ABNORMALITIES

A. ENUCLEATION AND ELECTROFUSION

Much of the research into genetic manipulation performed so far on animals has involved direct removal or transplantation of nuclei and pronuclei.[45,147] Zygotes can be manipulated in regard to either the paternal or maternal genome and can be reconstructed from different phenotypes. Manipulation techniques have been used, for example, to eliminate an extra pronucleus, thereby returning the triploid human zygote to its diploid status. Theoretically, zygote abnormalities such as diandry and digyny can be corrected in this way[80,114,128] while, conversely, a haploid egg could be brought to a diploid state by karyoplast reincorporation techniques (Figure 9.2).[72]

1. Procedure

Pronucleus removal from the zygote (enucleation) can be performed in different ways. The simplest approach incorporates ICSI settings and tools. The pronucleus to be aspirated must be positioned at the equatorial plane of the zygote. The periphery of the nuclear membrane and the tip of the enucleating tool should be brought to the same focal plane before penetration of the zona and oolemma. Advance the tip of the pipette to the center of the pronucleus, with aspiration of the nucleus slowly then from the oocyte (Figure 9.3). The nucleus farthest from the polar body is targeted in the case of a diandric zygote, whereas that closest to the polar body is chosen for correction of digyny.

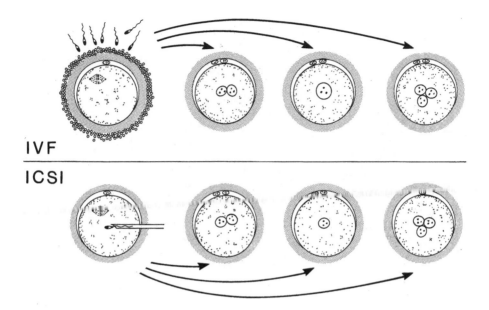

FIGURE 9.2 Fertilization patterns with IVF and ICSI. From left to right zygotes displaying 2, 1, and 3 pronuclei. The size of the single pronucleate oocyte in the IVF row is larger because of the often diploid constitution, while the ICSI one is often haploid. The three-pronucleate zygote in the ICSI row has only one polar body being the second polar body retained and decondensed in the ooplasm forming the additional pronucleus.

The technique of electrofusion requires the preparation of a karyoplast—a fragment of ooplasm surrounded by oolemma. To do this, a donor oocyte is incubated in 0.3% pronase for 5 to 10 minutes for zona removal, then in a medium containing 7 µg/ml cytochalasin B. A small portion of the oocyte, approximately 40 µm in diameter, is then drawn into a partitioning pipette whose tip is cut off and fire-polished to an inner diameter of 30 to 40 µm. That portion is then isolated by rubbing the oocyte against an intact egg fixed by a holding pipette. The process can be repeated to create additional membrane-bound cytoplasts, ideally of a 40 to 50 µm diameter. The latter can be exposed to spermatozoa or subjected to ICSI to produce male karyoplasts. Where used, for example, to restore a monopronucleate oocyte to diploidy, such a karyoplast is aspirated gently into a polished pipette with an inner diameter of 30 to 40 µm and then introduced through a slit in the zona to lie against the oocyte (Figure 9.4). Subsequently, the cell alignment and electrofusion is performed in a mannitol based medium.[72]

2. Tripronucleate Zygotes

Though seldom observed after ICSI, tripronucleate zygotes may arise either from dispermy or from failure of extrusion of the second polar body. Of the techniques that have been used to extract the extra pronucleus (enucleation), most have involved aspiration with a micropipette. However, Fulka et al. proposed a simplified technique

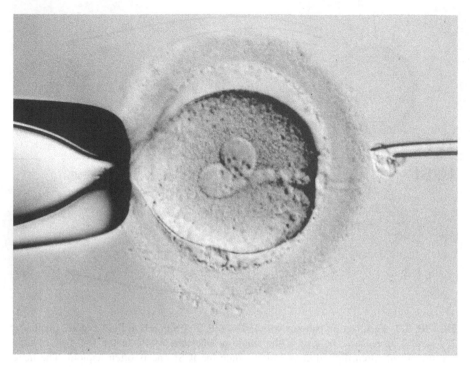

FIGURE 9.3 Enucleation procedure.

of chemical enucleation by exposure to cycloheximide and etoposide that does not require microsurgical skills.[35] Although this technique does not remove pronuclei selectively, it may be used to enucleate oocytes or obtain blastomeres for provision of host or donor nuclei. The challenge in such manipulation is to reestablish biparental diploidy.

Another central issue to consider in enucleation repair of dispermy or digyny is identification of the targeted pronucleus as being male or female, not least because diandric human embryos may develop as hydatidiform moles. The parental origin of a pronuclus is relatively clear in rodent zygotes where nuclear size, presence of the tail remnant, and position vis a vis the second polar body are all related to this. In humans, unfortunately, pronuclear size appears to be variable, and, as in the eggs of many mammals, the associated (fertilizing) sperm tail remnants cannot be identified by light microscopy.[80,145]

Since centrioles are absent in unfertilized but are present in fertilized human oocytes, the zygote centrosome must be paternally inherited in man,[117,118] and so the control of centrosome duplication and spindle formation during fertilization differs from that in somatic diploid cells. In the development of fertilized eggs, specific mechanisms must exist at the gamete or zygote level to control centrosome inheritance. If centrosomes from both gametes were retained and remained functional, the zygote would possess two sets of centrosomes and four centrioles, resulting in the generation of abnormal multipolar spindles and so aneuploidy and mosaicism at the first mitotic division.[125] In order to avoid this, the centrosome of one gamete

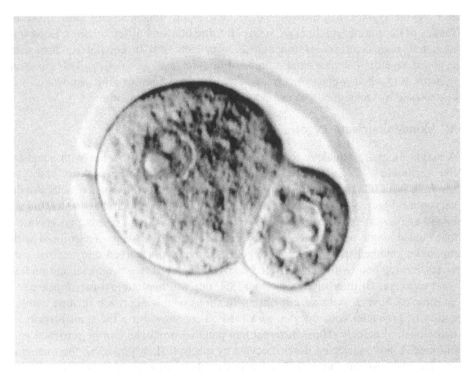

FIGURE 9.4 Following electrofusion a karyoplast is incorporated into a single pronucleate oocyte.

(usually of the oocyte) fails to develop, with the fertilizing spermatozoon introducing the functional centrosome in most of the species studied thus far.[109,119]

The way that the centrosome functions creates problems where attempts are made to correct polyploidy. For example, to assess whether the pronucleus farthest from the second polar body is consistently paternal in such zygotes, coamplification of X and Y probes using multiplex polymerase chain reaction (PCR) or simultaneous fluorescent *in situ* hybridization (FISH) was applied to a group of intact dispermic embryos and to other such embryos from which the distal pronucleus was removed.[93] Unfortunately, even when a single male pronucleus is removed successfully, such dispermic zygotes often later express a chromosomal mosaicism. This is because the extra sperm centrosome also contributes, resulting in the formation of abnormal or multipolar spindles. In contrast to dispermy, removal of one pronucleus from digynic zygotes restores the embryo to a diploid state compatible with normal development. As one caveat, while it is probably safe to replace enucleated embryos that began as digynic zygotes, further studies must determine the extent to which a female pronucleus can be selected with accuracy.

These are the principles that underlie the strategies aimed at reversing aneuploidy in human zygotes. Enucleation of one pronucleus from triploid zygotes may have several advantages. This may allow patients with only polyspermic or digynic zygotes to become pregnant. In addition, experimental enucleation of tripronucleate dispermic and digynic zygotes may provide androgenetic and gynogenetic cell lines of use in studies of imprinting, cell lineage, stem cell formation, and differentiation. However, as noted, both centrosomes function as organizers still in enucleated dispermic zygotes, resulting in abnormal spindle formation and mosaicism. The question remains as to whether embryo correction may become possible after removal of one centrosome by techniques that can label and identify the centrosome.[25]

3. Monopronucleate Zygotes

A single diploid pronucleus forms occasionally during fertilization with standard IVF techniques.[71,93] By contrast, the majority of the single-pronucleate embryos resulting from ICSI are haploid,[127] and these can be rescued by fusion with a male karyoplast (Figure 9.4). The latter generally result from insemination of a membrane-bound egg fragment or vesicles.[72] In a recent communication, researchers reported that human single pronucleate zygotes obtained after ICSI were electrofused with pronuclei obtained from polyploid zygotes. Three cryopreserved oocytes that survived thawing and two fresh activated oocytes displayed two pronuclei and underwent cleavage. Of three analyzable by FISH, one was haploid and two appeared to be diploid.[5] Several possible clinical applications of this approach include combination of pronuclei with oocytes as a method for preventing the transmission of mitochondrial defects. Thus, maternal and paternal pronuclei can be retrieved and introduced into enucleated donor oocytes by electrofusion, providing the maternal and paternal genome and mitochondria from a donor egg. In addition, the manipulation and cryopreservation of paternal and maternal haploid pronuclei may provide alternatives for future gene therapy and other genetic disease prevention technologies in instances where the DNA must be in a state capable of participation in fertilization.

IV. DIAGNOSIS OF GENETIC ABNORMALITIES

A. POLAR BODY BIOPSY

The risk of conceiving an aneuploid fetus increases from 6.8% at 35 to 39 years to 50% in women of 45 years or older.[51] Because most age-related aneuploidies originate during the first meiotic division of the oocyte,[3] first polar body chromosomes could be useful in determining its ploidy (Figure 9.5) as an anomaly in them will be a reflection of any anomaly existing in the egg. However, uncovering the consequences of errors in the second meiotic division, such as trisomy 18,[30] requires analysis of the second polar body.

Now, FISH can detect aneuploidy involving either an entire chromosome or one of the chromatids in the first and the second polar body.[31,89,142,143] Using this method in a small number of cases has produced no detrimental effects on embryo development or pregnancy rates.[144] As an additional possibility for the future, we may soon apply complete genome amplification to the polar body.

By now, pregnancies have been established after polar body biopsy for possible chromosome translocations.[91] If the first polar body can be biopsied immediately after oocyte retrieval, this allows sufficient time for analysis before embryonic

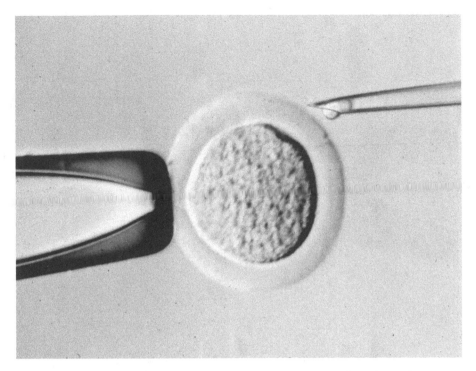

FIGURE 9.5 Polar body biopsy.

transfer. Biopsy of the first polar body has the advantage of being a pre-conception diagnosis method for the selection of genetically normal oocytes for ICSI. However, its usefulness is hampered by an inability to diagnose paternally derived chromosome abnormalities and those resulting at the second meiotic division.

1. Procedure

Polar body biopsy is performed with a beveled pipette of 12 to 15 µm inner diameter. The oocyte remains in place by the holding pipette with the polar body at 12 o'clock. The biopsy tool is inserted tangentially at approximately the 1 o'clock position into the perivitelline space adjacent to the polar body, which is aspirated gently and then allowed to recover its original shape before fixation for analysis by FISH.

B. EMBRYO BIOPSY

Embryo biopsy has been explored extensively in animals,[36,149] with its initial application in man being related to embryos at risk for X-linked diseases[47] and cystic fibrosis.[144] One can remove a blastomere without compromising development because all those in the 8 to 16-cell embryo are totipotent.[49] Thus, preimplantation diagnosis allows the replacement of presumably healthy embryos. Usually, embryo biopsy involves removal of one or more blastomeres at the 8-cell stage (Figure 9.6) and their assessment using FISH or PCR. However, the diagnosis must be highly

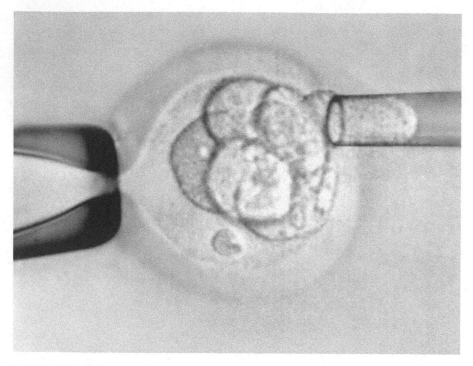

FIGURE 9.6 Embryo biopsy.

sensitive and specific and must be obtained within a few hours, in a time frame compatible with the embryo implantation schedule.

Both PCR and FISH can be used for sex determination where the parents are carriers of sex-linked diseases.[43,44,47] FISH can detect numerical chromosomal abnormalities in single blastomeres[44,94] and also is being used for the detection of maternally derived aneuploidies, i.e., chromosomes 13/21, 16, 18, and X and Y, in older women undergoing IVF.[90,92] However, PCR is the only method yet suitable for analysis of single gene diseases.[48,126]

Preimplantation diagnosis of inherited diseases currently is performed in at least 14 centers worldwide[50] with the largest number based on the identification of both X and Y chromosomes by FISH[13,44,47] for carriers of sex-linked disorders. Of those sexing cases in which embryos have reached the transfer stage, 26% of the PCR and 27% of the FISH cases have achieved a clinical pregnancy.[50] A negative aspect of this approach lies in the fact that approximately 50% of embryos of the undesired sex are discarded. Although most attempts at sex selection through separation of X and Y spermatozoa have not been successful, one approach that may prove to be realistic involves the use of X or Y populations selected by flow cytometry.[59,70] However, the possible mutagenic effect of the Hoechst dye used in flow sorting remains as one concern for man.

Preimplantation genetic diagnosis (PGD) is useful also for analysis of single gene defects, and 95% of cycles conducted so far have reached the embryo transfer stage, with a 34% pregnancy rate.[50] As of now, diagnostic methods developed for several gene defects include those for cystic fibrosis,[48] Duchenne muscular dystrophy,[76] Fragile X,[70] and Tay Sachs syndromes.[38,46]

In view of the fact that the incidence of oocyte aneuploidy increases significantly with maternal age,[51,88] routine selection of euploid embryos might improve delivery rates in older women dramatically. However, although this may minimize the need for invasive prenatal screening, PGD could have deleterious effects on embryos.[115] Other drawbacks of PGD include the possible failure to detect mosaicism since only one or two blastomeres are analyzed. In addition, FISH can uncover specific aneuploidies of only the few chromosomes (e.g., 13, 16, 18, 21, X, Y) for which specific markers currently are available.

Thus, attempts must be made to extend such analyses to a larger number of chromosomes and to maximize the possibility for diagnosis by means such as single cell recycling, use of primer extension preamplification (PEP), or comparative genome hybridization (CGH). Ultimately, PGD may identify couples at risk for transmitting some dominant single-gene disorders, including inherited cancer syndromes.

1. Procedure

Embryo biopsy is performed preferably at the 8-cell stage to allow analysis of one or preferably two blastomeres. The biopsy is a two-step procedure. When the embryo is secured with a holding pipette, a pipette of 10 µm inner diameter filled with acid Tyrode's solution is brought into tangential contact with the zona pellucida. Expulsion of a small volume of Tyrode's solution should create a discrete opening in the zona only large enough to allow introduction of the biopsy tool, a blunt aspiration pipette with an 18 to 20 µm inner diameter. After insertion of this into the perivitelline space, one or two blastomeres are then slowly sucked into it (Figure 9.6). On release from the glass pipette the biopsied blastomeres are allowed to recover their original shape prior to fixation for FISH or PCR analysis.

V. CORRECTION OF MEIOTIC ABNORMALITIES

A. CYTOPLASMIC TRANSFER

Although the embryo may carry chromosomal defects that can interfere with its development, several such abnormalities related to gamete defects have been corrected or overcome using micromanipulation techniques.

The oocyte can display a variety of defects ranging from single chromosomal aneuploidy to complete diploidy. Diploid oocytes, in addition to being larger, often extrude two first polar bodies on activation. However, as noted, the most common abnormality of the oocyte is either the retention or loss of both representatives of a particular chromosome during meiosis, an abnormality that appears increasingly with age. One solution to this involves transplantation of a GV nucleus from an egg of the older patient to an enucleated immature young oocyte.[154] In this case, the genome of the old egg may use the cytoplasmic infrastructure to haploidize normally. A type of manipulation that also involves this principle is the transfer of "young" ooplasm to putatively defective eggs.[24]

Cytoplasmic donation in human oocytes may have several benefits, ranging from avoidance of aneuploidy by correcting spindle behavior and nuclear division in oogonia, or germinal vesicle stage, to mitochondrial transfer for promotion of embryo growth. This may be performed either by fusion, by injection of selected organelles, or by transfer of anucleate cytoplasm (cytoplasmic transfer or donation). Such experimental reconstitution of oocytes and zygotes not only provides new therapeutic procedures but also helps in the study of fundamental processes.[23]

Control of nucleus behavior by the cytoplasm has been demonstrated by nuclear transplantation and cytoplasmic transfer in several animal species.[146,147] Specific cell cycle-related events related to cytoplasmic regulatory factors include germinal vesicle breakdown,[64,82] chromosome decondensation,[132] and metaphase arrest.[84,86] The ooplasm's ability to bring about sperm nucleus decondensation also depends on the stage of oocyte maturation.[133,139] Several other studies addressing the importance of cytoplasmic factors and organelles during meiosis and cleavage indicate that mitochondria are closely associated with the mitotic spindle in normally dividing blastomeres, but are absent in arrested ones. In this situation, resumption of normal mitosis and mitochondrial distribution occurred after transfer of G2 cytoplasm from normal blastomeres.[87] That cytoplasmic factors essential for developmental competence are absent in primate GV oocytes is suggested by their normal fertilization and development only after they receive mature oocyte cytoplasm.[34]

In three couples with previous implantation failure, cytoplasm transfer alone was performed by electrofusion prior to intracytoplasmic sperm injection and subsequent 4-day co-culture of embryos with epithelial cells.[23] When 21 of 22 recipient eggs were fused successfully with donor cytoplasts then subjected to ICSI, 8 had two pronuclei and 6 had one large pronucleus probably coming from the fusion of two normal pronuclei. Of the 14 embryos, 12 cleaved, 7 had compacted on day 4, and one appeared as an early blastocyst. At least three such embryos were transferred to each patient, but they did not implant. Two patients who returned for frozen donor embryos became pregnant, but one miscarried. The authors concluded that electrofusion of human oocytes with MII cytoplasm can favor normal fertilization, cleavage, and development. Recently, a 39-year-old woman suffering from poor embryo development in her previous IVF attempts had 14 recipient eggs injected with donor cytoplasm plus ICSI. Following this, 9 eggs showed signs of fertilization, 4 of 8 cleaved embryos were replaced and a single normal baby girl was carried to term.[24] Among the many issues that need to be resolved in this area occurs the possibility that embryos may be affected by the gaps in their zonae or by other unknown side effects of the treatments. Moreover, optimal timing of the procedure and the ideal amount and treatment of material transferred remain to be determined.[23]

1. Procedure

Germinal vesicles are removed from oocytes of older women by a glass tool similar to the one used for the production of cytoplasts before exposure to cytochalasin B. After mechanical breaching of the zona pellucida, the oocyte nucleus surrounded by a small amount of cytoplasm (karyoplast) is gently sucked out with an aspiration pipette of 20 µm inner diameter. At the same time the genomic material is removed from the young oocytes in the same fashion.

The GV karyoplast (from an aged oocyte) is then introduced into the perivitelline space of a previously enucleated young oocyte. Subsequently, the assembled oocytes in a mannitol-containing medium are aligned and subjected to AC pulses of 100 V/cm for 10 seconds followed by DC single pulse 1.3 KV/cm for 70 µ seconds, delivered by a BTX ECM 200 (Genetronics Inc., San Diego, CA). Then the treated oocytes are rinsed in fresh medium and cultured for approximately 15 min to allow fusion to occur. The success of the procedure can be confirmed by examination for extrusion of the polar body, which demonstrates the haploidization of the immature reconstituted oocyte.

VI. ENHANCEMENT OF IMPLANTATION

A. Assisted Hatching

One of the unsolved problems in IVF is the fact that a significant number of apparently normal embryos do not implant, possibly because of intrinsic embryo abnormalities and or defective uterine receptivity.[21] Recent attempts to improve the implantation rate include the application of better stimulation protocols to optimize follicular development,[75] modifications of the culture system such as co-culture,[10] and controlled incision of the zona pellucida, termed "assisted hatching."[16,21]

Assisted hatching (AH) is based on the hypothesis that weakening of the zona pellucida, either by drilling a hole through it, thinning it, or altering its stability, will promote hatching of embryos that are otherwise unable to escape from their zonae during blastocyst expansion.[21,62] This approach stemmed from the observation that cleaved embryos with a good prognosis for implantation had a reduced zona thickness and, presumably, the potential for escape from it[19] and particularly that microsurgically fertilized embryos with artificial gaps in their zonae appeared to have higher rates of implantation.[18]

Experimentally, researchers first observed that "drilled" mouse blastocysts shed the zona earlier than usual and through the artificial gap.[79] Whereas those with small holes in the zona tended to become trapped half within it in a characteristic figure-8 shape,[18] drilled holes of bigger size appeared to provide a better route to normal hatching. These observations encouraged the deliberate application of this as a possible way of enhancing the implantation rate of human embryos after transfer.

Although AH is applied widely now, its value is still debated. Objective analysis proves difficult due to the differences in study populations, in the performance of the procedure, in design of data analysis, and in the endpoints used to assess it. In addition, its implementation requires particular care during embryo replacement on day 3 using special catheters, and the administration of antibiotics and steroids. A summary of several studies of the clinical outcome of AH is presented in Table 9.5. Overall, it seems suited for patients with elevated basal FSH who are older than 38 years and, perhaps most important, for previous IVF failures whose eggs have a relatively thick (~17 µm) zona pellucida. Conversely, the outcome for patients whose eggs have thin zonae (<13 µm) may be jeopardized by it.[16] One should note that

TABLE 9.5
Clinical Studies on the Outcome of Assisted Hatching

Study Design	Study Population	Technique*	Implantation Rate (%)		p value	Ref.
			Control	Hatching		
Randomized	Normal basal FSH	ZD	21	28	NS	Cohen et al.[16]
Randomized	Poor prognosis embryos	ZD	18	25	p <0.05	Cohen et al.[16]
Randomized	High basal FSH	ZD	10	26	p = 0.05	Cohen et al.[16]
Retrospective	Poor prognosis patients	ZD	6.5	33	p <0.0001	Schoolcraft et al.[120]
Retrospective	Cryopreserved embryos	ZD	5.3	13.7	p <0.05	Check et al.[11]
Double-blinded Randomized	Patients ≥36 years	ZD	10.4	10.3	NS	Lanzendorf et al.[68]
Prospective	Cryopreserved embryos	PZD	9	16		Tucker et al.[136]
Randomized	Unselected group	PZD	17.1	17.9	NS	Hellebaut et al.[52]

* ZD = zona drilling; PZD = partial zona dissection.

zona thickness tends to correlate positively with the age of the patient, with day 3 FSH levels, and with preovulatory estradiol levels.[78]

A coincident advantage of zona opening is the access it allows for the removal of enucleated cell fragments and abnormal blastomeres. A 4% increase in implantation rate was noted when AH and fragment removal were applied in at least one embryo in a group of 234 patients. However, the rescue effect was more dramatic in patients whose embryos originally had 20% or more fragmentation.[14]

Several theories explain why AH may enhance the implantation rate. AH may overcome the effect of the zona "hardening" believed to occur in some poor-prognosis patients due to the culture conditions, particularly to protein supplementation. Researchers also have proposed that the implantation window moves forward in stimulated patients and, since hatching allows earlier implantation, that this may help to correct any temporal asymmetry between the embryo and the endometrium.[120]

Potential disadvantages of this approach include the possibility that excessive acid Tyrode's solution may adversely affect development, especially of embryos with thin zonae.[15] Investigators suggest that micromanipulation of the zona pellucida may favor monozygotic twinning,[17] though it is not yet clear if this does occur more commonly after hatching than after IVF alone. Another problem inherent in this technique is the possibility that embryos can escape from the zona prematurely during routine transcervical transfer.

The utility of assisted hatching really relates to the current less-than-optimal systems of embryo culture and the consequent need for embryo replacement after only 2 to 3 days. A reliable technique for culture of human embryos to the blastocyst stage may now be emerging, and since these implant at an extremely high rate,[83] this may soon make AH redundant.[6,37]

1. Procedure

Ideally, the embryo is positioned to present the zona above the larger perivitelline space not occupied with blastomeres or containing enucleated fragments. The microneedle is front-loaded in an adjacent droplet contained in the same dish, then acidic medium is expelled gently at 3 o'clock over a small area of zona of approximately 30 μm, while the needle presses slightly against it and at the same time is moved up and down in a limited pendular movement to avoid excess acid over any one point in the equatorial plane (Figure 9.7). Expulsion of the acidic Tyrode's medium should cease immediately when the innermost layer of the zona appears eroded. If embryo fragments are present these are removed, but this is best accomplished after moving the embryo to a fresh area of the droplet where the concentration of Tyrode's solution is minimal. The micromanipulated embryos should be rinsed quickly and placed in fresh culture medium until they are transferred.

VII. SUMMARY

Among the techniques designed to overcome an inability of spermatozoa to fertilize *in vitro*, ICSI is by far the most effective in that it leads to high rates of fertilization and pregnancy despite very low sperm numbers or extreme defects in sperm motility

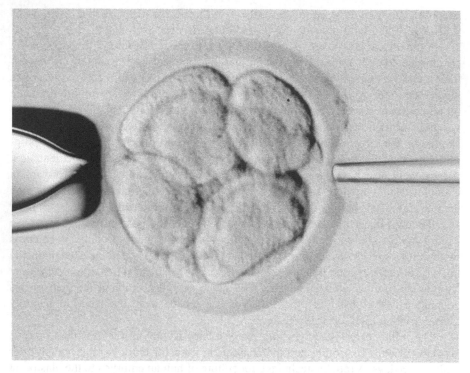

FIGURE 9.7 Assisted hatching.

and morphology. The only requirement is sperm viability, as reflected often in some form of sperm motion (though the sperm should be immobile at the time of injection). Because of its nature, the technique raised some justifiable concerns at first. However, several studies have demonstrated that babies born as a consequence of ICSI have a neonatal malformation rate within the range observed in newborns coming from standard IVF.[8,110] Because it permits high rates of fertilization and pregnancy and proved safe, ICSI is being used increasingly for non male-factor situations where any aspect of gamete function is in doubt. On the other hand, because ICSI may allow procreation by subfertile men, including some with no spermatogenesis in whose cases immature germ cells are used, the possibility exists that similar genetic abnormalities will be transmitted to and reflected postpubertally in some male babies. Therefore, couples treated by ICSI must be screened by chromosomal karyotype and, when oligo- or azoospermic, tested for cystic fibrosis carrier status or deletions present in the Y chromosome.[39]

Although the majority of zygotes created by IVF or by ICSI are quite normal, these techniques can produce a significant number of abnormal pronucleate stages. In the cases that display only one pronucleus, those created by IVF are genetically normal generally,[127] but those monopronucleate embryos that result after ICSI are haploid and so need to be brought to a diploid state.[104] The experience from correction of triploidy, in particular the outcome of persistent mosaicism where one of two male pronuclei are removed from dispermic eggs, supports the concept of paternal inheritance of the centrosome and its control of chromosomal distribution in the cleaving embryo.

Micromanipulation has helped other areas as well. Preimplantation diagnosis can be performed on the blastomeres of cleaved embryos and procedures such as polar body analysis are followed necessarily by ICSI so as to avoid any risk of polyspermy via the zona opening. However, in cases involving sex-linked genetic problems, such procedures may become redundant because of sperm separation techniques based on flow cytometry that promise a way to predetermine the sex of IVF- or ICSI-generated embryos accurately. An increasing need to correct zygote ploidy has stimulated various approaches to an ambitious project: the correction of meiotic abnormalities by the transplantation of oocyte nuclei and/or cytoplasm in an attempt to solve age-related aneuploidy. These and related procedures that until recently appeared to be science fiction, now find a credible foundation in the successful evidence of cloning from an adult mammal.[148]

Finally, we have focused on assisted hatching of the embryo from the enveloping zona, a technique that may enhance implantation. However, this technique may lose its usefulness as culture methods improve to a point that allows routine *in vitro* embryo development and embryo replacement at the expanded blastocyst stage.

REFERENCES

1. Alikani, M., Palermo, G., Adler, A., Bertoli, M., Blake, M., and Cohen, J., Intracytoplasmic sperm injection in dysmorphic human oocytes, *Zygote*, 3, 283–288, 1995.
2. Antinori, S., Versaci, C., Fuhrberg, P., Panci, C., Caffa, B., and Gholami, H., Seventeen live births after the use of an urbium-yttrium-aluminium-garnet laser in the treatment of male factor infertility, *Hum. Reprod.*, 9, 1891–1896, 1994.
3. Antonarakis, S. E. and the Down Syndrome Collaborative Group, Parental origin of the extra chromosome in trisomy 21 as indicated by analysis of DNA polymorphisms, *N. Engl. J. Med.*, 324, 872–876, 1991.
4. Avarbock, M. R., Brinster, C. J., and Brinster, R. L., Reconstitution of spermatogenesis from frozen spermatogonial stem cells, *Nat. Med.*, 2, 693–696, 1996.
5. Azambuja, R., Fugger, E. F., and Schulman, J. D., Human egg activation, cryopreservation and fertilization using a haploid nucleus, *Hum. Reprod.*, 9, 1990–1991, 1990.
6. Barnes, F. L., Crombie, A., Gardner, D. K., Kausche, A., Lacham-Kaplan, O., Suikkari, A. M., Tiglias, J., Wood, C., and Trounson, A. O., Blastocyst development and birth after *in vitro* maturation of human primary oocytes, intracytoplasmic sperm injection and assisted hatching, *Hum. Reprod.*, 10, 3243–3247, 1995.
7. Bedford, J. M. and Kim, H. H., Sperm/egg binding patterns and oocyte cytology in retrospective analysis of fertilization failure *in vitro*, *Hum. Reprod.*, 8, 453–463, 1993.
8. Bonduelle, M., Hamberger, L., Joris, H., Tarlatzis, B. C., and Van Steirteghem, A. C., Assisted reproduction by intracytoplasmic sperm injection: an ESHRE survey of clinical experiences until December 1993, *Hum. Reprod. Update*, 1, 3, CD-ROM, 1995a.
9. Bonduelle, M., Legein, J., Derde, M. P., Buysse, A., Schietecatte, J., Wisanto, A., Devroey, P., Van Steirteghem, A. C., and Liebaers, I., Comparative follow-up study of 130 children born after ICSI and 130 children born after IVF, *Hum. Reprod.*, 10, 3327–3331, 1995b.

10. Bongso, A., Ng, S. C., and Ratnam, S., Cocultures: a new lead in embryo quality improvement for assisted reproduction, *Hum. Reprod.*, 5, 893–900, 1990.
11. Check, J. H., Hoover, L., Nazari, A., O'Shaughnessy, A., and Summers, D., The effect of assisted hatching on pregnancy rates after frozen embryo transfer, *Fertil. Steril.*, 65, 254–257, 1996.
12. Chia, C. M., Sathananthan, H., Ng, S. C., Law, H. Y., and Edirisinghe, W. R., Ultrastructural investigation of failed *in vitro* fertilisation in idiopathic subfertility, *Proc. 18th Singapore-Malaysia Congr. Med.*, Singapore, Singapore: Academy of Medicine, 1984, 52.
13. Chong, S. S., Kristjansson, K., Kota, J., Handyside, A. S., and Hughes, M. R., Preimplantation prevention of X-linked disease: reliable and rapid sex determination of single human cells by restriction analysis of simultaneously amplified ZFX and ZFY sequences, *Hum. Mol. Genet.*, 2, 1187–1191, 1993.
14. Cohen, J., Alikani, M., Ferrara, T., Munné, S., Reing, A., Schattman, G., Tomkin, G., and Rosenwaks, Z., Rescuing abnormally developing embryos by assisted hatching, in Proceedings of the 8th World Congress on *In Vitro* Fertilization and Alternate Assisted Reproduction. September 12–15, 1993, Serono Symposium Review "Perspectives on Assisted Reproduction," 1993.
15. Cohen, J., Alikani, M., Reing, A. M., Ferrara, T. A., Trowbridge, J., and Tucker, M., Selective assisted hatching of human embryos, *Ann. Acad. Med. Singapore*, 21, 565–570, 1992.
16. Cohen, J., Alikani, M., Trowbridge, J., and Rosenwaks, Z., Implantation enhancement by selective assisted hatching using zona drilling of human embryos with poor prognosis, *Hum. Reprod.*, 7, 685–691, 1992.
17. Cohen J., Elsner, C., Kort, H., Malter, H., Massey, J., Mayer, M. P., and Wiemer, K., Impairment of the hatching process following IVF in the human and improvement of implantation by assisting hatching using micromanipulation, *Hum. Reprod.*, 5, 7–13, 1990.
18. Cohen, J. and Feldberg, D., Effects of the size and number of zona pellucida openings on hatching and trophoblast outgrowth in the mouse embryo, *Mol. Reprod. Dev.*, 30, 70–78, 1991.
19. Cohen, J., Inge, K. L., Suzman, M., Wiker, S. R., and Wright, G., Videocinematography of fresh and cryopreserved embryos: a retrospective analysis of embryonic morphology and implantation, *Fertil. Steril.*, 51, 820–827, 1989.
20. Cohen, J., Levron, J., Schimmel, T., and Willadsen, S., Cytoplasmic transfer, *Proc. 9th Annu. In Vitro Fertilization and Embryo Transfer*, Santa Barbara, CA, July 21–24, 1996.
21. Cohen, J., Malter, H., Elsner, C., Kort, H., Massey, J., and Mayer, M. P., Immunosuppression supports implantation of zona pellucida dissected human embryos, *Fertil. Steril.*, 53, 662–665, 1990.
22. Cohen, J., Malter, H., Fehilly, C., Wright, G., Elsner, C., Kort, H., and Massey, J., Implantation of embryos after partial opening of oocyte zona pellucida to facilitate sperm penetration, *Lancet*, ii, 162, 1988.
23. Cohen, J., Munné, S., and Palermo, G. D., Microsurgery in preimplantation embryology, in *Reproductive Endocrinology, Surgery and Technology*, Adashi, E. Y., Roch, J. A., and Rosenwaks, Z., Eds., Lippincott-Raven, Philadelphia, PA, 1996, 2374–2382.
24. Cohen, J., Scott, R., Schimmel, T., Levron, J., and Willadsen, S., Birth of infant after transfer of anucleate donor oocyte cytoplasm into recipient eggs, *Lancet*, 350, 186–187, 1997.

25. Colombero, L. T., Moomjy, M., Hariprashad, J., Oquendo, M., Rosenwaks Z., and Palermo, G. D., Labeling and localization of the centriole/centrosome in intact and dissected spermatozoa, *Fertil. Steril.*, (Suppl.), S122, 1996.

26. Craft, I., Bennett, V., and Nicholson, N., Fertilising ability of testicular spermatozoa, *Lancet*, 342, 864, 1993.

27. De Felici, M. and Siracusa, G., "Spontaneous" hardening of the zona pellucida of mouse oocytes during *in vitro* culture, *Gamete Res.*, 6, 107–113, 1982.

28. De Jonge, C. and Pierce, J., Intracytoplasmic sperm injection—what kind of reproduction is being assisted?, *Hum. Reprod.*, 10, 2518–2520, 1995.

29. deKretser, D. M., Yates, C. A., McDonald, J., Leeton, J. F., Southwick, G., Temple-Smith, P. D., Trounson, A. O., and Wood, E. C., The use of *in vitro* fertilization in the management of male infertility, in *Gamete Quality and Fertility Regulation*, Rolland, R., Heinemann, M. J., Hillier, S. G., and Vemer, M., Eds., Elsevier, Amsterdam, 1985, 213–223.

30. Delhanty, J. D. A. and Handyside, A. H., The origin of genetic defects in the human and their detection in the preimplantation embryo, *Hum. Reprod. Update*, 1, 201–215, 1995.

31. Dyban, A., Freidine, M., Severova, E., Cieslak, J., Ivakhnenko, V., and Verlinsky, Y., Detection of aneuploidy in human oocytes and corresponding first polar bodies by fluorescent *in situ* hybridization, *J. Assist. Reprod. Genet.*, 13, 73–78, 1996.

32. Feichtinger, W., Strohmer, H., Fuhrberg, P., Radivojevic, Antinori, S., Pepe, G., and Versaci, C., Photoablation of oocyte zona pellucida by erbium-yag laser for *in vitro* fertilisation in severe male infertility, *Lancet*, i, 811, 1992.

33. Fishel, S., Green, S., Bishop, M., Thornton, S., Hunter, A., Fleming, S., and Al-Hassan, S., Pregnancy after intracytoplasmic injection of spermatid, *Lancet*, 345, 1641–1642, 1995.

34. Flood, J. T., Chillik, C. F., Van Uem, J. F., Irritani, A., and Hodgen, G. D., Ooplasmic transfusion: prophase germinal vesicle oocytes made developmentally competent by microinjection if metaphase II egg cytoplasm, *Fertil. Steril.*, 53, 1049–1054, 1990.

35. Fulka, J. and Moor, R. M., Noninvasive chemical enucleation of mouse oocytes, *Mol. Reprod. Dev.*, 34, 427–430, 1993.

36. Gardner, R. L. and Edwards, R. G., Control of sex ratio at full term in the rabbit by transferring sexed blastocysts, *Nature*, 218, 346–348, 1968.

37. Gardner, D. K., Vella, P., Lane, M., Wagley, L., Schlenker, T., and Schoolcraft, W. B., Culture and transfer of human blastocysts increases implantation rates and reduces the need for multiple embryo transfers, *Fertil. Steril.*, (Suppl.) S1, 1997.

38. Gibbons, W. E., Gitlin, S. A., Lanzendorf, S. E., Kaufmann, R. A., Slotnick, R. N., and Hodgen, G. D., Preimplantation genetic diagnosis for Tay Sachs disease: successful pregnancy after pre-embryo biopsy and gene amplification by polymerase chain reaction, *Fertil. Steril.*, 63, 723–728, 1995.

39. Girardi, S. K., Mielnik, A., and Schlegel, P. M., Submicroscopic deletions in the Y chromosome of infertile men, *Hum. Reprod.*, 12, 1635–1641, 1997.

40. Gordon, J. W., Grunfeld, J., Garrisi, G. J., Talansky, B. E., Richards, C., and Laufer, N., Fertilization of human oocytes by sperm from infertile males after zona pellucida drilling, *Fertil. Steril.*, 50, 68–73, 1988.

41. Gordon, J. W. and Talansky, B. E., Assisted fertilization by zona drilling: A mouse model for correction of oligospermia, *J. Exp. Zool.*, 239, 347–354, 1986.

42. Goto, K., Kinoshita, A., Takuma, Y., and Ogawa, K., Fertilization by sperm injection in cattle, *Theriogenol.*, 33, 238, 1990.

43. Grifo, J. A., Tang, X. Y., Cohen, J., Gilbert, F., Sanyal, M. K., and Rosenwaks, Z., Pregnancy after embryo biopsy and coamplification of DNA from X and Y chromosomes, *JAMA*, 268, 727–729, 1992.

44. Griffin, D. K., Wilton, L. J., Handyside, A. H., Winston, R. M. L., and Delhanty, J. D. A., Dual fluorescent *in situ* hybridization for simultaneous detection of X and Y chromosome-specific probes for the sexing of human preimplantation embryonic nuclei, *Hum. Genet.*, 89, 18–22, 1992.

45. Gurdon, J. B., Laskey, R. A., and Reeves, O. R., The developmental capacity of nuclei transplanted from keratinized skin cells of adult frogs, *J. Embryol. Exp. Morph.*, 34, 93–112, 1975.

46. Handyside, A. and Delhanty, J. D. A., Preimplantation genetic diagnosis: strategies and surprises, *Trends Genet.*, 13, 270–275, 1997.

47. Handyside, A. H., Kontogianni, F. H., Hardy, K., and Winston, R. M. L., Pregnancies from biopsed human preimplantation embryos sexed by Y-specific DNA amplification, *Nature*, 244, 768–770, 1990.

48. Handyside, A. H., Lesko, J. G., Tarín, J. J., Winston, R. M. L., and Hughes, M. R., Birth of a normal birth after *in vitro* fertilization and preimplantation diagnostic testing for cystic fibrosis, *N. Engl. J. Med.*, 327, 594–598, 1992.

49. Hardy, K., Martin, K. L., Leese, H. J., Winston, R. M., and Handyside, A. H., Human preimplantation development *in vitro* is not adversely affected by biopsy at the 8-cell stage, *Hum. Reprod.*, 5, 708–714, 1990.

50. Harper, J. C., Preimplantation diagnosis of inherited disease by embryo biopsy: an update of the world figures, *J. Assist. Reprod. Genet.*, 13, 90–95, 1996.

51. Hassold, T. and Chiu, D., Maternal age-specific rates of numerical chromosome abnormalities with special reference to trisomy, *Hum. Genet.*, 70, 11–17, 1985.

52. Hellebaut, S., De Sutter, P., Dozortsev, D., Onghena, A., Qian, C., and Dhont, M., Does assisted hatching improve implantation rates after *in vitro* fertilization or intracytoplasmic sperm injection in all patients? A prospective randomized study, *J. Assist. Reprod. Genet.*, 13, 19–22, 1996.

53. Hiramoto, Y., Microinjection of the live spermatozoa into sea urchin eggs, *Exp. Cell Res.*, 27, 416–426, 1962.

54. Hoshi, K., Yanagida, K., and Sato, A., Pretreatment of hamster oocytes with Ca^{2+} ionophore to facilitate fertilization by ooplasmic microinjection, *Hum. Reprod.*, 7, 871–875, 1992.

55. Hosoi, Y., Miyake, M., Utsumi, K., and Iritani, A., Development of rabbit oocytes after microinjection of spermatozoa, *Proc. 11th Int. Congr. Anim. Reprod. Artif. Inseminat.*, Dublin, 1988, 331.

56. In't Veld, P., Brandenburg, H., Verhoeff, A., Dhont, A., and Los, F., Sex chromosomal abnormalities and intracytoplasmic sperm injection, *Lancet*, 336, 773, 1995.

57. Iritani, A. and Hosoi, Y., Microfertilization by various methods in mammalian species, in *Development of Preimplantation Embryos and Their Environment*, Yoshinaga, K. and Mori, T., Eds., Alan R. Liss, New York, 1989, 145–149.

58. Iritani, A., Current status of biotechnological studies in mammalian reproduction, *Fertil. Steril.*, 50, 543–551, 1988.

59. Johnson, L. A., Welch, G. R., Keyvanfar, K., Dorfman, Afugger, E. F., and Schulman, J. D., Gender preselection in humans? Flow cytometry separation of X and Y spermatozoa for the prevention of X-linked disease, *Hum. Reprod.*, 8, 1733–1739, 1993.

60. Keefer, C. L., Fertilization by sperm injection in the rabbit, *Gamete Res.*, 22, 59–69, 1989.

61. Keefer, C. L., Younis, A. I., and Brackett, B. G., Cleavage development of bovine oocytes fertilized by sperm injection, *Mol. Reprod. Dev.*, 25, 281–285, 1990.
62. Khalifa, E. A. and Tucker, M. J., Cruciate thinning of the zona pellucida for more successful enhancement of blastocyst hatching in the mouse, *Hum. Reprod.*, 7, 532–536, 1992.
63. Kimura, Y. and Yanagimachi, R., Development of normal mice from oocytes injected with secondary spermatocyte nuclei, *Biol. Reprod.*, 53, 855–862, 1995.
64. Kishimoto, T., Microinjection and cytoplasmic transfer in starfish oocytes, in *Methods in Cell Biology*, Prescott, D. M., Ed., Academic Press, 1986, 1379–1392.
65. Lalonde, L., Langalis, J., Antaki, P., Chapdelaine, A., Roberts, K. D., and Bleau, G., Male infertility associated with round-headed acrosomeless spermatozoa, *Fertil. Steril.*, 49, 316–321, 1988.
66. Lanzendorf, S. E., Maloney, M. K., Ackerman, S., Acosta, A., and Hodgen, G., Fertilizing potential of acrosome-defective sperm following microsurgical injection into eggs, *Gamete Res.*, 19, 329–337, 1988.
67. Lanzendorf, S. E., Maloney, M. K., Veeck, L. L., Slusser, J., Hodgen, G. D., and Rosenwaks, Z., A preclinical evaluation of pronuclear formation by microinjection of human spermatozoa into human oocytes, *Fertil. Steril.*, 49, 835–842, 1988.
68. Lanzendorf, S. E., Nehchiri, F., Butler, L., Ohehninger, S., and Muasher, S., A prospective, randomized, double-blind study for evaluation of assisted hatching in an *in vitro* fertilization program, *Fertil. Steril.*, (Suppl.) S61, 1996.
69. Laws-King, A., Trounson, A. O., Sathananthan, H., and Kola, I., Fertilization of human oocytes by microinjection of a single spermatozoon under the zona pellucida, *Fertil. Steril.*, 48, 637–642, 1987.
70. Levinson, G., Keyvanfar, K., Wu, J. C., Fugger, E. F., Fields, R. A., Harton, G. L., Palmer, F. T., Sisson, M. E., Starr, K. M., Dennison-Lagos, L. et al., DNA-based X-enriched sperm separation as an adjunct to preimplantation genetic testing for the prevention of X-linked disease, *Hum. Reprod.*, 10, 979–982, 1995.
71. Levron, J., Munné, S., Wiladsen, S., Rosenwaks, Z., and Cohen, J., Male and female genomes associated in a single pronucleus in human zygotes, *Biol. Reprod.*, 52, 653–657, 1995.
72. Levron, J., Willadsen, S., Munné, S., and Cohen, J., Formation of male pronuclei in partitioned human oocytes, *Biol. Reprod.*, 53, 209–213, 1995.
73. Liebaers, I., Bonduelle, M., Van Assche, E., Devroey, P., and Van Steirteghem, A., Sex chromosome abnormalities after intracytoplasmic sperm injection, *Lancet*, 346, 773, 1995.
74. Lin, T. P., Microinjection of mouse eggs, *Science*, 151, 333–337, 1966.
75. Liu, H.-C., Jones, G. S., Jones, H. W., Jr., and Rosenwaks, Z., Mechanisms and factors of early pregnancy wastage in *in vitro* fertilization-embryo transfer patients, *Fertil. Steril.*, 50, 95–101, 1988.
76. Liu, J., Lissens, W., Van Broeckhoven, C., Logfren, A., Camus, M., Liebaers, I., and Van Steirteghem, A. C., Normal pregnancy after preimplantation DNA diagnosis of a dystrophin gene deletion, *Prenatal Diagn.*, 15, 351–358, 1995.
77. Liu, J., Nagy, Z., Joris, H., Tournaye, H., Devroey, P., and Van Steirteghem, A. C., Successful fertilization and establishment of pregnancies after intracytoplasmic sperm injection in patients with globozoospermia, *Hum. Reprod.*, 10, 626–629, 1995.
78. Loret de Mola, J. R., Garside, W. T., Bucci, J., Tureck, R. W., and Heyner, S., Analysis of the human zona pellucida during culture: correlation with diagnosis and the preovulatory hormonal environment, *J. Assist. Reprod. Genet.*, 14, 332–336, 1997.

79. Malter, H. E. and Cohen, J., Blastocyst formation and hatching *in vitro* following zona drilling of mouse and human embryos, *Gamete Res.*, 24, 67–80, 1989.

80. Malter, H. E. and Cohen, J., Embryonic development after microsurgical repair of polyspermic human zygotes, *Fertil. Steril.*, 52, 373–380, 1989.

81. Markert, C. L., Fertilization of mammalian eggs by sperm injection, *J. Exp. Zool.*, 228, 195–201, 1983.

82. Masui, Y. and Markert, C. L., Cytoplasmic control of behavior during meiotic maturation of frog oocytes, *J. Exp. Zool.*, 177, 129–136, 1971.

83. Menezo, Y., Hazout, A., Dumont, M., Herbaut, N., and Nicollet, B., Coculture of embryos on Vero cells and transfer of blastocysts in humans, *Hum. Reprod.*, 7 (Suppl. 1), 101–106, 1992.

84. Meyerhof, P. G. and Masui, Y., Properties of a cytostatic factor from Xenopus laevis eggs, *Dev. Biol.*, 72, 182–186, 1979.

85. Morton, P. C., Yoder, C. S., Tucker, M. J., Wright, G., Brockman, W. D. W., and Kort, H. I., Reinsemination by intracytoplasmic sperm injection of 1-day-old oocytes after complete conventional fertilization failure, *Fertil. Steril.*, 68, 488–491, 1997.

86. Muggleton-Harris, A., Whittingham, D. G., and Wilson, L. Cytoplasmic control of preimplantation development *in vitro* in the mouse, *Nature*, 299, 460–461, 1982.

87. Muggleton-Harris, A. L. and Brown, J. J. G., Cytoplasmic factors influence mitochondrial reorganization and resumption of cleavage during culture if early mouse embryos, *Hum. Reprod.*, 3, 1020–1028, 1988.

88. Munné, S., Alikani, M., Tomkin, G., Grifo, J., and Cohen, J., Embryo morphology, developmental rates and maternal age are correlated with chromosome abnormalities, *Fertil. Steril.*, 64, 382–391, 1995.

89. Munné, S., Dailey, T., Sultan, K. M., Grifo, J., and Cohen, J., The use of first polar bodies for preconception diagnosis of aneuploidy, *Hum. Reprod.*, 10, 1014–1020, 1995.

90. Munné, S., Lee, A., Rosenwaks, Z., Grifo, J., and Cohen, J., Diagnosis of major chromosomes aneuploidies in human preimplantation embryos, *Hum. Reprod.*, 8, 2185–2191, 1993.

91. Munné, S., Scott, R., Bergh, J., and Cohen, J., First pregnancies after polar body biopsy for testing chromosome translocations, *Fertil. Steril.*, (Suppl) S1, 1996.

92. Munné, S., Sultan, K. M., Weier, HUG, Grifo, J., Cohen, J., and Rosenwaks, Z., Assessment of numerical abnormalities of X, Y, 18 and 16 chromosomes in preimplantation embryos prior to transfer, *Am. J. Obstet. Gynecol.*, 172, 1191–1201, 1995.

93. Munné, S., Tang, Y. X., Grifo, J., and Cohen, J., Origin of a single pronucleated human zygotes, *J. Assist. Reprod. Genet.*, 10, 276–279, 1993.

94. Munné, S., Weier, H. U. G., Stein, J., Grifo, J., and Cohen, J., A fast and efficient method for simultaneous X and Y *in situ* hybridization of human blastomeres, *J. Assist. Reprod. Genet.*, 10, 82–90, 1993.

95. Nagy, Z. P., Staessen, C., Liu, J., Joris, H., Devroey, P., and Van Steirteghem, A. C., Prospective, auto-controlled study on reinsemination of failed-fertilized oocytes by intracytoplasmic sperm injection, *Fertil. Steril.*, 64, 1130–1135, 1995.

96. Naish, S. J., Perreault, S. D., and Zirkin, B. J., DNA synthesis following microinjection of heterologous sperm and somatic cell nuclei into hamster oocytes, *Gamete Res.*, 18, 109–120, 1987.

97. New York State Department of Health. Congenital Malformations Registry: Annual Report 1990, Albany, New York.

98. Ng, S.-C., Bongso, A., and Ratnam, S. S., Microinjection of human oocytes: a technique for severe oligasthenoteratozoospermia, *Fertil. Steril.*, 56, 1117–1123, 1991.

99. Odawara, Y. and Lopata, A., Zona cracking: a new technique for assisted fertilization, *Proc. Aust. Fertil. Soc. Meet.*, Sidney, 1987, 073.

100. Ogura, A., Matsuda, J., and Yanagimachi, R., Birth of normal young after electrofusion of mouse oocytes with round spermatids, *Proc. Natl. Acad. Sci. USA*, Developmental biology, 91, 7460–7462, 1994.

101. Palermo, G., Joris, H., Derde, M. P., Camus, M., Devroey, P., and Van Steirteghem, A. C., Sperm characteristics and outcome of human assisted fertilization by subzonal insemination and intracytoplasmic sperm injection, *Fertil. Steril.*, 59, 826–835, 1993.

102. Palermo, G., Joris, H., Devroey, P., and Van Steirteghem, A. C., Induction of acrosome reaction in human spermatozoa used for subzonal insemination, *Hum. Reprod.*, 7, 248–254, 1992.

103. Palermo, G., Joris, H., Devroey, P., and Van Steirteghem, A. C., Pregnancies after intracytoplasmic injection of single spermatozoon into an oocyte, *Lancet*, 340, 17–18, 1992.

104. Palermo, G., Munné, S., and Cohen, J., The human zygote inherits its mitotical potential from the male gamete, *Hum. Reprod.*, 9, 1220–1225, 1994.

105. Palermo, G. and Van Steirteghem, A. C., Enhancement of acrosome reaction and subzonal insemination of a single spermatozoon in mouse eggs, *Mol. Reprod. Dev.*, 30, 339–345, 1991.

106. Palermo, G. D., Cohen, J., Alikani, M., Adler, A., and Rosenwaks, Z., Intracytoplasmic sperm injection: a novel treatment for all forms of male factor infertility, *Fertil. Steril.*, 63, 1231–1240, 1995.

107. Palermo, G., Alikani, M., and Bertoli, M., Oolemma characteristics in relation to survival and fertilization patterns of oocytes treated by ICSI, *Hum. Reprod.*, 61, 265–268, 1996.

108. Palermo, G. D., Cohen, J., and Rosenwaks, Z., Intracytoplasmic sperm injection: a powerful tool to overcome fertilization failure, *Fertil. Steril.*, 65, 899–908, 1996.

109. Palermo, G. D., Colombero, L. T., and Rosenwaks, Z., The human sperm centrosome is responsible for normal fertilization and early embryonic development, *Rev. Reprod.*, 2, 19–27, 1997.

110. Palermo, G. D., Colombero, L. T., Schattman, G. L., Davis, O. K., and Rosenwaks, Z., Evolution of pregnancies and initial follow-up of newborns delivered after intracytoplasmic sperm injection, *JAMA*, 276, 1893–1897, 1996.

111. Patrizio, P., Intracytoplasmic sperm injection (ICSI): potential genetic concerns, *Hum. Reprod.*, 10, 2520–2, 1995.

112. Perreault, S. D., Wolf, R. A., and Zirkin, B. R., The role of disulfide bond reduction during mammalian sperm nuclear decondensation *in vivo*, *Dev. Biol.*, 101, 160–167, 1984.

113. Perreault, S. D. and Zirkin, B. R., Sperm nuclear decondensation in mammals: role of sperm associated proteinase *in vivo*, *J. Exp. Zool.*, 224, 252–257, 1982.

114. Rawlins, R. G., Binor, Z., Radwanska, E., and Dmowski, W. P., Microsurgical enucleation of tripronuclear human zygotes, *Fertil. Steril.*, 50, 266–272, 1988.

115. Reubinoff, B. E. and Schushan, A., Preimplantation diagnosis in older patients. To biopsy or not to biopsy?, *Hum. Reprod.*, 11, 2071–2075, 1996.

116. Sathananthan, A. H., Ng, S. C., Trounson, A. O., Bongso, A., Laws-King, A., and Ratnam, S. S., Human micro-insemination by injection of single or multiple sperm: ultrastructure, *Hum. Reprod.*, 4, 574–583, 1989.

117. Sathananthan, A. H., Kola, I., Osborne, J., Trounson, A. O., Ng, S. C., Bongso, A., and Ratnam, S. S., Centrioles in the beginning of human development, *Proc. Natl. Acad. Sci. USA*, 88, 4806–4810, 1991.

118. Sathananthan, A. H., Ratnam, S. S., Ng, S.-C., Tarin, J. J., Gianaroli, L., and Trounson, A. O., The sperm centriole: its inheritance, replication and perpetuation in early human embryos, *Hum. Reprod.*, 11, 345–356, 1996.

119. Schatten, G., The centrosome and its mode of inheritance: the reduction of the centrosome during gametogenesis and its restoration during fertilization, *Dev. Biol.*, 165, 299–335, 1994.

120. Schoolcraft, W. B., Schlenker, T., Gee, M., Jones, G. S., and Jones, H. W., Assisted hatching in the treatment of poor prognosis *in vitro* fertilization candidates, *Fertil. Steril.*, 62, 551–554, 1994.

121. Schoysman, R., Vanderzwalmen, P., Nijs, M., Segal, L., Segal-Bertin, G., Geerts, L., van Roosendaal, and Schoysman, D., Pregnancy after fertilization with human testicular spermatozoa, *Lancet*, 342, 1237, 1993.

122. Schoysman, R., Vanderzwalmen, P., Zech, H., Yemini, M., Birkenfield, A., Chan, M., Vandamme, B., and Lejeune, B., Results of spermatid injection in human oocytes in relation to previous testis biopsy and oocytes treatment, *Fertil. Steril.*, (Suppl), S529, 1996.

123. Silber, S. J., Devroey, P., Nagy, Z., Liu, J., Tournaye, H., and Van Steirteghem, A. C., ICSI with testicular and epididymal sperm, *Proc. ESHRE Workshop*, Brussels, 1994, 36–41.

124. Silber, S. J., Ord, T., Borrero, C., Balmaceda, J., and Asch, R., New treatment for infertility due to congenital absence of the vas deferens, *Lancet*, 2, 850–851, 1987.

125. Sluder, G., Miller, F. J., Lewis, K., Davison, E. D., and Rieder, C. L., Centrosome inheritance in starfish zygotes: selective loss of the maternal centrosome after fertilization, *Dev. Biol.*, 131, 567–579, 1989.

126. Strom, C. M., Rechitsky, S., and Verlinsky, Y., Reliability of gender determination using polymerase chain reaction for single cells, *J. In Vitro Fert. Embryo Transfer*, 8, 225–229, 1991.

127. Sultan, K., Munné, S., Palermo, G., Alikani, M., and Cohen, J., Chromosomal status of uni-pronuclear human zygotes following *in vitro* fertiliztion and intracytoplasmic sperm injection, *Hum. Reprod.*, 10, 132–136, 1995.

128. Tang, Y. X., Munné, S., Reing, A., Schattman, G., Grifo, J., and Cohen, J., The parental origin of the distal pronucleus in dispermic human zygotes, *Zygote*, 2, 79–85, 1994.

129. Temple-Smith, P. D., Southwick, G. J., Yates, C. A., Trounson, A. O., and de Kretser, D. M., Human pregnancy by *in vitro* fertilization (IVF) using sperm aspirated from the epididymis, *J. In Vitro Fert. Embryo Transfer*, 2, 119–122, 1985.

130. Tesarik, J., Mendoza, C., and Testart, J., Viable embryos from injection of round spermatids into oocytes, *N. Engl. J. Med.*, 333, 525, 1995.

131. Thadani, V. M., A study of oocyte interactions using *in vitro* fertilization and sperm microinjection, Ph.D. thesis, Yale University, New Haven, CT, 1981.

132. Thadani, V. M., Injection of sperm heads into immature rat oocytes, *J. Exp. Zool.*, 210, 161–168, 1979.

133. Thibault, C. and Gerard, M., Cytoplasmic factor necessary for formation of male pronucleus in rabbit oocyte, *CR Hebd. Seances Acad. Sci. Paris*, 270, 2025–2026, 1970.

134. Tournaye, H., Deveroey, P., Liu, J., Nagy, Z., Lissens, W., and Van Steirteghem, A., Microsurgical epididymal sperm aspiration and intracytoplasmic sperm injection: a new effective approach to infertility as a result of cogenital bilateral absence of vas deferens, *Fertil. Steril.*, 61, 1045–1051, 1994.

---

135. Tsunoda, Y., Yasui, T., and Nakamura, K., Effect of cutting the zona pellucida on the pronuclear transplantation in the mouse, *J. Exp. Zool.*, 240, 119–125, 1986.
136. Tucker, J. M., Cohen, J., Massey, B. J., Mayer, P. M., Wiker, R. S., and Wright, G., Partial dissection of the zona pellucida of frozen-thawed human embryos may enhance blastocyst hatching, implantation, and pregnancy rates, *Am. J. Obstet. Gynecol.*, 165, 341–345, 1991.
137. Uehara, T. and Yanagimachi, R., Behavior of nuclei of testicular, caput and cauda epididymal spermatozoa injected into hamster eggs, *Biol. Reprod.*, 16, 315–321, 1977.
138. Uehara, T. and Yanagimachi R., Microsurgical injection of spermatozoa into hamster eggs with subsequent transformation of sperm nuclei into male pronuclei, *Biol. Reprod.*, 15, 467–470, 1976.
139. Usui, N. and Yanagimachi, R., Behavior of hamster sperm nuclei incorporated into eggs at various stages of maturation, fertilization, and early development. The appearance and disappearance of factors involved in sperm chromatin decondensation in egg cytoplasm, *J. Ultrastruct. Res.*, 57, 276–288, 1976.
140. Van Blerkom, J. and Henry, G., Oocyte dysmorphism and aneuploidy in meiotically mature human oocytes after ovarian stimulation, *Hum. Reprod.*, 3, 379–390, 1992.
141. Veeck, L. L., Oehnninger, S., Acosta, A. A., and Muasher, S. J., Sperm microinjection in a clinical *in vitro* fertilization program, *Proc. 45th Ann. Congr. Am. Fertil. Soc.*, San Francisco, CA, 50, 1989.
142. Verlinsky, Y., Cieslak, J., Freidine, M., Ivakhnenko, V., Wolf, G., Kovalinskaya, L., White, M., Lifchez, A., Kaplan, B., Moise, J., Valle, J., Ginsberg, N., Strom, C., and Kuliev, A., Polar body diagnosis of common aneuploidies by FISH, *J. Assist. Reprod. Genet.*, 13, 157–162, 1996.
143. Verlinsky, Y., Cieslak, J., Freidine, M., Ivakhnenko, V., Wolf, G., Kovalinskaya, L., White, M., Lifchez, A., Kaplan, B., Moise, J. et al., Pregnancies following preconception diagnosis of common aneuploidies by fluorescent *in situ* hybridization, *Hum. Reprod.*, 10, 1923–1927, 1995.
144. Verlinsky, Y., Cieslak, J., Wolf, G., Rechitsky, S., Strom, C., White, M., Lifchez, A., Ginsberg, N., and Applebaum, M., Polar body sampling, *Prenatal Diag.*, (Suppl. 12) 37, 1992.
145. Wiker, S., Malter, H., Wright, G., and Cohen, J., Recognition of paternal pronuclei in human zygotes, *J. In Vitro Fertil. Embryo Transfer*, 7, 33–37, 1990.
146. Willadsen, S. M., Cloning of sheeps and cows embryos, *Genome*, 31, 956–963, 1989.
147. Willadsen, S. M., Nuclear transplantation in sheep embryos, *Nature*, 320, 63–65, 1986.
148. Wilmut, I., Schieke, A. E., McWhir, J., Kind, A. J., and Campbell, K. H. S., Viable offspring derived from fetal and adult mammalian cells, *Nature*, 385, 810–813, 1997.
149. Wilton, L. J. and Trounson, A. O., Biopsy of preimplantation mouse embryos: development of micromanipulated embryos and proliferation of single blastomeres *in vitro*, *Biol. Reprod.*, 40, 145–152, 1989.
150. World Health Organization, Task Force on the Diagnosis and Treatment of Infertility, Towards more objectivity in diagnosis and management of male infertility, prepared by Comhaire, F. H., de Kretser, D., Farley, T. M. M., and Rowe, P. J., *Int. J. Androl.*, (Suppl) 7, 1–53, 1987.
151. Yanagida, K., Bedford, J. M., and Yanagimachi, R., Cleavage of rabbit eggs after microsurgical injection of testicular spermatozoa, *Hum. Reprod.*, 6, 277–279, 1991.
152. Younis, A. I., Keefer, C. L., and Brackett, B. G., Fertilization of bovine oocytes by sperm injection, *Theriogenol*, 31, 276, 1989.

153. Yovich, J. L. and Stanger, J. D., The limitations of *in vitro* fertilization from male with severe oligospermia and abnormal sperm morphology, *J. In Vitro Fert. Embryo Transfer*, 1, 172–179, 1984.

154. Zhang, J., Grifo, J., Blaszczyk, A., Meng, L., Adler, A., Chin, A., and Krey, L., *In vitro* maturation (IVM) of human preovulatory oocytes reconstructed by germinal vesicle (GV) transfer, *Fertil. Steril.*, (Suppl.) S1, 1997.

10 Quality Control: A Framework for the ART Laboratory

Kathryn J. Go

CONTENTS

0-8493-1677-4/00/$0.00+$.50
© 2000 by CRC Press LLC

I. INTRODUCTION

Quality control (QC) is a goal realized through a program for the routine inspection of a system to ensure that a product or service is delivered under optimal conditions. When applied to a clinical laboratory, the QC program addresses both tangible elements, such as instrumentation, equipment, and supplies and intangible elements, such as the qualifications and expertise of personnel, protocols, and record-keeping. In this chapter, the components comprising a program for quality control in the assisted reproductive technologies (ART) laboratory will be described. Such a program is the underpinning for a quality awssurance (QA) program,[1] the mission of which is to offer the consumer, or patient in this case, optimal care through constant surveillance of the system in which the patient's care is delivered.

This author would be presumptuous to *prescribe* a quality control program for the ART laboratory. As the myriad of procedures included in ART has evolved and expanded, so has a range of technical and managerial styles as well as laboratory designs. Rather, this chapter is intended to identify the elements that should receive attention within the framework of a quality control program for an ART laboratory and to suggest some approaches in pursuit of that goal. A subtext of common sense will pervade, for the cornerstone of achieving good results in a laboratory is having the right people do the right things in the right environment.

II. THE ASSISTED REPRODUCTIVE TECHNOLOGIES (ART)

A compendium of procedures and techniques comprising ART is provided in Table 10.1. Evolving from the foundation of *in vitro* fertilization (IVF), an array of additional and related methodologies to deliver gametes or embryos to the female reproductive tract to initiate pregnancy, accomodate supernumerary zygotes or embryos from a stimulation cycle, and achieve fertilization in cases of severe male factor infertility have been developed. The contemporary ART laboratory is challenged to acquire new technologies as they arise and are refined in its mission to offer effective state-of-the-art therapy to patients.

TABLE 10.1
The Assisted Reproductive Technologies (ART)

In vitro fertilization (IVF)
Gamete intra-fallopian transfer (GIFT)
Zygote intra-fallopian transfer (ZIFT)
Tubal embryo transfer (TET)
Cryopreservation of zygotes and embryos
Intracytoplasmic sperm injection (ICSI)
Assisted hatching
Preimplantation genetic diagnosis (blastomere biopsy)

ART is a multi-disciplinary approach to treating infertility, requiring expertise from clinical personnel, physicians, and nurses, and from the scientists, embryologists, and technologists specializing in the culture of human gametes and embryos. The success of a clinic is similarly multifactorial. Some of the effectors of an ART program's pregnancy rate are patient selection (age and indication for infertility), clinical expertise and experience, and the performance of the ART laboratory.[2] Unlike some clinical laboratories that perform routine bioassays, the ART laboratory cannot construct standard curves values for, as an example, the fertilization rate, as this parameter depends on various factors including the quality of the oocytes obtained during the patient's ovulation induction or the presence of a male fertility factor. Each clinic and laboratory will, in the course of its experience, appraise the characteristics of its own ART program and assess the factors influencing its clinical outcomes.

The ART laboratory has a critical and integral role in the clinic. Within this cooperative effort to help a patient couple achieve a pregnancy, the laboratory should strive to ensure that its individual operating systems conserve, both quantitatively and qualitatively, the gametes and embryos in its care and provide conditions under which they can realize their full developmental potential. Both the reporting of clinical outcome data and the development of a model program for laboratory accreditation are the provisions of the Fertility Clinic Success Rate and Certification Act, passed in 1992, to oversee ART in the U.S. The model program for the ART laboratory was foreseen by early attention directed to quality control as reflected by the provisions of guidelines[3] and a voluntary laboratory inspection program.[4]

III. THE GOALS OF QUALITY CONTROL (QC)

Table 10.2 encapsulates the objectives of a quality control program for the ART laboratory. Each objective must be met to fulfill the mission of the laboratory and its QC program. Together, these objectives account for all the operating components of the laboratory, both tangible (personnel, instruments, etc.) and intangible (techniques, documentation, record-keeping, etc.). In the chapter sections that follow, each objective will be addressed and folded into the context of the operation of the laboratory as a unit.

TABLE 10.2
Elements of a Quality Control (QC) Program

Appropriately educated and trained laboratory personnel.
Correct operation and calibration of all instruments.
Consistent and proper execution of appropriate techniques and methods.
Procedure and policy manuals.
Documentation and record-keeping.
System for patient sample collection and management.
System for the appraisal of performance, correction of deficiencies, and implementation of advances and improvements.

In acknowledgment that the pursuit of quality control begins at the planning and inception of a laboratory, the subject of laboratory design will be considered first. Those who use and benefit from it will appreciate the attention to rational design and laboratory configuration.

IV. LABORATORY DESIGN

A. PERSPECTIVES ON PHYSICAL PLANT

The ART laboratory is unique. Its work transcends the usual assay/diagnostic role played by a clinical laboratory although data of that nature also result. The ART laboratory is entrusted with the task of producing human embryos for transfer to the uterus to a achieve a much-sought implantation and pregnancy.

Despite the magnitude of this responsibility, there are, no doubt, many embryologists who remember establishing their laboratories in spare rooms supplied by hospitals, and who might regale us with anecdotes of laboratories installed in closets and storage rooms. We hope that we live in more enlightened times and that administration recognizes the critical importance of the physical plant, layout, and special support considerations for the ART laboratory.

ART laboratories historically were located in hospitals. The advent of ultrasonically guided, transvaginal follicular aspiration for oocyte collection obviated the laparoscopic approach and the attendant requirement for an operating room, paving the way for office-based ART programs.

Another permutation on availability of ART services is the centralized laboratory to which eggs retrieved off-site are transported under controlled physiologic conditions for IVF or intracytoplasmic sperm injection (ICSI). This modality relieves the infertility center of the considerable expense of having its own ART laboratory and personnel or allows access by multiple infertility centers to specialized techniques not offered in their own ART laboratories, such as micromanipulation.

B. REQUIREMENTS

There could be as many architectural/engineering designs for an ART laboratory as there are embryologists who would design them. Some general principles have been described[5,6] and a list of common denominators in the organization of an ART laboratory is presented in Table 10.3.

Design should provide adequate space for:

- Instruments and equipment
- Separation of tasks
- Mobility of laboratory workers
- Storage of supplies and reagents

All surfaces in the ART laboratory must lend themselves to cleaning and sterilization.

TABLE 10.3
Physical Plant Requirements
of the ART Laboratory

Adequate space
Appropriate location
Rational design
Control of cleaning and maintenance
Control over air quality
Security

C. Location

Establishing an appropriate location for the ART laboratory is often a luxury, given the premium on hospital space, surgical centers, and office suites. Ideally, locate the laboratory in a protected, sheltered part of the facility where traffic is minimal and there is more control over the immediate environment.

Procedure rooms for egg retrievals or embryo transfers and the ART laboratory should be contiguous or only a short distance apart. One would not want to traverse great distances holding tubes of follicular fluid or a catheter loaded with embryos. In cases in which distance is unavoidable, isolettes equipped with temperature control and carbon dioxide infusion help. The principle of maintaining a suitable environment for gametes and embryos is at the foundation of ART.

D. Environs

In consideration of ventilation in the ART laboratory, positive pressure coupled with atmospheric particle filtration [High Efficiency Particulate Air filtration (HEPA) filters] ensures that air quality protects the gamete and embryo cultures. One should reduce incident odors, noxious fumes, or vapors. And, colognes, scented lotions, or cosmetics on both personnel and patients should be prohibited.

Additional means of filtering or treating the air in the ART laboratory through placement of intra-incubator filtration devices and free standing air handlers may be necessary. These may be particularly useful when location of the ART laboratory makes it susceptible to sources of volatile solvents or atmospheric agents commonly found in healthcare facilities, e.g., anesthetic gases, disinfectants, and cleaning agents, isopropyl alcohol.[7] However, initial design of the ART laboratory should address locational considerations that minimize exposure to atmospheric agents.

E. Configuration

Careful design of the ART laboratory, as with any working environment, will enhance efficiency. Thoughtful placement of related instruments, e.g., laminar flow hood and incubator, will minimize embryologist movement and allow shortest times of exposure of gametes and embryos.

F. SECURITY

For both security and maintenance, one must limit access to the ART laboratory. This eliminates tampering through incidental or accidental contact with any of the patient samples, instruments, supplies, or equipment in the ART laboratory or the introduction of a potential toxicant to the area. Both the Security Department and the Environmental and Engineering services in the hospital or office building should receive written notification of the special requirements and conditions for the ART laboratory. An embryologist should never have to worry about entering the laboratory and finding a crew applying a fresh coat of paint to the walls!

Maintenance and repair work should be planned in advance at appropriate times with an embryologist present to ensure that any questions about moving instruments or modifying some aspect of the laboratory's structural organization can be answered.

V. PERSONNEL

A. HISTORICAL PERSPECTIVE

IVF is only two decades old as a clinical technique, and an "original cast" of embryologists is likely to still be in the work force. These pioneers came from both clinical and basic science research laboratories and assembled a practical knowledge gleaned from backgrounds in tissue culture, embryology, agricultural science, microbiology, genetics, and clinical chemistry.

To answer the demand for workers in the expanding number of infertility centers offering ART, individuals often received training "on-the-job," in an apprentice relationship with an experienced embryologist. Training resulted from observation, reading, review of current literature, and hands-on practice. Another expedient route to obtain training was to visit an established laboratory and receive the tutelage of the presiding embryologist. Inevitably, a host of styles for performing the various ART techniques evolved with different emphases, points of attention, and levels of acceptance of various tasks, materials, and instruments. Although this can be interpreted as a lack of standardization, it also can be viewed, reasonably, as a variety of techniques, which differ in style, but are founded on the same solid principals of good laboratory practice and scientific intuition.

B. TRAINING

ART training still occurs through the tutelage by an experienced embryologist, but it now has been supplemented by formal courses offering both didactic and practical approaches. These tend, however, to focus on recently developed or emerging techniques that require both extensive experience in ART and previous specialized training. An example of the latter is ICSI for which workshops proliferated for the embryologist already familiar with IVF and micromanipulation. The foundation of training in ART is likely to still be acquired in the workplace, which offers the benefit of the accumulated experience, the guidance of an experienced embryologist, and exposure to a variety of circumstances sometimes requiring innovation and creative solutions.

For the uninitiated, the handling of gametes and embryos can be daunting. The mouse embryo biosassay (see section VIII of this chapter) serves as a valuable teaching tool, providing practice in all the fundamentals of ART: manipulation of cells, sterile technique, preparation of the culture system, and a global understanding of the reproductive biology underlying the technique, including its kinetics and endpoints for assessing outcome. Because parallel culture systems can be run by trainer and trainee, a comparison of results is possible, providing some insight into where potential deficiencies exist.

The laboratory director or manager determines the completion of training and the attainment of a skill level by an individual and permits subsequent unsupervised work in the ART laboratory. A combination of indices helps make this determination including the evaluation of results from bioassays conducted as part of the practice of a technique (in which a biological or development end-point is reached and can be quantified), supervised clinical experience, and the self-evaluated confidence level of the trainee.

Documentation of an embryologist's proficiency should be recorded and updated as new or specialized techniques such as micromanipulation are added to the individual's repertoire in ART.

C. CONTINUING EDUCATION

Maintenance and honing of skills in the ART laboratory are essential. One must remain proficient as this facilitates optimal patient care and inspires confidence in the ART practitioner at the laboratory level. Acquisition of new skills is desirable and necessary to remain competitive in this rapidly evolving field infused with high expectations from all participants—patients, clinicians, and embryologists.

Professional education continues through enrollment in formal courses and the reading of peer-reviewed scientific literature. Memberships in professional organizations can provide interaction with peers, with the attendant benefit of a network providing exposure to new ideas and exchange of information.

D. CERTIFICATION

With the appropriate academic preparation and professional experience, certification may be desirable for career development or required for employment in some laboratories. In accordance with educational background and work experience, certification as a laboratory director or manager, technical consultant or supervisor, general supervisor, or clinical consultant can be obtained through the American Board of Bioanalysis.

E. EXTRAMURAL SUPPORT

The ART laboratory may use support services provided by hospitals or outpatient surgi-centers. These may include the participation of and assistance from operating room nurses or technicians during procedures or the provision or processing of supplies, equipment, or instruments.

Because these services can assist, increase efficiency, or even fulfill certain ART laboratories' operational requirements, one should ensure that the providers of such services understand the special requirements of ART. Education through in-service presentations to operating room or central suppliers within the facility help in understanding issues of toxicity. Many products used routinely in operating rooms are potent embryotoxins, e.g., talc, iodine, alcohol, etc.

ART procedures may require dispensation from normal operating room routine. The requirements for special handling and processing should be outlined in policies specific for ART procedures.

The embryologist may wish to perform as much as possible of the processing or preparation of materials used in the ART laboratory, such as washing, packaging, and labeling of equipment before delivery to extramural processing, such as sterilization. Periodic correspondence with any centralized processing unit handling ART laboratory materials will provide constant surveillance and a channel for making any amendments to processing protocols.

VI. PATIENT SAMPLE MANAGEMENT

A. SAMPLE IDENTIFICATION

Paramount among QC issues in an ART program are the systems employed to ensure patient identification and patient sample identification. Although obvious, it bears stating explicitly that an ART laboratory must have absolute certainty when combining gametes and when transferring embryos to a patient. The embryologist must verify, with documentation, and with a witness if necessary, the sources of the gametes and the identities of embryos and the corresponding recipient.

The ART laboratory must establish with clarity the name, or unique identification number or code, with which the labeling of patient materials will proceed. The last name of the female patient frequently is used. Once the unique identifier is established, it must be used uniformly and consistently. This identification will be used for the labeling of all culture dishes, the husband or partner's semen specimen container, and all laboratory records. More exacting strategies must be employed for more common surnames, such as inclusion of initials or supplementary coding. All labeling should be permanent so that it is legible and cannot be obliterated through handling.

B. CHAIN OF CUSTODY

Laboratories should implement a system by which the embryologist is required to document his/her performance of every significant laboratory event such as receipt of a semen sample, preparation of sperm from a semen sample, egg insemination, or transfer of zygotes to growth medium. This safety redundancy and similar methods of double-checking and cross-checking with documentation must comprise a system that ensures correct matching of gamete sources and matching of embryos and recipient. One cannot overestimate the anxiety that patients may harbor about this issue.

VII. WRITTEN PROCEDURES AND POLICIES

A requisite component of the ART laboratory is the written procedure manual. For each procedure or technique, complete details are provided on the requirements of supplies, instruments, and method. The clarity and precision of the manual should allow the embryologist to perform any of the recorded techniques in a consistent, reproducible fashion with understanding of each method and its objectives.

A poignant example of the importance of a clear procedure description is provided by inter-laboratory transfer of cryopreserved embryos. The laboratory of origin must provide to the receiving laboratory the appropriate thawing procedure. The necessity for well-written, organized descriptions of a procedure is appreciated by laboratories who must share them.

The policies governing the procedures also should be outlined. These will provide some consistency in decision-making processes, e.g., at what stage should cryopreservation occur, how many eggs should be inseminated if cryopreservation is declined, how many embryos should be transferred to the patient? Of course, policies may require modification as clinical and laboratory experience accumulates, must be flexible to accommodate special circumstances, and should consider ethical and legal principles.

VIII. QUALITY CONTROL ASSAYS

A. INTRODUCTION

The assisted reproductive techniques, particularly the cornerstone technique of IVF, have a dual nature: the process is both therapeutic and diagnostic. The therapeutic role is realized in the provision of the embryos that may give rise to the desired pregnancy. The diagnostic role is fulfilled by the data generated from observations of the gametes and embryos. These can provide information at the cellular level and result from the semen analysis, maturation assessment of eggs, and developmental and morphologic status of the embryos.

B. OBJECTIVES OF THE QC BIOASSAY

A QC assay for the ART laboratory entails the routinely scheduled survey of the culture system utilized in the ART laboratory for gametes and embryos. In this section, the assays and what they are designed to demonstrate will be discussed.

One cannot overstate the central importance of the culture media that support gametes and embryos and the materials to which they are exposed. While culture media of various formulations, in conjunction with a variety of protein sources, are utilized routinely, all must provide an environment that will support fertilization and early embryo development. The embryologist must be confident that these media are free from toxins, contaminants, or inhibitors of these processes and that the ambient conditions provided by contact materials such as culture vessels, incubator and its gas supply, and ultimately, the embryo transfer catheter, are similarly pristine.

C. Types of Bioassay

Researchers invest much effort in developing sensitive assays that assess prospective culture media for ability to support mammalian embryo development or that identify embryotoxins in culture supplements or contact materials. The merits and disadvantages of these assays have long been the subject of peer-reviewed articles in the scientific literature illustrating the evolving nature of this topic.

Time-honored and commonly used systems for the detection of embryotoxicity use the following as bioassays:

- Support of *in vitro* development to hatching blastocyst
  - Mouse 1-cell (zygote) assay[8,9,10]
  - Mouse 2-cell embryo assay[11,12,13]
- Sustaining of motility and forward progression *in vitro*
  - Hamster sperm motility assay[14]
  - Human sperm motility assay[15]
- Growth of a somatic cell line[16]

The ART laboratory must determine which assay(s) it will incorporate into its QC program. Underlying this decision will be the factors of convenience, cost, and desired sensitivity.

For those ART laboratories without access to facilities providing animal housing and maintenance, the availability of cryopreserved mouse zygotes and embryos through commercial suppliers is an enormous convenience. This offers economic savings and alleviates the added effort of hormonal preparation of the animals and embyro harvesting.

In incorporating a bioassay into the QC program, one must understand the individual characteristics of the system. Factors that may influence the bioassay and its sensitivity follow:

- The strain of the animal and the specific metabolic requirements of the embryos[17,18]
- Configuration of the culture: Are embryos cultured in individual culture droplets or are they pooled?[19]
- Use of oil overlays:[20] These may serve as a sink for some potential toxins
- Environmental stresses on the embryos[21]

Once the specific type of bioassay is selected and theprotocol for its use is established, it can fulfill a range of functions for the ART laboratory: (a) testing of new media and media supplements, (b) screening of new lots of disposable culture ware and equipment, such as embryo transfer catheters, (c) practice for new laboratory protocols, (d) training tool for embryologists for techniques such as cryopreservation, and (e) routine check of the laboratory culture system.

D. PROFICIENCY TESTING AND LABORATORY SURVEYS

Proficiency testing programs provide some context to interpret the relevance of a given bioassay. While a laboratory faithfully submits all culture media, culture supplements, and supplies to evaluation using a selected bioassay and obtains levels of blastocyst development or sperm motility that inspire confidence, the knowledge that colleagues in other ART centers obtain the same results under the same conditions will be both useful and reassuring. Disparate results, conversely, should inspire critical appraisal of the entire bioassay and its ability to uncover potential ramifications affecting the system. Proficiency testing achieves the goal of education, reinforces technical and methodological skill, and encourages examination of a system and all of its components.

A proficiency testing program using these bioassays in a survey of participating ART laboratories was first introduced through the combined efforts of the College of American Pathologists (CAP) and the American Society for Reproductive Medicine (ASRM). The Reproductive Biology Resource Committee formed from representatives of both organizations and formulated the Reproductive Laboratory Accreditation Program (RLAP) which outlined, on a checklist, the requirements for an ART laboratory. Proficiency testing involved the distribution of culture media to the participants who utilized these in their QC bioassays. The results of the bioassays in conjunction with a questionnaire concerning the specific features of each laboratory's bioassay comprised the database. The effects of various culture conditions and styles, as well as insight into the knowledge base from which participants were operating, were uncovered by this survey.

Recently, the American Association of Bioanalysts (AAB) assumed the administration of the RLAP survey. The interest of this organization in fostering excellent laboratory practice and its general interest in laboratory function makes it an excellent candidate to provide this service.

IX. RECORD-KEEPING AND DOCUMENTATION

Even in this era of the "paperless" office and computerized databases, written records as a permanent history of a patient's treatment and as a material insurance against loss of the electronic database should be maintained. The written ART laboratory chart records the patient's identity, the type of ART procedure performed, the date, the identities of clinical and laboratory personnel who presided over individual events of the patient's treatment, and the data and results derived from the procedure. Pertinent data include the number of eggs collected at ovarian follicular aspiration, the maturational status of each egg, the results from the semen analysis for the sample used for IVF or ICSI, the number of fertilized eggs and embryos, the stages of embryonic development, and the disposition of the embryos. Accountability is the cornerstone of record-keeping and documentation. A detailed history of each egg and embryo and the role of team members in the provision of care are key components in these records.

The written record can be transcribed or encoded in an electronic database to generate clinical outcome reports and to analyze data with the program. The provision of clinical data, particularly pregnancy rates, is required by the Fertility Clinic Success Rate and Certification Act and for periodic analysis of data within the program as part of its QA/QC program. The laboratory record also can be incorporated into the permanent patient's file or kept in a permanent repository specifically maintained by the ART laboratory. The same legal rules governing clinical records apply to laboratory records: they must not be altered. Amendments can be made by notations, such as crossing out of incorrect information and the entry of correct information accompanied by the signature or initials of the person making the amendment.

X. INSTRUMENTS, EQUIPMENT, AND SUPPLIES

All instruments and equipment in the ART laboratory should have the appropriate design and quality of manufacture consistent with their tasks. Written records detailing purchase, regular maintenance and calibration, and any repairs or modifications should be kept by the ART laboratory for the following:

- Incubators
- Laminar flow hoods
- Microscopes
- Centrifuges
- Micromanipulators
- Refrigerators and freezers
- Cell freezers
- Cryopreservation storage tanks
- Water purification systems
- Heating units, e.g., stage warmers
- Suction pumps for aspiration
- Balances
- pH meters
- Osmometers
- Pipettors

Regular maintenance within the ART laboratory includes cleaning and checking that operation is within the appropriate parameters. In addition, scheduled examinations of instruments such as the incubator, laminar flow hood, microscopes, cell freezer, balances, and water purification system must be performed by qualified individuals or companies who can certify that the unit is functioning according to specification, and who can provide service, repairs, and parts authorized by the unit's manufacturer.

Systems providing for continuous energy (electricity), such as emergency power generators, and alarms to alert personnel to malfunction or departure from proper function should be installed in equipment such as incubators, refrigerators, freezers, and cell freezers.

Managers should have a method and routine for surveillance of all the pertinent instruments in the ART laboratory. This ensures that on a regular basis, the embryologist inspects each instrument and its settings, and either confirms its correct operation or makes appropriate adjustments with documentation. A checklist of instruments and the parameters for QC focus is provided in Table 10.4 as an example of the daily inspection of the ART laboratory.

TABLE 10.4
Daily Systems Checklist for the ART Laboratory

I. Incubators
  A. Temperature
    – Chamber thermometer reading
  B. % CO_2
    – Fyrite reading
  C. CO_2 tank gas levels and regulator setting
  D. % Relative humidity
    – Check water level
II. Microscopes
  Heated stage temperature setting and reading
III. Heated working surfaces
  Temperature setting and reading for:
    – Slide warmers
    – Culture tube holders
IV. Refrigerator
  Temperature setting and reading
V. Cryopreserved sample storage tanks
  Liquid nitrogen level
VI. Laminar flow hood
VII. Suction pump for ovarian follicular aspiration

Although instruments such as incubators will provide read-out values on exterior panels, e.g., carbon dioxide level, temperature, and relative humidity, one must use independent methods for validating these parameters. Fyrite is a commonly used indicator for percentage of carbon dioxide in an incubator chamber air sample. Certified thermometers in all heated chambers or surfaces ensure correct temperature of these sites for cell cultures and samples.

Stringent standards of quality in materials and manufacture should be applied in selecting the array of disposable instruments and laboratory culture ware used in the ART laboratory. These include follicular aspiration systems, embryo transfer catheters, and tissue culture dishes and tubes. The application of a bioassay, as discussed previously, to individual lots or batches of materials can be made prior to their introduction into clinical use.

A burgeoning marketplace of supplies and equipment appeared as ART expanded in both volume of patients and number of clinics and laboratories. We have come a long way from the early days in which equipment was co-opted from other laboratories and supplies were often adapted to ART from other research or clinical uses. An array of manufacturers and suppliers now stand at the ready to provide virtually every conceivable item required in an ART laboratory from capital equipment to the most common disposable accessory.

For marketing to the ART laboratory, manufacturers remain sensitive to the embryotoxicity screening that must accompany the appraisal of anything introduced into clinical use. Mouse embryo QC assay results, for instance, will often accompany culture media products prepared industrially. Some ART laboratories will still conduct its own appraisal using its own QC assays.

The use of commercially available materials carries with it some disadvantages. Product recalls or product withdrawals may occur, resulting in the need to identify a substitute component rapidly. Suppliers will often seek to fill any gaps in the marketplace.

XI. SAFETY

A. UNIVERSAL PRECAUTIONS FOR BLOOD-BORNE PATHOGENS

The nature of ART requires working with bodily fluids, including blood, follicular aspirates, semen, testicular tissue, aspirates collected from the epididymis or vas deferens, cervical and uterine fluids. To prevent the transmission of any potential infectious agent from these materials to the embryologist, an Exposure Control Plan should be incorporated into the ART laboratory lexicon.

Exposure can occur during procedures and processing and requires the education and advising of the ART laboratory staff on the following:

- An understanding of the identity and infectious nature of blood-borne pathogens
- Training in exercising universal precautions for handling bodily fluids
- Correct disposal of all exposed materials
- Documentation of and procedure for handling an unprotected exposure event
- Post-exposure follow-up

The ART laboratory must provide the appropriate protective equipment to its workers for exercising universal precautions, including scrub suits, latex gloves, masks, eye-shields, and any other devices to prevent contact with the biologic specimens. An appropriate method for cleaning and disinfecting contaminated equipment and workspace must be identified and implemented. In addition, appropriate disposal containers for sharp material, such as follicular aspiration needles, or contaminated labware and instruments, such as embryo transfer catheters, must be available in the laboratory.

Some preemptive steps can be provided. Embryologists should know about the availability and efficacy of vaccinations against infections such as Hepatitis B that are transmitted through blood. Documentation of such a vaccination program should appear in the embryologist's medical/personnel file.

B. CHEMICAL HAZARDS

Some of the individual techniques in ART require the use of potentially hazardous chemicals. The laboratory staff should be aware of the hazards involved with handling liquid nitrogen, for instance, and implement the use of protective gear for hands and eyes.

With respect to some of chemicals used in the preparation of gamete or embryo cultures, the embryologist should learn protocols for the following:

- Labeling
- Handling and application
- Storage
- Disposal after use or expiration date

Some of the chemicals commonly used in the ART laboratory include those for semen processing and sperm isolation (Percoll™), preparation of gametes for ICSI (hyaluronidase and polyvinyl pyrrolidone), and cryopreservation of embryos (propanediol, glycerol, or dimethylsulfoxide). While none of these present an obvious hazard in its application, proper treatment of all agents used in a laboratory is an essential element of good practice.

XII. SUMMARY

The design and implementation of a QC program for the ART laboratory ensures a consistent set of appropriate conditions will facilitate the goals of optimal gamete and embryo culture and that every effort is made to conserve these specimens both quantitatively and qualitatively. The QC program underlies a calibrated, regularly surveilled system for patient care using these unique ART techniques for the treatment of infertility.

REFERENCES

1. Byrd, W., Quality assurance in the reproductive biology laboratory, *Arch. Pathol. Lab. Med.*, 116, 418, 1992.
2. Bustillo, M., Imposing limits on the number of oocytes and embryos transferred: is it necessary/wise or naughty/nice?, *Hum. Reprod.*, 12, 1616, 1997.
3. Guidelines for human embryology and andrology laboratories, *Fertil. Steril.*, 58 (Suppl. I), 1S, 1992.
4. Visscher, R. D., Partners in pursuit of excellence: development of an embryo laboratory accreditation program, *Fertil. Steril.*, 56, 1021, 1991.
5. May, J. V. and Hanshew, K., Organization of the *in vitro* fertilization and embryo transfer laboratory, in *Handbook of the Laboratory Diagnosis and Treatment of Infertility*, Keel, B. A. and Webster, B. W., Eds., CRC Press, Boca Raton, FL, 1990, 291–327.

6. Ball, G. D., ART laboratory organization: size, layout, personnel and equipment, in *Assisted Reproduction: Laboratory Considerations*, May, J. V., Ed., Infertility and Reproductive Clinics of North America, Diamond, M. P. and DeCherney, A., Eds., vol. 9, W.B. Saunders, Philadelphia, PA, 1998, 275–283.

7. Cohen, J., Gilligan, A., Esposito, W., Schimmel, T., and Dale, B., Ambient air and its potential effects on conception *in vitro*, *Hum. Reprod.*, 12, 1742, 1997.

8. Quinn, P., Warnes, G. M., Kerin, J. F., and Kirby, C., Culture factors in relation to the success of human *in vitro* fertilization and embryo transfer, *Fertil. Steril.*, 41, 202, 1984.

9. Rinehart, J. S., Bavister, B. D., and Gerrity, M., Quality control in the *in vitro* fertilization laboratory: comparison of bioassay systems for water quality, *J. In Vitro Fert. Embryo Transf.*, 5, 335, 1988.

10. Fleetham, J. A., Pattinson, H. A., and Mortimer, D., The mouse embryo culture system: improving the sensitivity for use as a quality control assay for human *in vitro* fertilization, *Fertil. Steril.*, 59, 192, 1993.

11. Ackerman, S. B., Swanson, G. K., Stokes, R. J., and Veeck, L. L., Culture of mouse preimplantation embryos as a quality control assay for human *in vitro* fertilization, *Gamete Res.*, 9, 145, 1984.

12. Naz, R. K., Janousek, J. T., Moody, T., and Stillman, R., Factors influencing murine embryo bioassay: effects of proteins, aging of the medium, and surgical glove coatings, *Fertil. Steril.*, 46, 914, 1986.

13. Davidson, A., Vermesh, M., Lobo, R. A., and Paulson, R. J., Mouse embryo culture as a quality control for human *in vitro* fertilization: the one-cell versus the two-cell model, *Fertil. Steril.*, 49, 516, 1988.

14. Gorrill, M. J., Rinehart, J. S., Ramhane, A. C., and Gerrity, M., Comparison of the hamster sperm motility assay to the mouse one-cell and two-cell embryo bioassays as quality control tests for *in vitro* fertilization, *Fertil. Steril.*, 55, 345, 1991.

15. Critchlow, J. D., Matson, P. L., Newman, M. C., Horne, G., Troup, S. A., and Lieberman, B. A., Quality control in an *in vitro* fertilization laboratory: use of human sperm survival studies, *Hum. Reprod.*, 4, 545, 1989.

16. Bertheussen, K., Holt, N., Forsdahl, F., and Hoie, K. E., A new cell culture assay for quality control in IVF, *Hum. Reprod.*, 4, 531, 1989.

17. Dandekar, P. V. and Glass, R. H., Development of mouse embryos *in vitro* is affected by strain and culture medium, *Gamete Res.*, 17, 279, 1987.

18. Scott, L. F., Sundaram, S. G., and Smith, S., The relevance and use of mouse embryo bioassays for quality control in an assisted reproductive technology program, *Fertil. Steril.*, 60, 559, 1993.

19. Lane, M. and Gardner, D. K., Effect of incubation volume and embryo density on the development and viability of mouse embryos *in vitro*, *Hum. Reprod.*, 7, 558, 1992.

20. Hammitt, D. G., Rogers, P. R., Ruble, K. A., Syrop, C. H., and Hood, C. C., The human sperm-survival, two-cell zona-free, and one-cell zona-intact assays for IVF quality control, *Int. J. Fertil.*, 38, 347, 1993.

21. Jackson, K. V. and Kiessling, A. A., Fertilization and cleavage of mouse oocytes exposed to the conditions of human oocyte retrieval for *in vitro* fertilization, *Fertil. Steril.*, 51, 675, 1989.

11 Internal and External Quality Control in the Andrology Laboratory

Matthew J. Tomlinson and Christopher L. R. Barratt

CONTENTS

I. INTRODUCTION

An effective system for assessing the quality of testing procedures in the andrology laboratory is essential if meaningful clinical information is to be obtained. The clinical value of semen analysis relies wholly on the laboratory methods employed and the operator's technical competence. In general, many andrology laboratories still ignore the need for rigorous quality control (QC) and quality assurance (QA) procedures despite data that show considerable variation among technicians in the same laboratory and significant differences between laboratories.[5,7,17] However, with the increasing requirement for laboratory accreditation and the emphasis placed on QA and QC measures by the World Health Organization,[25,26] a comprehensive QA and QC program in the andrology laboratory is mandatory.[6] In this chapter, we discuss several issues essential in the development of a comprehensive and effective QA and QC program:

1. Detailed standard operating procedures (SOPs)
2. The use of standardized laboratory methods that minimize error
3. Training of technicians to high levels of competence
4. Quality control measures and assessment of data produced by each technician in a laboratory and among laboratories, i.e., internal and external QC
5. Continuous assessment of the "clinical value" of the output from the laboratory

II. STANDARD OPERATING PROCEDURES

Quality control in the andrology laboratory begins before sample collection and ends with the presentation of results and communication to the clinician. Detailed SOPs for sample collection, analysis, and reporting of results must be established and enforced if reliable information is to be obtained. Failure to achieve this will lead to inconsistency and errors in diagnosis. In general, the technical staff in consultation with the clinicians (end users) should develop SOPs. The technical staff must understand what information the clinicians require for the suitable management of the couple. Equally, the clinician must understand the diagnostic limitations (and confidence limits) of each of the semen parameters. SOPs must be working documents, not texts written by administrators who only see the daylight when inspectors or visitors arrive in the laboratory. They must be updated regularly and modified if any problems occur. Staff find that discussing aspects of the SOPs at each laboratory meeting ensures that protocols are effective. Numerous protocols exist for the standardization of semen sample collection and presentation of results, but the most widely accepted are those published by the World Health Organization.[25,26] Such guidelines are recommended by many national societies, e.g. British Andrology Society (BAS), British Fertility Society (BFS), and the European Society for Human Reproduction and Embryology (ESHRE).

III. STANDARD MANUAL SEMEN ANALYSIS

The WHO[25,26] recommended that the standard semen analysis should include the assessment of liquefaction, appearance, volume, consistency, pH, agglutination, cellular elements other than spermatozoa, sperm concentration, motility, morphology, and antisperm antibodies. Other tests on the semen sample are considered optional, e.g., semen culture. A plethora of methods can determine the above. The WHO recommends some methods in preference to others, e.g., use of an improved Neubauer counting chamber to determine sperm concentration. If alternative methods to the WHO are used they must have equivalent accuracy, precision, and clinical relevance.

IV. THE ROLE OF COMPUTER ASSISTED SPERM ANALYSIS (CASA)

The difficulties associated with using CASA to achieve repeatable and reliable results has led to a paucity of studies that critically evaluate the use of CASA. Several long-term follow up studies have evaluated the predictive value of CASA for *in vivo* fertility.[2,13,22] These studies show that parameters such as the concentration of progressively motile cells are significantly related to time to conception. The concentration of progressively motile cells can be determined accurately using CASA provided that adequate care is taken in specimen preparation and instrument use.[5] User training is fundamental to the effective use of CASA, and guidelines for the introduction of CASA into the laboratory and for technician training have been developed.[8] Although CASA's primary purpose is to determine sperm motion, advances in technology, particularly with fluorescent DNA stain (IDENT stain [Hoechst 33342 dye] using a Hamilton Thorne IVOS CASA), allow repeatable and reliable determinations of sperm concentration.[9,28] In addition, one can estimate both sperm motility and concentration in the same aliquot thus reducing time in preparing the samples.[10]

A major advantage of CASA is the potential ability to analyze the morphology of spermatozoa. Examination of sperm morphology by a trained observer provides important diagnostic and prognostic clinical information; however, such analysis is subjective and difficult to standardize.[11,19] One might believe that a computerized image analysis system would be an ideal method to standardize the assessment of sperm morphology, generate quantitative data about sperm shape, and, at the same time, provide objective criteria. Yet, significant problems with the technology, preparation of spermatozoa for analysis, and, of course, the inherent pleomorphic nature of human spermatozoa have hindered developments in this field. Over the last several years an increasing number of studies suggest that assessment of sperm morphology using computerized methods does provide clinically useful information.[14,15] Preparation of the semen smears for analysis is of critical importance. Factors such as different fixation protocols and staining methods can affect the dimensions of the spermatozoa; thus standardization of these factors is important.[12,16] The routine analysis of sperm morphology using CASA is now close to reality. Hopefully, this will minimize the significant problems involved in the subjective assessment of sperm morphology.

V. TECHNICIAN TRAINING FOR HIGH LEVELS OF COMPETENCE

For semen analysis tests to be performed with accuracy and precision a suitable degree of formal instruction and training must occur. The "goal-oriented" approach recently described by Mortimer[18] is one such structured method for organizing training. This method is used widely and well proven. Briefly, experienced staff present new staff with laboratory methodology and reference material. Subsequently, each method is explained in detail by the experienced personnel. Following a period of induction, the trainee performs an assessment on each aspect of the semen analysis and compares his or her result to that of the experienced technician. These results are analyzed to detect difference between observers. The results provide useful feedback for the trainee and a record to monitor improvements in performance. In general, Mortimer recommends duplicate assessments are performed and analyzed in groups of 30. The competence of the trainee determines how many groups of 30 are performed. When the difference between the trainee and the experienced technician is within acceptable limits the training period is complete (see Mortimer[18] for detailed description of method).

A large number of "approved" semen assessment training courses, e.g., organized by ESHRE, exist that technicians can attend. These courses complement the "goal-oriented" method of training and are especially useful when no trained technicians are available to instruct (and compare with) the trainee. Technicians must perform a basic semen assessment before the course starts and at the end of the course. Interestingly, considerable data now show a reduction in the variability of semen parameters as the courses progress, highlighting the effectiveness of organized training.[3,20,24] Structured courses provide a theoretical background to the subject (encompassing reproductive physiology), details of health and safety standards, and particulars of regulatory/legislative issues. If technicians do not attend structured training courses and are trained in-house, they must be armed with a sound theoretical knowledge base of the subject. Often, the latter is ignored when in-house methods of training are used. Interestingly, technicians who attend ESHRE-approved basic semen analysis training courses show reduced variability in their semen assessments in external QC schemes compared to technicians that have not been in such courses (Vreeburg unpublished observations). Possibly, in the near future, computer assisted learning techniques specifically developed for semen assessment may enhance technicians' learning ability.

VI. QUALITY CONTROL MEASURES

A. INTERNAL QUALITY CONTROL (IQC)

A variety of techniques exist for assessing IQC.[5,7,18] In devising a system, one must determine the objective of each technique; for example, different technicians reading the same counting chamber will not detect errors in preparation of the chamber.[7] Therefore, the system adopted must test all aspects of sample analysis, e.g., dilution, pipetting, incorrect identification of spermatozoa, arithmetic ability, etc. We suggest the following series of points to consider:

1. Samples—Well-mixed, low viscosity semen samples should be used. In addition, a wide range should appear in the quality of these samples so as to reflect the workload of the laboratory. It is possible to pool samples and analyze aliquots from the pool. Analysis of the sample by each operator will determine inter-operator variation. Repeat readings will determine operator precision.
2. Sperm concentration—Each operator should prepare and read both sides of an improved Neubauer chamber according to the WHO.[25,26] This should be repeated several times and coefficients of variation (CVs) calculated.
3. Sperm motility—Sperm should be assessed by each operator and categorized according to the WHO.[25,26] Each uses a separate 10 µL aliquot and repeats the measurement several times. Video recordings of motile spermatozoa are a valuable resource both for QA and QC. Usually, errors in defining spermatozoa according to the WHO gradings (a,b,c,d)[25] can be addressed easily using a video.[27]

4. Sperm morphology—Each operator should prepare his or her own slide from the same sample and assess the percentage of ideal forms. This should be repeated several times and CVs calculated for precision. A batch of prepared slides can be examined routinely to determine if the definition of normal has changed over time.[5]

5. Antisperm antibodies—The ability of each operator to perform and read an antibody test also must be assessed. In addition, regular testing using known positive and negative control sera will ensure reagent sensitivity. An indirect test using stored test serum/seminal plasma (previously shown to be ASA positive and ASA negative) is logistically the best way to do this. A stock of frozen test serum/seminal plasma should be kept specifically for this purpose. Each operator should prepare his or her own ASA test and read the slide several times.

Once a month, the in-house scheme may be run in conjunction with the external quality assurance scheme (see below). Individuals within a laboratory can then compare their own values with those values formed by national consensus.

B. Recording and Analyzing IQC

Several statistical techniques analyze QC and QA data.[5] Each technician must know the basic methods to record and analyze the data, e.g., construction of control charts[5] and monthly means.[4] As with all aspects of good laboratory practice, regular checking and maintenance of laboratory equipment ensures validity of quality assurance procedures. Methodology for each semen analysis test may be followed with care but if, for example, pipettes are inaccurate, the results will be meaningless.

C. External Quality Assessment—United Kingdom National External Quality Assurance Scheme (UKNEQAS)*

The UKNEQAS scheme specifically addresses issues of quality in diagnostic andrology, providing a national framework to encourage standardization and improvements in semen analysis. The basic aims of the scheme are to minimize inter-laboratory variation with regard to laboratory methodology and to encourage accuracy and precision in the application of those methods. Participants in the scheme receive periodic distributions of semen samples (for assessment of sperm concentration and morphology), serum samples (assessment of antibodies), and videotapes (assessment of sperm motility). The results are returned to the scheme organizers for detailed analysis and comparison to "target values" usually calculated from a consensus achieved by six "reference" laboratories, known only to the scheme organizer. Each laboratory is encouraged to use the WHO[25,26] standard methods of assessment. At present, participation in the UKNEQAS is optional, but mandatory if a laboratory wishes to apply for accreditation (Clinical Pathology Accreditation) and strongly recommended if the laboratory is part of a HFEA-licensed center. In addition to sending out samples, the NEQAS scheme organizes an annual one day symposium that presents seminars on

---

* For further details on the UKNEQAS scheme contact A. Atkinson, Sub Fertility Laboratory, St. Mary's Hospital, Manchester, UK M13 OJH. Email: anna@labmed.cmht.nwest.nhs.uk

all aspects of semen assessment. During the annual symposium small group teaching schemes allow participants to discuss particular problems. The interaction, on both a formal and informal level, between the organizers, participants, and steering committee is a critical component in the success of the scheme.

D. ORGANIZATION OF UKNEQAS

Sperm Concentration and Morphology: Pooled semen samples are distributed to approximately 140 centers within the U.K. and Europe. Concentration and morphology are assessed using differing methodologies, although the vast majority use WHO criteria.[25] Mean, standard deviation, and coefficients of variation (CVs) are reported to individual participating centers including their own score and bias. .

Antisperm Antibody Detection: Serum samples are sent for antibody testing. The most common testing methods include the tray-agglutination test, indirect immuno-bead test or MAR test, although a number of others also are employed, e.g., gelatin agglutination test (GAT), immunofluorescence (IF), enzyme linked immunosorbent assay (ELISA). Intended results are compared to actual results, with any false positives and false negatives reported back to participating centers.

Sperm Motility: Participating centers analyze four samples by video. Sperm are categorized according to WHO criteria.[25] Means, standard deviation, and CVs are reported to individual participating centers including their own score and bias.

The scheme is popular and appears to be effective as a variation in the assessment of sperm concentration has decreased since the scheme was initiated. However, the scheme highlights a number of key issues:

1. Despite having clear guidelines for semen analysis from the WHO, many centers fail to follow them, do not understand them, and/or prefer to use local in-house methodology. Standardization of the assessments throughout the U.K. remains a significant problem.
2. Particularly poor agreement arises over what constitutes normal/abnormal spermatozoa, thus, sperm morphology is particularly prone to error. Administrators now send standardized prepared slides to help users identify normal spermatozoa. In addition, at the training courses run by the British Andrology Society (BAS), instructors place specific emphasis on the identification of normal spermatozoa.
3. The lack of internal quality control measures at many centers compounds the problems raised in points 1 and 2. Remarkably, many centers are unaware of comprehensive internal QC and QA measures or are unwilling to perform them.[21]
4. How should target values be derived? To date, several reference laboratories determine the correct sperm concentration. What should be used? What is the role of CASA? The use and construction of target values remains a critical issue on their agenda.
5. What constitutes poor performance? In general, laboratories outside the 10 and 90 centiles are encouraged to make informal contact with the scheme organizers so that outstanding issues can be addressed. Other assessments of poor performance are now being explored.

An external quality control scheme such as UKNEQAS helps evaluate the performance of many centers. The major drawback is lack of consensus with regard to methodology. A true comparison of participants can occur only if testing methods are consistent and are performed with appropriate in-house quality control measures. Interestingly, purchasers can ask each laboratory for the results of its performance in the external QC scheme and thus evaluate the effectiveness of each laboratory performing semen assessments. In reality, without such financial influence, many laboratories who perform badly have no incentive to improve.

The UKNEQAS is one of the few national schemes operating throughout the world. The high degree of variability among centers examining the same semen sample is not particular to the U.K. The issues raised by NEQAS are international, and hopefully the problems identified can be used as a basis for improving the quality of semen assessments worldwide.

VII. ASSESSMENT OF CLINICAL VALUE

Many laboratories appear to neglect self-appraisal of their service in terms of their ability to provide both diagnostic and prognostic information. In many cases, the semen analysis results dictate the chances of conception either naturally or using assisted reproductive techniques. Often the suitability of various forms of assisted reproduction depends on the results of the semen analysis, e.g., choice between IUI, IVF, or ICSI. Therefore, the laboratory must contact its end users (clinicians) to determine if the results provided are of clinical significance. This is relatively easy if the laboratory is associated with an infertility clinic as the results can be cross checked with fertilization rates and/or pregnancies. Examples of how to perform this type of analysis abound, e.g., logistic regression.[1,2,23] The assessment of seminal parameters in relation to fertilizing potential should be seen as a quality control measure and not simply a research exercise. In cases where the laboratory is not associated with an infertility center, relevant information may not be easy to access, but such information should be sought.

VIII. CONCLUSIONS

A comprehensive program of measures ensures quality. These measures include standard operating procedures, standardized techniques for semen analysis, comprehensive staff training, internal and external quality control measures, and assessment of the clinical value of tests of the laboratory. The demand increases for andrology laboratories to implement comprehensive QC measures, e.g., compliance with the HFEA Code of Practice (HFEA licensed centers). Monitoring and presentation of QC results on a regular basis is a basic requirement for laboratories providing a diagnostic andrology service and not an optional extra.

ACKNOWLEDGMENTS

The authors would like to thank The University of Birmingham and The Birmingham Women's Hospital U.K. for financial support of their research.

REFERENCES

1. Barratt, C. L. R., Naeeni, M., Clements, S., and Cooke, I. D., Clinical value of sperm morphology measurements for *in vivo* fertility: comparison between World Health Organisation (WHO) criteria of 1987 and 1992, *Hum. Reprod.*, 10, 2096–2106, 1995.
2. Barratt, C. L. R., Tomlinson, M. J., and Cooke, I. D., The prognostic significance of computerised motility analysis for *in vivo* fertility, *Fertil. Steril.*, 60, 520–525, 1993.
3. Bjorndahl, I. and Kvist, U., Basic semen analysis courses: experience in Scandinavia, in *Modern ART in the 2000s. Andrology in the Nineties*, Ombelet, W., Bosmans, E., Vandeput, H., Vereecken, A., Renier, M., and Hoomans, E., Eds., Parthenon Publishing Group, London, U.K., 1998, 91–102.
4. Clarke, G. N., A simple monthly means chart system for monitoring sperm concentration, *Hum. Reprod.*, 12, 2710–2712, 1997.
5. Clements, S., Cooke, I. D., and Barratt, C. L. R., Implementing comprehensive quality control in the andrology laboratory, *Hum. Reprod.*, 10, 2096–2106, 1995.
6. De Jonge, C. J., Total quality management and the clinical andrology laboratory: essential partners, in *Modern ART in the 2000s. Andrology in the Nineties*, Ombelet, W., Bosmans, E., Vandeput, H., Vereecken, A., Renier, M., and Hoomans, E., Eds., Parthenon Publishing Group, London, U.K., 1998, 55–60.
7. Dunphy, B. C., Kay, R., Barratt, C. L. R., and Cooke, I. D., Quality control during conventional analysis of semen: an essential exercise, *J. Androl.*, 10, 378–385, 1989.
8. ESHRE Andrology Special Interest Group, Guidelines on the application of CASA technology in the analysis of spermatozoa, *Hum. Reprod.*, 13, 142–145, 1998.
9. Farrell, P. B., Foote, R. H., and Zinaman, M. J., Motility and other characteristics of human sperm can be measured by computer-assisted sperm analysis of samples stained with Hoechst 33342, *Fertil. Steril.*, 66, 446–453, 1996.
10. Farrell, P. B., Foote, R. H., McArdle, M. M., Trouern-Trend, V. L., and Tardif, A. L., Media and dilution procedures tested to minimize handling effects on human, rabbit and bull sperm for computer-assisted sperm analysis (CASA), *J. Androl.*, 17, 293–300, 1996.
11. Freund, M., Standards for the rating of human sperm morphology. A cooperative study, *Int. J. Fertil.*, II, 97–118, 1966.
12. Katz, D. F., Overstreet, J. W., Samuels, S. J., Niswander, P. W., Bloom, T. D., and Lewis, E. L., Morphometric analysis of spermatozoa in the assessment of human male fertility, *J. Androl.*, 7, 203–210, 1986.
13. Krause, W., Computer-assisted sperm analysis system: comparison with routine evaluation and prognostic value in male fertility and assisted reproduction, *Modern Androl.*, 10, 1, 60–66, 1995.
14. Kruger, T. F., du Toit, T. C., Franken, D. R., Menkveld, R., and Lombard, C. J., Sperm morphology: assessing the agreement between the manual method (strict criteria) and the sperm morphology analyzer IVOS, *Fertil. Steril.*, 63, 134–141, 1995.
15. Kruger, T. F., Lacquet, F. A., Sarmiento, C. A. S. et al., A prospective study on the predictive value of normal sperm morphology evaluated by computer (IVOS), *Fertil. Steril.*, 66, 285–291, 1996.
16. Lacquet, F. A., Kruger, T. F., Du Toit, T. C., Lombard, C. J., Sanchez Sarmiento, C. A., De Villiers, A., and Coetzee, K., Slide preparation and staining procedures for reliable results using computerized morphology, *Arch. Androl.*, 36, 133–13, 1996.
17. Matson, P. L., External assessment for semen analysis and sperm antibody detection: results of a pilot scheme, *Human Reprod.*, 10, 620–625, 1995.

18. Mortimer, D., *Practical Laboratory Andrology*, Oxford University Press, New York, 1994, 337–347.
19. Ombelet, W., Pollet, H., Bosmans, E., and Vereecken, A., Results of a questionnaire on sperm morphology assessment, *Hum. Reprod.*, 12, 1015–120, 1997.
20. Punjabi, U. and Spiessens, C., Basic semen analysis courses: experience in Belgium, in *Modern ART in the 2000s. Andrology in the Nineties*, Ombelet, W., Bosmans, E., Vandeput, H., Vereecken, A., Renier, M., and Hoomans, E., Eds., Parthenon Publishing Group, NY, 1998, 107–113.
21. Souter, V. L., Irvine, D. S., and Templeton, A. A., Laboratory techniques for semen analysis: a Scottish survey, *Health Bull.*, (*Edinb.*), 55, 140–149, 1997.
22. Tomlinson, M. J., Barratt, C. L. R., and Cooke, I. D., Prospective study of leukocytes and leukocyte subpopulations in semen suggests they are not a cause of male infertility, *Fertil. Steril.*, 60, 1069–1075, 1993.
23. Tomlinson, M. J., Amissah-Arthur, J. B., Thompson, K. A., Kasraie, J. A., and Bentick, B., Prognostic indicators for intra-uterine insemination: statistical model for IUI susccess, *Hum. Reprod.*, 11, 1892–1896, 1996.
24. Vreeburg, J. T. M. and Weber, R. F. A., Basic semen analysis courses: experience in the Netherlands, in *Modern ART in the 2000s. Andrology in the Nineties*, Ombelet, W., Bosmans, E., Vandeput, H., Vereecken, A., Renier, M., and Hoomans, E., Eds., Parthenon Publishing Group, London, U.K., 1998, 103–107.
25. World Health Organization, *WHO Laboratory Manual for the Examination of Human Semen and Semen - Cervical Mucus Interaction*, 3rd ed., Cambridge University Press, Cambridge, 1992.
26. World Health Organization, *WHO Laboratory Manual for the Examination of Human Semen and Semen - Cervical Mucus Interaction*, 4th ed., Cambridge University Press, Cambridge, 1998.
27. Yeung, C. H., Cooper, T. G., and Nieschlag, E., A technique for standardisation and quality control of subjective sperm motility assessments in semen analysis, *Fertil. Steril.*, 67, 1156–1158, 1997.
28. Zinamen, M. J., Uhler, M. L., Vertuno, E., Fisher, S. G., and Clegg, E. D., Evaluation of computer-assisted semen analysis (CASA) with IDENT stain to determine sperm concentration, *J. Androl.*, 17, 288–292, 1996.

12 Quality Assurance in the Embryology, Andrology, and Endocrine Laboratories

Chad A. Johnson, Theresa A. Kellum, and Jeffrey P. Boldt

CONTENTS

I. INTRODUCTION

A. BACKGROUND

The sum of all our efforts in the field of reproductive medicine, both clinically and medically, is to provide the highest level of care for the patients that are served. In order to optimize care, one must first understand what makes a lab efficient, makes it reliable, and allows accurate and precise reporting of results. Andrology and IVF labs include a component directly related to patient outcomes, and although equally important, this is more difficult to quantitate. This therapeutic component does not always give a specific endpoint that can be used to judge the quality of care provided by the lab. As will be discussed later, multiple factors contribute to the therapeutic aspect of an ART lab. In this chapter, we attempt to define quality assurance (QA) and the role it plays in the embryology, andrology, and endocrine labs. While the approaches taken for each lab may differ, the basic tenets addressed should be constant.

In the following sections (embryology, andrology, and endocrine) each author will present different approaches to and applications of QA. This illustrates that many ways to implement QA in a lab abound, and that while every QA program will have similar requirements, each lab must identify a system that works best for them.

B. DEFINITION

While the issue of quality control (QC) has been addressed in many venues, including the chapters preceding this, the assisted reproductive technology (ART) laboratories have had little introduction in the area of QA. Quality assurance has many components, and QC is the most recognizable aspect of QA to those working in ART labs. One author stressed the need for ART labs to become familiar with QA and implement policies addressing these issues in their labs.[1] For many years, the terms quality control and quality assurance were used interchangeably. Because they are not the same, we will attempt to define the terms used in discussing this subject. One must realize that establishing and administering a QA program is not optional. The Clinical Laboratory Improvement Act of 1988 (CLIA '88) describes in detail the requirement for QA and sets forth guidelines on implementing QA for moderate and high complexity labs.[2,5] QA may be a foreign concept to embryology labs that have not voluntarily submitted to inspection by an agency utilizing CLIA '88 guidelines (e.g., College of American Pathologists, Commission on Laboratory Accreditation, state boards of health). To date, IVF labs remain unregulated and while many labs have undergone inspection voluntarily, others have not. While inspection does not ensure that a lab will be successful, it does ensure that policies and procedures have been established and provides the tools needed to determine deviations from normal and a means to address any discrepancies.

Many definitions for QA exist. Several that give a general meaning of QA follow:

1. QA is the sum of all activities in which a laboratory is engaged. A QA program is an essential part of a sound analytical protocol used by the laboratory to detect and correct problems in analytical and interpretational processes.[3]
2. QA involves preventive activities undertaken prior to the examination of samples which are intended to establish systems conducive to accuracy in analytical testing.
3. QA is an administrative program that systematically monitors the effectiveness of quality control throughout the life cycle of a service or product.[4]

From these definitions we find that, in essence, *all* aspects of laboratory operations fall under QA. Inherent in these definitions are the tasks of reducing errors, both clinical and clerical, and providing a clinical outcome that will be useful to the patient in either diagnosis or treatment. In monitoring lab quality, we can differentiate testing and procedural events as preanalytical, analytical, and postanalytical, keeping in mind that for IVF, we do not perform analysis but provide treatment. Note that analysis is only a small part of the entire process and that the events leading up to and following analysis all start and end with the patient.

C. Description

The events leading up to and following an analysis (procedure) are as critical as the event itself. In describing QA, we can partition the tasks involved in a comprehensive program into three general categories.

1. **Preventative activities,** such as quality control, stringent adherence to protocol manuals, preventive maintenance, instrument calibration, and appropriate personnel training, can help establish a baseline for overall performance of equipment and personnel.
2. **Monitoring activities** ensure that testing and procedures are performing as expected. These include the use of standards, controls, quality control review, and proficiency testing.
3. **Corrective actions** occur when we detect errors or abnormalities in laboratory functions. Activities include equipment repair or recalibration, troubleshooting, personnel reassessment or retraining, etc.

D. CLIA '88 QA Standards

Taken together, these activities not only allow the lab to optimize outcomes (testing and procedures), but also provide a mechanism to review events when problems occur. The standards issued in the Federal Register give us a basic structure upon which to build our QA program. Below are the standards addressed by CLIA '88[2] and each is described briefly to provide background on the issues each standard must address. Specific examples of each standard can be found in the subsequent sections of this chapter.

1. **Patient test management assessment:** The lab must have in place a method to monitor and evaluate all aspects of patient information from pre-test information gathering to results reporting. The lab must ensure that samples are identified correctly, that appropriate patient information is collected, and that the appropriate testing or procedure is implemented. The lab must report results accurately and rapidly, and must store results for easy access.
2. **Quality control assessment:** Every lab should have ongoing quality control measures to ensure reliability in equipment and to identify abnormal trends in lab function so that corrective action may be taken.

3. **Proficiency testing assessment:** As part of any lab QC program, routine proficiency testing enables the lab to determine the accuracy and precision of their testing and/or procedures. By assessing unknown samples provided by an external source, the lab can evaluate how well their methods allow them to judge the actual value of the unknown (accuracy). Repeated measures of these samples can determine repeatability of the test result (precision). Precision describes the ability to test and find the same result over repeated measures. Determining if we are accurate and precise, simultaneously, is one of the main goals of a proficiency testing program. This gives the lab confidence they can determine the true value of the unknown and can perform this function repeatedly.

4. **Comparison of test results:** For labs performing tests in different locations, using different methodologies for the same unknown, or performing a test that has no proficiency testing application, comparisons of the same sample must be made to ensure accuracy of the methodologies.

5. **Relationship of patient information to patient test results:** The lab must have a mechanism for identifying a lab result that appears incongruous with patient information available to the lab (e.g., a patient evaluated for presence of sperm following vasectomy, several million sperm detected, identify and report the incongruity).

6. **Personnel assessment:** Each lab needs an ongoing method of assessing staff competency in terms of their clinical and clerical skills.

7. **Communications:** A mechanism must exist to reduce the risk of miscommunication and to provide corrective action if needed.

8. **Complaint investigation:** Labs must maintain a system for addressing and documenting complaints (patient, co-worker, director, etc.).

9. **Quality assurance review with staff:** In order to be effective, QA policies and procedures must be evaluated and revised constantly. All staff, clinical and clerical, must participate in preventative and corrective activities.

10. **Quality assurance records:** The lab must maintain QA records, including problems identified and the corrective actions taken.

E. THE ROLE OF QA IN ART LABORATORIES

Why is QA important to ART labs? Embryology, andrology, and endocrine labs are defined by CLIA '88 as "a facility for the biological, microbiological, serological, chemical, immunohematological, biophysical, cytological, pathological, or other examination of materials derived from the human body for the purpose of providing information for the diagnosis, prevention, or treatment of any disease or impairment of, or the assessment of, the health of human beings."[5] Given this definition, the ART labs certainly fall in one, if not all, of these categories. All labs are expected to meet the CLIA '88 requirements, and in order to accomplish this we must first understand the role QA plays in the ART lab.

One aspect of QA in the ART labs that is different than, for example, a clinical chemistry lab, is the disparity in how each lab ascertains outcomes. The endocrine lab has a well-defined endpoint—a specific value for a given analyte of unknown quantity, such as a hormone. For every sample analyzed, we obtain a numeric value that we can use to assist in clinical decision making. To obtain this value, we can run both a standard curve and a control value so that unknown to known sample levels can be compared directly. This is not true for andrology labs, as we do not run controls with conventional semen analysis. Semen analysis is more subjective than an endocrine assay, and we have greater room for error without controls and with technician variation.[6-8] In the embryology lab, and also the andrology labs performing sperm washes, the final outcome anticipated is an ongoing pregnancy. Herein lies one of the difficulties in assessing QA in these labs.

Unlike the endocrine lab where the outcome is based on a testing analyte, establishing pregnancies in the ART labs entails numerous components that are out of the control of the laboratory. An embryology lab can only work with the oocytes provided by the clinician. Controlled ovarian hyperstimulation (COH), when performed and monitored properly, can provide the lab with oocytes that have an excellent prognosis for fertilization, cleavage, and pregnancy. Unfortunately, COH, when mismanaged, is capable of producing inferior quality oocytes that even the best labs cannot rescue. Also, many patients do not respond to gonadotropins and at best give small numbers of poor quality oocytes. Equally important to the IVF process is the embryo transfer. Once embryos are given to the physician, the physician then has the responsibility to perform an atraumatic and successful transfer. Difficult or traumatic transfers may impinge on the uterine milieu, negatively affecting implantation and pregnancy. Many patients simply have a very poor prognosis even with optimal care provided by the physician and laboratory. These factors establish how vital QA is in the ART lab. Because we must consider many variables in the ART lab, many of which are beyond laboratory control, QA can assist us by ensuring that the basic principles and practices of the lab are being carried out and monitored closely. When troubleshooting a problem, it is much easier to rule out factors that are known to be correct because of up-to-date QA.

The lack of control over the inherent quality of patient gametes makes the need for ongoing QA paramount. QA provides a means of constant oversight and evaluation and facilitates the monitoring of quality of all aspects of our labs. Given the cost of the ARTs to patients, both financial and emotional, an established QA program adds value by optimizing the likelihood of a positive outcome for patients.

II. QA IN THE EMBRYOLOGY LAB

A. INTRODUCTION

In order to achieve and maintain success in the embryology lab it important to establish a comprehensive quality assurance program. The main goal of this program is to monitor and evaluate the ongoing and overall quality of the IVF process and all the events leading up to and after the actual procedure. The plan is designed to evaluate the effectiveness of policies and procedures, identify and correct problems, assure the accuracy and precision of procedures, and monitor the performance and competency of the lab staff.

A description follows a QA plan currently in use in an active IVF program. This plan's outline that may be different from other labs and illustrates one approach to establishing a QA plan. The QA plan will help set forth guidelines the lab staff may follow and use to help coordinate QA activities and day-to-day lab procedures. One must realize that QA policies are not set in stone and that as the lab changes, so should the QA plan. The lab director should establish regular QA meetings to discuss policies and occurrences in the lab and to decide how to implement policies and procedures. Also, as the dictum goes, "if it isn't written down, it wasn't done," documentation of all steps in the lab is imperative, from changes in policy to taking minutes at QA meetings. When the lab is under scrutiny for accreditation or in case any procedure is in question, documentation is crucial, even if simple notes are taken and maintained in a notebook. The QA plan discussed below has been adapted from an existing QA manual, and therefore may be useful as an outline for those looking to establish a QA manual.

B. QA PLAN

1. Scope of Practice

In attempting to establish a QA plan, first define the lab's scope of practice. This will help define the role of the lab and what the lab hopes to achieve as an outcome. Below are two examples of simple statements that address the scope of practice.

a. Provide patients with the highest quality IVF and related procedures. Procedures are employed to maximize the possibility of a positive outcome.

b. Quality control procedures are routinely performed to ensure that patient gametes are exposed to only the highest quality supplies and equipment. Daily monitoring of IVF equipment is performed to optimize proper operation.

While the intention of these statements seems obvious, it does help establish a set of goals that may lead to a positive attitude about the lab and its goals.

2. QA Goals

The QA plan evaluates and monitors the quality and appropriateness of its services on an ongoing basis. Its goal is to assure the accuracy and precision, as well as the reliability, of the results produced. Managerial, administrative, statistical, investigative, preventative, and corrective techniques will be employed to maximize the reliability of all data. The emphasis of the QA plan should be the *prevention* of problems rather than the detection and correction of problems after they occur.

a. *Responsibility for QA activities*: The lab director is responsible for ensuring the quality of services provided by the lab. The director may delegate both administrative and clinical responsibilities provided appropriate documentation is included.

b. *Definition of procedures*: List the procedures performed routinely in the lab and how frequently they occur.
c. *QA indicators*: This will define areas that are subject to scrutiny in QC and QA. By defining these indicators, routine monitoring will be established since these indicators are crucial to the scope of care. These will be described in detail separately.
d. *Ongoing review of lab events and outcomes*: Information should be summarized for monthly and yearly meetings to help evaluate outcomes and establish trends.
e. *Corrective action*: When problems occur, they must be evaluated for cause and corrective action taken. Preventative measures are then discussed to avoid future occurrences.

3. QA Indicators

In order to provide optimal care in the lab, one must first define the areas that require monitoring on an ongoing basis. This provides for review of these practices and their outcomes. From these reviews, changes or corrective actions can be implemented when necessary or decisions regarding procedures can be made. Only by monitoring these indicators can we evaluate the need for action.

a. *QC parameters*: Constant surveillance of QC parameters permits a certain comfort level that the system into which we expose patient gametes has been thoroughly tested and monitored to ensure the highest chance for a positive outcome. Such vigilance also prevents any unwanted changes in environment during gamete culture. The preceding chapters discuss the role and implementation of QC in the embryo lab and give examples of the QC parameters that would be monitored and evaluated in the embryo lab.
b. *Proficiency testing results*: Analysis of results determines how well the lab can evaluate the quality of unknown culture media.
c. *IVF procedure outcomes*: In the embryology lab, outcomes manifest themselves in stages. The most apparent indicators are percent fertilization, cleavage and embryo quality, and, of most concern, pregnancy rate. Knowledge of expected values for these outcomes helps determine when abnormal occurrences or trends are developing.
d. *Patient/physician complaints*: Identify cause and effect, then take corrective action.
e. *Accident/illness reports*: Monitor number and type of occurrences.

4. Quality Control

The purpose of an established QC program is to monitor and evaluate the level of quality of care provided for patient gametes. The QC requirements include standards for maintaining acceptable media testing, equipment, reagents and materials, guidelines for procedure manuals, calibration and control procedures, corrective action, and QC records.

a. *Methods and performance*: The lab must use culture methods that provide reliable results with expected rates of fertilization, cleavage and embryo quality, and pregnancy. Because patients vary in their fertility status, we must monitor not only individual patients, but results and trends over time.

b. *Equipment*: The lab must perform and document equipment maintenance and function checks within the frequency period recommended by the manufacturer.

c. *Reagents and supplies*: The lab should define and maintain written criteria essential for proper preparation, storage, and handling of reagents and supplies. A method for testing these materials should be established and performed prior to the use of newly introduced materials. As no mandate exists for testing products each lab must establish policy on product reagent and supply testing.

d. *Procedure manuals*: All lab personnel should have and follow a written procedure manual for the preparation for and performance of IVF culture procedures. Manuals should include detailed information on all aspects of the embryo lab, including all procedures performed in the lab. Quality control issues such as equipment maintenance also should be included. Procedures and any changes to these procedures must be approved, signed, and dated by the laboratory director. Written procedures addressing clerical tasks also should appear in the procedure manual as they relate to specimen handling. Other clerical tasks can be addressed in the policy guidelines (see Lab Policies). Procedures will be reviewed annually by the director. Discontinued procedures will be retained for two years. A description for formatting a manual is available.[9]

e. *Tolerance limits*: Procedure results are expected to fall within a given set of criteria. Up to a given value may be considered normal, but exceeding that value represents data out of the norm. Tolerance limits provide preset acceptable limits. Data beyond these limits warrant investigation. Setting tolerance limits can help determine if an individual or group is producing acceptable outcomes. Below are several examples of tolerance limits in an IVF setting (minimal expected values):

- incubator $CO2 \pm 0.5\%$ based on gas analysis
- 85% of two-cell mouse embryos develop to expanded blastocyst
- fertilization >60% of mature human oocytes
- >50% of embryos at 8-cell stage by 72 hours post-insemination
- >80% of frozen embryos survive thaw
- >30% ongoing pregnancy rate

Each lab should set tolerance limits based upon its experience with each parameter established. While monitoring the tolerance limits by looking for values outside of normal is critical, one must realize that patient variation, as well as other clinical variables, contribute to the overall performance of the embryo lab.

f. *Patient and data certification*: Patient worksheets containing IVF data should be monitored for clinical and clerical error. Any errors should be corrected by drawing a line through the incorrect entry and writing the corrected information in. This must be initialed by the person making the correction.

5. Accreditation

Presently no mandate exists for human IVF (embryo) labs to undergo scrutiny by any of the accrediting agencies. Since inspection is voluntary, labs can decide whether or not to seek accreditation. More than half of the IVF labs in the U.S. have been inspected, and we can anticipate that mandatory regulation of some form is imminent. Labs that have passed inspection must notify their accrediting agency within 60 days of any change in laboratory management staff.

While voluntary, inspection can be a useful exercise for any lab as no conflict of interest occurs for the inspectors sent to review the lab. In many cases, the inspection is an educational opportunity for both the inspector and the lab staff. Many innovative ways of approaching QA can be gleaned from inspectors who have visited many labs and been through inspection themselves.

6. Proficiency Testing

The lab should subscribe to proficiency testing (PT) made available through the American Association of Bioanalysts. PT for the embryo lab consists of two unknown culture media and two unknown protein sources. Testing of all combinations of media and protein is expected. A lab can test its ability to discern if one or all of the components for testing will support sperm survival or embryo growth. Testing must occur within two weeks of receipt of unknowns.

1. Surveys are sent twice annually and should be alternated so that the same person does not always perform the assays. Also, sufficient media are sent to allow multiple participants to compare results with the same batch of unknowns.
2. When results are returned, they should be analyzed by the lab director and reviewed with staff. Any abnormal results will be addressed with discussion focused on resolution of the aberrant results.
3. Results from several tests done over time should be compared and reviewed for unusual trends. One could expect that control results remain similar over time. Any marked changes warrant investigation.

7. Personnel

Detailed, written job descriptions should exist for all employees. Job standards attesting to the expectations of each employee should be developed for each position and are useful for employee review. All hands-on laboratory personnel should comply with guidelines for human embryology established by the American Society for Reproductive Medicine.[10]

Yearly review of personnel is recommended and, in many institutions, mandatory. The review process is important for evaluating skills and, when warranted, adding new responsibilities as personnel gain experience and skills. Verification of training must appear in each employee file, with continuing education and training updates included.

8. Lab Policies

Lab policies change continually as new methods and situations develop. All lab policies should be reviewed annually and updated as needed. The lab director must review and approve in writing all changes in lab policy. A notebook containing lab policies should be maintained in the lab in the event discussion over policy occurs.

9. Occurrence Reports

Documentation of any errors or unusual events occurring in the lab is important. Document the occurrence and how the situation was remedied, and keep this information on file as part of the QA manual. Because errors and mishaps occur, it is best to document them in detail, making sure that the entire staff knows of the incident. The lab director must verify in writing that the error occurred, that it was addressed, and that an attempt was made to correct it. In this same context, labs should maintain an adverse reaction file to avoid repeating an avoidable situation.

10. Continuing/Corporate Education

Staff members involved in continuing education learn new skills and maximize their abilities. Attending meetings or lectures helps keep staff up to date on the latest procedures and techniques, as well as the basic principles of the embryo lab. Continuing education may be required in future regulation; therefore, documentation of such education should be included in each employee's personnel file.

11. Annual QA Review

Obtaining and compiling QA data is of little use without extensive review. The lab should include all staff for data and procedural review. Many insights come from those with the most hands-on time in the lab. While monthly QA meetings can address immediate issues, the lab director must spend time reviewing QC and QA data to look for trends or problems. Positive trends also emerge that can lead to improvements in other areas, can initiate changes in procedures that may be useful to other labs, or can warrant more detailed investigation, such as initiation of a research project.

Each of the sections discussed above may have changes that are imperceptible when viewed on a weekly or monthly basis, but that are readily apparent when data covering 12 months are reviewed. Even when no deviations from normal appear, analysis can confirm that all systems appear to be functioning normally.

In the embryology lab, the most obvious and critical factors are fertilization, cleavage, embryo grading, pregnancy, and implantation rates. Other factors for evaluation might include number of embryos transferred, percent of multiple pregnancies, and quality of embryo transfer techniques by physician. Also, managers must evaluate any changes made in the lab during the last year under review. For example, if a change in culture media occurred in May, then evaluating the January to May vs. the June to December pregnancy rates can help ascertain if the change had any positive or negative consequences. In some cases, statistical analysis will determine if enough data exists to make meaningful conclusions. Because all aspects of the lab are under scrutiny in a QA review, one must evaluate all QA indicators, including the mundane but equally important tasks of patient and specimen identification, reporting of results, and patient/staff communication. Analysis should establish clearly that observed differences are significant and not just trends that, over time, have no real clinical value in the QA process, and therefore in our embryology lab.

III. QA IN THE ANDROLOGY LAB

A. INTRODUCTION

Quality assurance in andrology testing should enable the laboratory to meet, at minimum, standards outlined under CLIA '88 for test management. CLIA requires that a QA program monitor and evaluate ongoing and overall quality of the testing processes used by the laboratory. The QA policies should address the pre-analytic, analytic, and post-analytic phases of the testing procedures used. Information in a comprehensive QA program should include the following categories: patient test management assessment, quality control assessment, proficiency testing assessment, comparison of test results if using differing test methods, relationship of patient information to patient test results, personnel assessment, communications, complaint investigations, staff review, and maintenance of appropriate QA records. Different laboratories will meet these requirements in different ways, as dictated by factors such as the number of procedures performed, the specific tests offered, number of testing personnel, extent of referral services, and others. An effective QA program for an in office andrology laboratory that performs semen analysis only for patients requiring inseminations will be different from that required for a high volume reference laboratory that provides a range of tests (such as antisperm antibodies, sperm penetration assays, etc). In this section, an overview of QA procedures will be presented followed by a specific andrology lab at Indianapolis Andrology and Laboratory Services, Inc. Not all of the procedures will apply to all laboratories, and, in fact, one could take issue with some of the procedures in use at this facility. Nevertheless, a description of this system, which has met with approval under several CLIA inspections, should provide a reasonable basis for comparison. Other published model systems for andrology lab QA may also prove useful to the reader.[11]

B. QA PLAN

1. Patient Test Management

Patient test management (as in all phases of QA) must have methods in place to assess pre-analytic, analytic, and post-analytic phases of the testing procedure. Several QA indicators ensure that all of these phases of patient test management are addressed. For *pre-analytic* phases of testing, the following are examined:

a. A written order for the appropriate test must be obtained before the lab accepts any specimen. Lab supervisors conduct a monthly random audit of patient charts, using 100% agreement as the threshold.
b. When arriving for testing, patients are asked to fill out a form with appropriate demographic information including the name of the patient and partner, social security number, time and method of collection, and other information. Records are audited randomly every month to ensure that all requested information is completed.
c. Patient waiting times are monitored by monthly random audit to ensure that samples are processed in a timely fashion.

For the *analytic* phase of test management, the following parameters are examined:

a. Turn-around times from receipt of sample to return of washed specimens for IUI are monitored, with a threshold of 90% of specimens returned within 70 minutes considered suitable. Again, this is monitored by random chart reviews conducted monthly. We feel this is a useful indicator from several standpoints. First, if turn-around time takes too long it could indicate a scheduling problem or a staffing problem that needs to be addressed. In either case, failure to achieve this goal could result in a sample mix-up, which, of course, is probably the primary concern for any laboratory director and staff. Second, because it is a reference lab, patients must transport specimens to their physician office for insemination. Holding processing time to a minimum will save the patient time, thereby helping maintain client satisfaction.
b. A log book is kept in the lab and monitored monthly to ensure that the test ordered is actually that which was run on the specimen, with a threshold of 100%. Other mechanisms such as bar coding of samples can be used to ensure correct testing procedures are performed.
c. All specimens are transported to the lab from the collection area for testing, and must be labeled with the patient name as well as a unique identifier (e.g., social security number) before testing proceeds. This ensures that the specimen can be appropriately labeled throughout all phases of testing, and is again monitored randomly on a monthly basis.

Post-analytic phases of test management comprise the following:

a. All specimens for IUI are given directly to the female partner for transport to the physician office. Each specimen is labeled with date, patient initials, and social security number, and the patient must sign that the specimen is the correct specimen before the sample is released. This information is monitored monthly to ensure that 100% of specimens have been signed out appropriately.
b. Before releasing results to the physician office, the lab supervisor or director compares results from the hand-written worksheet prepared during actual testing to the typed report to be sent to the physician to ensure that no clerical errors have occurred. This is also monitored monthly by random audit.
c. The percentage of reports sent to the referring physician office on time (within 48 hours of testing) is also monitored monthly, with a threshold of 90%. All of the above patient test management data are compiled monthly by the lab supervisor and reviewed with the director. Any necessary corrective actions are then discussed and relayed to testing personnel.

2. Quality Control Assessment

Quality control (QC) and QA are commonly confused terms. Our view of QA relative to QC is that QA should provide the means to document the effectiveness of your QC procedures. QC for andrology lab testing has been reviewed elsewhere in this text. We utilize several means to assess our QC procedures. For semen analyses, records are examined by random audit to ensure that duplicate counts for sperm concentration are recorded for each analysis. In addition, all personnel performing semen analyses do triplicate counts of sperm concentration and sperm motility (graded as rapid progressive, slow progressive, nonprogressive, and immotile) on the same semen specimen. This is done monthly, and the inter- and intra-assay coefficients of variation calculated. A CV of <15% is expected, and these records are reviewed each month as part of the QA plan. If results exceed this threshold corrective actions are necessary including equipment checks and retraining of personnel if required. A similar approach addresses strict morphology assessment and, in fact, can be applied to any andrology test. Thus, this QA program analyzes the data obtained from standard QC policies to ensure that results are within acceptable limits and that corrective actions can be taken if QC limits are exceeded. In addition, for tests that require use of positive and negative controls such as antisperm antibody tests, the lab supervisor reviews all results to ensure that all QC parameters are met prior to release of results to the referring physician. Any results not within QC are not released, and such incidences are discussed and reviewed by the director and supervisor on a monthly basis.

3. Proficiency Test Assessment

Under CLIA guidelines, laboratories performing high complexity testing must participate in a proficiency testing program. One of the historical problems for andrology testing labs is that, until recently, no programs existed that could make interlaboratory comparisons on identical samples. This problem has been alleviated somewhat, with several companies or organizations (including the American Association of Bioanalysis and Fertility Solutions) offering samples for interlaboratory comparisons for semen analysis and sperm antibody testing. Labs can, for a fee, obtain specimens on a periodic basis and obtain data on performance relative to other labs using similar methodology. Records must be obtained for all PT procedures indicating that testing was performed using standard testing methods by the lab in question. In other words, one cannot use CASA for all regular testing, but use a Makler chamber for testing PT samples. Documentation of corrective actions taken as a result of unacceptable PT samples also must be kept and proven effective through successful participation in subsequent PT challenges. In our laboratory, we are enrolled in PT programs for semen analysis and sperm antibody testing, in which samples are obtained twice yearly. All PT records are reviewed by the lab director and supervisor to ensure that results fall within acceptable levels. For our lab, we consider results within two standard deviations of the sample mean acceptable. Corrective actions include examination of counting chambers, calibration of pipettors, and retraining of personnel. Note that CLIA does not exempt a lab from performing PT testing if a program for such testing is not available. If tests are done that do not "fit" under approved CLIA programs, CLIA mandates that the lab have a system for verifying the accuracy and reliability of testing results at least twice yearly. In such instances, labs must devise their own plan for sharing samples with other labs for purposes of comparison. A good example of such a situation would be sperm penetration assays. In such cases, labs could score the same micrographs for numbers of penetrated sperm. Each lab also would have to develop its own mechanisms for distinguishing between positive vs. negative performance in comparative testing under such a circumstance.

4. Comparison of Test Results

This part of QA refers to comparison of testing where the same test is done with different methods or where the same test is performed at multiple sites. In such situations, CLIA dictates that QA involves assessing different testing methods for sources of variation, if such variation actually exists. A scenario that could affect andrology testing would be the use of different counting chambers (e.g., Makler vs. CASA) for routine semen analysis. In such a case, labs must have mechanisms that evaluate the relationship between the different methods to ensure that accurate results are provided to the lab's clients. For example, if PT samples show that a consistently accurate count is provided by one testing system, but not another, the lab must document and take steps to correct such discrepancies.

5. Relationship of Patient Information to Patient Test Results

CLIA requires that labs have mechanisms to identify and evaluate patient test results that appear inconsistent with relevant patient criteria. For example, if a patient who has had a vasectomy provides a specimen demonstrating sperm, something is obviously wrong. On the other hand, we have seen several cases where men who had normal analyses in the past provided specimens of extremely poor quality. In such cases, the lab should have mechanisms to identify such outliers and to evaluate possible reasons for the discrepancy. Our laboratory attempts to deal with this QA requirement by having the patient fill out a brief history (problems with erection, ejaculation, regularity of intercourse), history of any testicular trauma (including injury or delayed testicular descent), any recent medical problems, use of any medications, or information on any other medical problems. If patients have an abnormal outcome, then the questionnaire is reviewed to determine a possible cause. In this manner, we have identified several problems that might have resulted in adverse, unexpected outcomes. As an example, one patient with severe oligospermia was found to have been placed on high doses of testosterone for impotence, which may have affected spermatogenesis. For "panic" situations (i.e., the couple scheduled for IUI with no sperm in the sample), the referring physician is contacted immediately to discuss options with the couple. As with all QA parameters, such cases are discussed routinely to document if there was any information that would be useful in the diagnosis of the problem.

6. Personnel Assessment

An effective QA program has ongoing methods to evaluate the effectiveness of its policies for demonstrating employee competence. Note again, this is not QC—QC actually provides one with mechanisms to determine competence by such approaches as PT tests or, in our cases, routine assessment of inter- and intra-observer variability. The QA part of the process deals with determining the effectiveness of the competency assessment program. This can be done on a yearly, or even more frequent, basis if deemed necessary. For our lab, the director routinely reviews QC data to ensure that all testing personnel fall within established limits. Part of an ongoing assessment for QA should be whether or not the limits established are appropriate. For example, the cutoff for intra-assay variation for semen analysis had been 20%, but at that level no one had ever exceeded the limit. One must then question whether the limit is appropriate and determine whether new QA guidelines should be established. This is, in fact, a good rule of thumb for any QA procedure. If, for example, a QA indicator is set such that, over an extended time period, it is never violated (for example, QA indicator is that all semen analyses are processed within 3 hours, when, in fact, none ever exceed 2 hours), then clearly this is an inappropriate QA parameter to measure and should be adjusted.

7. Communications

The laboratory must have a mechanism to document problems occurring as a result of communication errors between the lab and its clients and must also document corrective action. This kind of communication will vary depending on the particular situation. For in-house labs such communication can involve direct one-on-one communication, staff meetings, etc., whereas for large reference labs with multiple clients, other procedures must prevail. In our lab, we hold monthly QA meetings with referring physicians and their office staff during which any communication problems are discussed and documented. The laboratory director and supervisor then formulate corrective actions and distribute them to physician offices. Follow-up at subsequent QA meetings reviews the success or failure of the corrective actions.

8. Complaint Investigation

The laboratory should have a system to document that any complaints (patient or physician) received by the lab are reviewed with necessary corrective actions taken. This is best achieved by maintaining a complaint log, with instruction to lab personnel that any complaints must be logged in with date, person lodging the complaint, and the nature of the complaint. Complaints are then reviewed monthly by the director and supervisor, and appropriate corrective actions taken and relayed to all lab personnel.

9. Staff Reviews

All the QA plans in the world are useless if the information gained by the QA program is not shared with laboratory staff. In our case, the supervisor and director meet weekly and review QA data monthly. Any changes in lab policies are then shared by written memo with lab staff who sign off on any changes in protocol. Any changes must of course be documented and maintained in your record.

10. Maintenance of QA Records

One must remember the motto, "if it isn't written down, it wasn't done." Each lab must develop a clearly written and focused QA plan that meets the needs of its testing capacity. Labs should keep records for test management assessment, PT, QC, and the other parameters discussed above and the QA plan should be reviewed at least yearly to ensure that the procedures actually assure quality. QA is more than determining whether you do a semen analysis correctly. It is a comprehensive evaluation of the effectiveness of everything the lab does, from providing precise and accurate results to providing clients with prompt, professional, and courteous service. Without record maintenance on all these phases of QA, one cannot ensure that such goals are, in fact, being met.

IV. QA IN THE ENDOCRINE LAB

A. INTRODUCTION

The purpose of an endocrine laboratory is to provide information that aids clinicians in confirming or rejecting a diagnosis and to monitor current or follow-up therapy. Close adherence to a quality assurance program fulfills this purpose. An effective quality assurance program encompasses proper specimen collection, handling, and processing. It is also concerned with personnel qualifications, training and continuing education, result reporting, information management, and implementation of a quality control program. Federal regulations (CLIA '88) detail standards to be followed by the laboratory. Each laboratory must be able to provide documentation that complies with the rules and regulations stipulated by CLIA 88. Our laboratory operates within the state of New York. Laboratories operating in New York are regulated thoroughly by our State Health Department and we are, therefore, exempt from CLIA '88. However, the following section summarizes both the New York State and the CLIA '88 regulations, both of which, in essence, outline a quality assurance program.

B. QA PLAN

1. Accession Systems

The endocrine laboratory must maintain records that contain the following:

  a. The accession number or other identification of the specimen
  b. The name or other identification of the person from whom the specimen was taken
  c. The date the specimen was received
  d. The tests requested
  e. The date the specimen was tested
  f. The date the result was reported
  g. The name of the licensed physician or other authorized person or entity submitting the specimen

2. Reports

The reports generated by the endocrine laboratory must contain all of the above information in addition to normal values, reference intervals, or similar methods for identifying abnormal values.

3. Record Retention

Endocrine laboratories should retain documentation of laboratory operations for varying times depending on the type of information contained within the specific document. In New York State test results, requests, and accession records must be retained for 7 years. CLIA requires that labs retain these same records for 2 years. Quality control records must be retained for 2 years for labs operating under CLIA or New York State. Preventative maintenance, service, and repair records must be retained for as long as the instrument remains in use.

4. Personnel Qualifications

According to CLIA, endocrine tests are classified at a moderate complexity level if performed by automated or semi-automated assay systems and are considered high complexity if performed by manual methods such as radioimmunoassay (RIA). Personnel requirements for endocrine laboratories vary with the level of complexity and the position held. Specific requirements exist for directors, technical supervisors, clinical consultants, general supervisors, and testing personnel. Personnel files should contain documentation of each individual's qualifications in the form of copies of degrees, transcripts, certificates, resumés, and curriculum vitae.

5. Training and Continuing Education

All personnel should undergo a defined training procedure that includes instruction in testing, quality control, safety requirements (universal precautions), chemical hygiene plans, hazardous waste disposal, confidentiality, communication with physicians and nurses, and other areas necessary in individual laboratories. Documentation for the completion and comprehension of all procedures should be maintained in the personnel file.

A regular program of continuing or in-service education should be conducted and documented. The educational component should be broad and include topics such as the use of new equipment, changes in standard operations, and the physiology behind disease states and treatment protocols.

6. Problems and Resolutions

When problems occur in any aspect of laboratory function, the problem as well as the resolution should be documented in a problem log. The log should include how the problem was discovered, by whom, what the problem concerned, and the corrective action taken. This log should also document the action taken to prevent further recurrence of the problem.

7. Quality Control

The heart of a good quality assurance program is quality control. Two basic forms of quality control exist in the endocrine laboratory, namely internal and external. Internal quality control monitors **precision** through daily examination of laboratory tests. External quality control monitors the **accuracy** of laboratory tests usually through a proficiency testing (PT) program provided by your state health department or other paid programs.

Endocrine laboratories must strive for both accuracy and precision. Accuracy in the laboratory is the extent to which the measured value is close to the true value.

It is monitored through the assay of control or reference specimens of known concentration. Precision is the measure of random variability, and describes the reproducibility of a measurement when it is run repeatedly under identical conditions. Precision is independent of accuracy. An analyte may be measured any number of times with a similar result obtained each time; however, those measurements, although close to one another could be far from the true measurement and thus they are inaccurate but precise.

8. Internal Quality Control

Internal quality control is monitored using a variety of statistical formats, all of which encompass plotting control data as a function of time. One of the earliest statistical methods utilized in the endocrine laboratory, and widely in use today is the Levey-Jennings chart.[12] Other less frequently used methods are the analysis of variance, the mean and range, and trend analysis. In order to provide data points for quality control analysis, laboratories run control samples and patient samples under identical conditions on a daily basis. Control samples may come with the kits purchased to assay samples or may be purchased separately from unrelated manufacturers. In either case, manufacturers provide target ranges and individual laboratories should establish their own ranges every 30 days based on monthly statistical analysis of the data obtained from daily runs. Control samples purchased from commercial suppliers provide a large pool of material in which the analytes are stable in storage for long periods of time, the levels of analytes are nearly equivalent to one another, and the material is abundant enough to be used by many laboratories. Over time this allows for comparisons among laboratories and various assay systems. Commercial suppliers provide controls with target values that fall within the ranges at which clinical decisions will be made based on the hormone levels reported by the laboratory.

Precision, when expressed in terms of standard deviation (SD), can be calculated with the following formulas:

$$SD = (\Sigma\,((\overline{X}) - X)^2 / (n{-}1))^{1/2},$$

where $\overline{X}$ = mean of all observed values

$$= \Sigma X/n,$$

where X = observed values and n = number of observations.

SD can be converted to the coefficient of variance (CV) and both parameters can be used to monitor assay performance. CV is calculated as follows:

$$CV = (SD/X) \times 100,$$

where X = concentration of the analyte in question.

Both SD and CV indicate the accuracy and precision of a particular assay system. For example, laboratories that use radioimmunoassays will pipette the standard curve, control samples, and patient samples in duplicate. Control samples will be examined to determine whether they fall within 2 SD of the mean control value, and the duplicates will be examined for precision by determining whether or not the CV of the duplicates is less than a predetermined percentage (usually 20 to 25%).

Most laboratories define their control limits as ± 2 SD and will thus operate within a 95% confidence limit. Distribution of results of an assay repeatedly performed can be depicted graphically by a frequency curve. Statistical analysis assumes that the distribution is symmetric and bell shaped. When the total area under the curve is equal to all the plotted results, 68% of the measurements will fall within one SD around the mean and 95.5% of the measurements fall within 2 SD around the mean.

9. Analysis of Accuracy and Precision

The most commonly used tool to track quality control are Levey-Jennings charts. Software programs usually accompany automated assay systems, and gamma counters used in radioimmunoassays (RIA) allow the user to monitor these programs' assay performance. Values for control samples are plotted on the ordinate (y-axis) against the days of the month on the abscissa (x-axis). The expected mean value is drawn as a solid line in the center of the chart while the range (2 SD) above and below the mean is indicated by dashed lines (Figure 12.1). The chart is interpreted by examining whether control values fall within 2 SD (between the dashed lines). The run is considered to be "out of control" when the values fall outside of the dashed lines. The goal is an equal distribution of values above and below the mean and within 2 SD of the mean.

All laboratory personnel who run assays need experience examining these charts in order to identify subtle changes occurring in control values. Personnel will find helpful the ability to classify the type of error as random or systematic once a problem is identified. Random error appears as a wide range of scatter on the Levey-Jennings chart termed dispersion (Figure 12.1A). Systematic error is indicated when a shift or sudden change from the mean occurs and persists (Figure 12.1B), or when a trend, a more gradual change from the mean is observed (Figure 12.1C).

Once errors appear, the cause of the problem must be determined. A single value falling outside of a laboratory's chosen control limits does not indicate that the entire assay should be rejected. Laboratories often adopt less stringent rules for rejecting a run. Commonly, each daily assay has three control values, and the laboratory rule for accepting the run may be that two of the three controls fall within the accepted range. This is not a bad rule; however, the lab should question the validity of patient results that are found to fall in the same area at which a control sample was determined to be out of range. Care must be taken not to rely solely on once a month analysis of Levey-Jennings charts. Assay performance should be monitored daily. The laboratory supervisor or director should be notified when control values fall outside of acceptable limits for a daily assay. The supervisor or director can then make the decision to accept or reject an assay.

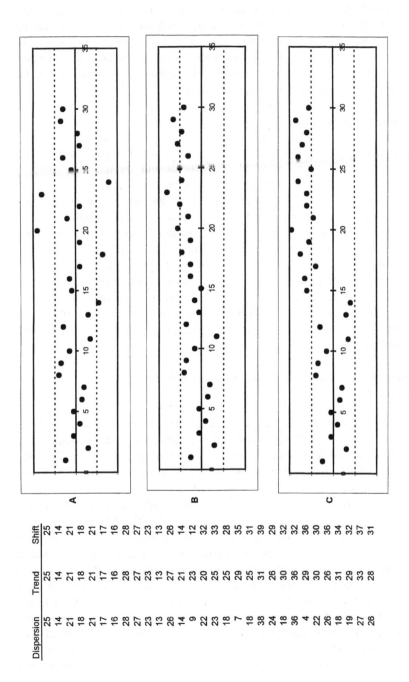

Dispersion	Trend	Shift
25	25	25
14	14	14
21	21	21
18	18	18
21	21	21
17	17	17
16	16	16
28	28	28
27	27	27
23	23	23
13	13	13
26	27	26
14	21	14
9	23	12
22	20	32
23	25	33
18	25	28
7	29	35
18	25	31
38	31	39
24	26	29
18	30	32
36	36	32
4	29	36
22	30	30
26	26	36
18	31	34
19	29	32
27	33	37
26	28	31

FIGURE 12.1 Three patterns of control data illustrating random or systematic error: (A) dispersion, (B) trend, (C) shift.

Busy laboratories can be lulled easily into relying too heavily on automated assay systems to eliminate errors in the laboratory. One must remember that machines can fail. Automated assay systems rarely break down completely; their failures usually begin with slow, subtle changes. Additionally, humans run the automated assay systems, and even experienced technicians may formulate "operational short-cuts" they feel will not make a difference in assay validity. The laboratory director has the responsibility to observe subtle deviations from standard operating procedures and correct them prior to reporting results.

10. External Quality Control

The most frequently used form of external quality control is participation in a proficiency testing (PT) survey program. Nationwide and abroad, large numbers of laboratories analyze the same specimens three times a year and send the results of these blind samples back to the program to obtain an unbiased, critical assessment of their analyses in comparison to peer laboratories. Additionally, regional or state PT programs may originate from state health departments or organized laboratory groups. The College of American Pathologist (CAP) Survey Program offers the largest program in the country and currently has 16,170 clinical laboratory subscribers. The number of participants in the various endocrinology programs is 7299. CLIA '88 requires all laboratories to participate in an accredited PT survey program. The Health Care Financing Administration (HCFA) has set forth criteria for laboratory accreditation. Laboratories must achieve an 80% pass rate for successful performance.

C. Implementing a Quality Control Program in the Endocrine Lab

The first step in implementing a quality control program in the endocrine laboratory is to have a written protocol that details the laboratory's daily, weekly, and monthly quality control requirements. This protocol should specify which individuals are responsible for each component and the corrective action to initiate when problems arise.

Endocrine laboratories use assay kits and automated analyzers that are purchased or leased from any number of commercial suppliers. RIA kits also are used widely in many laboratories. Implementing a quality control program involves daily, weekly, and monthly maintenance of equipment used to run commercial assays. Automated analyzers have varying levels of maintenance that must occur at time intervals indicated by the manufacturers. A detailed description of these maintenance programs is beyond the scope of this discussion. It suffices to say that manufacturers provide detailed instructions and schedules for equipment maintenance and these should be strictly adhered to and well documented. Laboratories that use RIAs will not have the same types of equipment schedules, but all laboratories have common components (small equipment) that must be monitored and maintained.

1. Temperature Checks

Temperature control and recording is essential for refrigerators/freezers that store assay reagents and patient serum samples. Water baths used to incubate RIAs also require such monitoring. Temperature charts should be placed on or near all refrigerators/freezers and waterbaths, and individual pieces of equipment should be permanently equipped with thermometers. Thermometers should be placed such that technicians do not have to touch or move them in order to take a reading. Take temperature readings daily before using the equipment. Record readings on the temperature charts along with the date and name or initials of the technician taking the recordings. The laboratory's acceptable temperature limits should be displayed clearly on the chart, and if the daily reading deviates from the range, the technician must inform the supervisor or director prior to using the equipment for assays. Waterbaths also should have water level checks on a daily or weekly basis as necessary. If water needs to be added this should be done in the evening to allow the temperature to equilibrate overnight. Ideally, thermometers should be placed with the area from which the reading is taken extending beyond the lid of the waterbath; water temperature falls rapidly (within seconds) when the lid is removed from the waterbath. Thermometers used for monitoring equipment should themselves be calibrated against thermometers certified for accuracy by the National Institute of Standards and Technology (NIST). These thermometers are available for purchase from most laboratory product suppliers.

2. Pipette Checks

Automated assay systems often include self-contained dilution schemes that virtually eliminate the need for pipettes in the endocrine laboratory, but some systems still require manual dilutions to be carried out by technicians. Laboratories that use RIA systems must have confidence that the pipettes are accurate. Pipettes can be checked for accuracy by weighing volumes of water equal to the volumes used for pipetting the laboratory's assays. A milliliter (ml) of water weighs 1 gram (g), 0.5 ml weighs 0.5 g, 0.1 ml weighs 0.1 g and so on. When checking the accuracy of a pipette, a technician should make at least ten consecutive measures at each chosen setting and record these measures for later analysis. All pipettes should be checked at several measurement levels encompassing the range for which that particular pipette performs in the laboratory. Once all measurements are recorded they should be examined for accuracy to the true value. Laboratory personnel can calculate the percent difference between the desired and actual measurements. The laboratory supervisor or director must determine the acceptable limits of inaccuracy (usually 5%). Pipettes that exceed these limits should go back to the manufacturer for calibration, or if this is not possible they should be discarded. Not all pipettes can be calibrated and this fact should be kept in mind when purchasing them.

3. Balance Checks

Balances are used for checking pipette accuracy, balancing opposing centrifuge buckets, and weighing assay reagents. Balances can be checked for accuracy using a universal set of weights that can be purchased from most laboratory products suppliers. The process for checking a balance is similar to that described for pipettors. A technician will take several consecutive weight measurements, record them, and determine the percent difference between the expected and measured reading. When a balance's accuracy falls outside acceptable limits, corrective action must be taken. Frequently, the problem can be resolved by adjusting the plane in which the balance sits. All balances come with a bubble-float device that adjusts so that the center of the balance lies in a plane of 180°. The float device consists of a small enclosed plastic chamber containing a liquid and a small amount of air that forms a bubble. The "feet" of the balance can be raised or lowered until the bubble in the float device lies directly in the center of the circle. Once the balance is adjusted the accuracy check should be repeated, and if the values continue to be outside acceptable limits, the balance should be serviced by the manufacturer or other qualified technician.

In summary, quality control in the endocrine laboratory is a goal all laboratories can reach without great difficulty. The key is to have a written plan with strict adherence to the protocol. All members of the lab should participate in the quality control process at some level, but one person ultimately must be responsible for implementing and overseeing the quality control program. Adhering to a quality control protocol will assure that the laboratory provides the highest level of quality care to patients and will circumvent any crisis situations.

REFERENCES

1. Byrd, W., Quality assurance in the reproductive biology laboratory, *Arch. Pathol. Lab. Med.*, 116, 418, 1992.
2. Code of Federal Regulations (CFR), Quality assurance for moderate or high complexity testing, or both, *Fed. Regist.*, Vol. 57, No. 40, Subpart P, 7002, 1992.
3. National Fish and Wildlife Forensic Laboratory, Quality Assurance Manual, Introduction, Webpage http://olmec.lab.labr1.fws.gov/qaqc/qaqc1.html.
4. Clark, G. B., Quality assurance, an administrative means to a managerial end: part I, *Clin. Lab. Manag. Rev.* 4, 1, 1990.
5. Code of Federal Regulations (CFR), Summary, Clinical Laboratory Improvement Amendments of 1988, *Fed. Regist.*, Vol. 57, No. 40, 7002, 1992.
6. Dunphy, B. C., Kay, R., Barratt, C. L. R., and Cooke, I. D., Quality control during the conventional analysis of semen: an essential exercise, *J. Androl.*, 10, 378, 1989.
7. Mortimer, D., Shu, M. A., and Tan, R., Standardization and quality control of sperm concentration and motility counts in semen analysis, *Hum. Reprod.*, 1, 299, 1986.
8. Menkveld, R., Stander, F. S. H., Kotze, T. Jv. W., and Kruger, T. F., The evaluation of morphological characteristics of human sperm according to stricter criteria, *Hum. Reprod.*, 5, 586, 1990.
9. National Committee for Clinical Laboratory Standards, Clinical laboratory procedure manuals, GP2-A (NCCLS), Villanova, Pennsylvania, 1994.
10. American Society for Reproductive Medicine, Guidelines for human embryology and andrology laboratories, Vol. 58, No. 4, Suppl. 1, 1992.
11. Muller, C. H., The andrology laboratory in an assisted reproductive technology program: QA and lab methodology, *J. Androl.*, 13, 349, 1992.
12. Barger, J. D., Levey and Jennings revisited, *Arch. Path. Lab. Med.*, 116, 799, 1992.

13 Quality Control, Quality Assurance, and Management of the Cryopreservation Laboratory

Grace M. Centola

CONTENTS

0-8493-1677-4/00/$0.00+$.50
© 2000 by CRC Press LLC

I. INTRODUCTION

Cryobanking of reproductive tissue is now an accepted option for couples proceeding with assisted reproductive technologies (ART). Semen banking is an option for patients prior to cancer treatments or vasectomy as a form of "fertility insurance." Most recently, cryopreservation of epididymal aspirates and testicular tissue has been used to store sperm cells for later use in ART.[1-4] Cadaveric or posthumous retrieval of sperm or testicular tissue, with cryopreservation and storage until subsequent use, has been performed in a few selected medical centers (Schlegel, personal communication). Since 1988 the law mandates that donor semen be cryopreserved and quarantined for a minimum of six months, with initial and pre-release donor infectious disease testing. Although successful oocyte cryopreservation with subsequent fertilization *in vitro* has occurred only in a few cases (Tucker, M. J., personal communication, 1997), embryo cryopreservation is rapidly becoming routine for the ART lab.[5,6] In recent years, investigators have cryopreserved ovarian tissue, albeit as a research tool, with the potential clinical application to store ovarian tissue prior to cancer therapy, for example (Fugger, personal communication).

In the past several years, reports of errors in reproductive laboratories demonstrate the need for strict quality control procedures for all reproductive laboratories, including, but not limited to, those performing reproductive tissue cryopreservation and storage. Recognition of the possible catastrophic consequences of poor quality control procedures has led to a realization that quality control, quality assurance and management, competency testing, and process validation are critical components of reproductive tissue banks.[7] This chapter will discuss quality control (QC) and quality assurance (QA) procedures for the reproductive tissue bank. For purposes of clarity, the term "reproductive tissue" will be used to indicate both semen and embryos unless there is a difference between the two, when the terms will be used individually. For purposes of discussion, the topics will be divided into QC, which includes equipment maintenance and validation, and QA, which includes process validation and procedural assessments. Laboratories must comply with state regulations, if available, and with federal regulations, which include the Clinical Laboratory Improvement Act of 1988, and Food and Drug Administration (FDA) rules. The FDA recently published a proposal that includes mandates for disease testing and quality control procedures for facilities involved in donated reproductive tissue.[8,9] Furthermore, the College of American Pathologists (CAP) Reproductive Laboratory Accreditation Program (RLAP) also mandates minimum QC and QA procedures in andrology and embryology laboratories, including cryopreservation laboratories.

II. BACKGROUND AND TERMINOLOGY

Total quality management (TQM) has three components: quality control (QC), quality assurance (QA), and quality improvement (QI). The goal of any TQM program is to provide the optimum product or service possible, in the most efficient and cost-effective way. QC considers a single item, whereas QA is generally process oriented. Quality control and quality assurance refer to the control of the testing process to ensure that test results meet quality requirements.[10] Examples of TQM are shown in Table 13.1. QC includes establishing specifications for each aspect of the testing process, assessing the procedures to determine conformance with specifications, and taking corrective action to bring the procedures into conformance.[10] Laboratories must establish and follow written policies and procedures for QC. The goal of the QC program is to follow a written protocol and monitor the quality of the analytical testing process of each method to assure the accuracy, precision, and reliability of the test results and reports. This process includes checking the performance of equipment and personnel. The frequency of QC checks should be determined by the individual laboratory standard operating protocol (SOP), but should be based on the following: instrument/reagent stability, frequency with which the test is performed, how strongly the method is technique dependent, frequency of QC failure, and experience and training needed by testing personnel (Dasuray, personal communication). The QA program reviews and analyzes data in order to identify problems related to the quality of care provided by the laboratory. The QA program also *prevents* problems. QA data should be assessed on a regular basis and the information used to identify and resolve problems. The laboratory director is responsible for setting the QC and QA guidelines and ensuring implementation of the QC/QA program.

TABLE 13.1
Examples of Total Quality Management (TQM)

Quality Control	Quality Assurance	Quality Improvement
Accuracy of test method	Adverse reaction file	Turn around time for test results
Precision of test method	Specimen/vial ID; verification/labeling	Smoother workflow
Temperature verification	Analysis of PT vial; cryosensitivity testing	Inter-technician variability
Fluid contaminant check	Assessment of pregnancy rates; outcome indicators	Intra-technician variability
Proficiency testing		# vials/specimen
Instrument function verification; calibration		Pregnancy outcomes
Liquid nitrogen levels		Donor samples rejected

III. LABORATORY MANAGEMENT

The Clinical Laboratory Improvement Act of 1988 (CLIA '88) mandates that all laboratories "that examine human specimens for the diagnosis, prevention or treatment of any disease or impairment of, or the assessment of the health of, human beings" must be accredited, which involves registration of the laboratory, inspection, and proficiency testing (where one exists).[10–13] Reproductive laboratories, particularly andrology, embryology, and cryopreservation laboratories are classified into moderate and high complexity testing laboratories under CLIA '88.[11,13] Performance of sperm concentration, motility, and morphology is classified as high complexity, whereas determination of the presence or absence of sperm only is considered moderate complexity.[11,13] Classification of embryology laboratories as high complexity laboratories is still subject to final determination.[13] The Centers for Disease Control and Prevention (CDC) is also in the process of developing a model program for certification of embryo laboratories. This is part of the implementation of the Fertility Clinic Success Rate and Certification Act of 1992.[14,15] In view of the definitions under CLIA '88, as well as the model certification program developed by the CDC, it seems appropriate that cryopreservation laboratories would come under the purview of CLIA '88 and the CDC model system, as well as any state department of health regulations where those might exist.[15]

Laboratory classification under the high complexity rating as determined by CLIA '88[10–13] will determine laboratory personnel[13] and quality control/quality assurance requirements.[13,16] The phase-in period for implementation of these personnel requirements lasted for several years, with final implementation mandated for July, 1998. Under CLIA '88, the laboratory director must be a pathologist, M.D., or D.O. with specific clinical laboratory training during residency, 2 years supervisory experience, or certification in a laboratory specialty. The laboratory director also can be a Ph.D., with a minimum of 4 years clinical laboratory experience and board certification in a laboratory subspecialty (i.e., andrology, embryology). Specific training requirements also exist for technical supervisor, clinical consultant, general supervisor, and testing personnel under CLIA '88.[13,15] Currently, board certification in the specialty of andrology and embryology is available through the American Board of Bioanalysis (ABB).

Tissue banks, i.e., cryopreservation laboratories, including reproductive tissue banks, should follow the personnel requirements under CLIA '88.[10–13,15] The laboratory director must be an M.D. or D.O. or a Ph.D. with appropriate experience. A technical supervisor is required only if the laboratory director is not a pathologist, and can be a pathologist, M.D., Ph.D., M.S., or B.S..

The laboratory director oversees the general operation of the laboratory, including development and implementation of a Standard Operating Procedure Manual (SOPM) and Technical Procedure Manual. The SOPM contains the personnel policy, safety policy, biohazard waste removal, exposure control plan, and quality control/quality assurance manuals. The Technical Procedure Manual contains the actual procedure manual outlining the various laboratory procedures utilized in the clinical laboratory services. The laboratory director not only develops the SOPM and procedure manual, but is responsible for periodic review of the manuals, updating the manuals, and ensuring that the personnel follow the policies and procedures. The laboratory supervisor can be designated by the laboratory director to assist in the periodic review of the policy and procedure manuals. The laboratory director also will review QC and QA records, implement changes in policies and procedures, and keep appropriate records of this review.

Often, the laboratory director is not involved in the day-to-day operation of the laboratory or in the actual laboratory benchwork. However, the laboratory director does enforce the accurate and safe implementation of the laboratory procedures. The laboratory director also ensures that appropriate physician requisitions are in place for each requested laboratory procedure, in this case gamete cryopreservation. Furthermore, the laboratory director must sign all laboratory reports and records of completion of the laboratory procedure (i.e., gamete cryopreservation and storage).

In summary, management of the cryopreservation laboratory is much the same as management of any clinical laboratory. The only difference may lie in the type of records, the QC/QA methodology, and the type of technical lab procedures employed. All laboratories must undergo certain QC and QA procedures, and these are designed specifically for the type of laboratory, i.e., the specifics for a cryopreservation laboratory would differ from those for an endocrine or microbiology laboratory. Yet, all labs are managed similarly using the principles of QA/QC.

IV. QUALITY ASSURANCE IN THE CRYOPRESERVATION LABORATORY

Quality assurance is test-result and patient-care outcome driven, and, together with quality control, is essential to quality laboratory service.[14] The laboratory's customers reap the benefits of a good QA program. Customers comprise the recipients of the cryopreserved gametes or tissue, the requesting health care professionals, and other laboratories or tissue banks that might receive gametes or tissues from the facility. Regulatory agencies also must be assured that the facility meets minimum standards. The quality assurance program should be constant. It should reach beyond minimum regulatory compliance and strive for excellence. The QA program provides a system of operations monitoring of corrective actions and continuous improvement. This establishes that the cryopreserved gametes/tissue meet quality standards. The QA program assures quality for legal as well as technical requirements, emphasizing the technical prowess of the organization. This system has a "zero tolerance" for defects. It discovers and eliminates defects in the cryobank's operation before they become catastrophic. The quality assurance program should contain both an internal (in-house) evaluation and an external, impartial assessment of the facility. The American Association of Tissue Banks (AATB) requires an external audit of the cryobank to comply with the organization's standards for accreditation.[17] The QA program should include monitoring, inspecting, auditing, scheduling, reporting/record keeping, documenting, evaluating, and advising to facilitate proactive improvements in the laboratory techniques and services.

Monitoring is the direct observation, testing, and assessment of operations and personnel for independent evaluation of regulatory compliance, quality, and integrity. Quality assurance meetings should occur at least quarterly. The laboratory can devise in-house forms for monitoring quality assurance. Sample forms for documentation of QA minutes can be found in Appendix A (see also Chapter 15). Monitoring involves patient test management assessment, that is, review of criteria for patient preparation, specimen collection, chain of custody, labeling, preservation and transportation, and review of test requisitions. Problems should be identified, and means for correcting such problems must be outlined. Actual patient information/charts should be randomly chosen and reviewed. Corrective action and follow-up should be documented. The laboratory director and supervisor ensure that appropriate actions are taken and that policies and procedures are modified as necessary. Auditing within the cryopreservation laboratory is the process of method-ical examination to verify raw and derived or transformed data, protocols, reports, standard operating procedures, personnel records, notes, electronic records, and related documentation for accuracy, integrity, and adequacy for regulatory compli-ance. This is the heart of process validation.

Scheduling is a management tool for controlling the flow of work in the quality assurance unit. Scheduling provides a mechanism for identifying and tracking the status of tasks, functions, and responsibilities. Organizational functions such as managing workload and planning audits/inspections and follow-up are advanced by the use of this tool. Periodically, personnel require training in appropriate scheduling techniques.

Reporting and record keeping are processes for physically capturing, document-ing, and communicating the observations, comments, findings, recommendations, and activities of the QA program (Appendix A). Once the assessment is done, the data are evaluated. Evaluation is the critical assessment of the nature, significance, adequacy, value and/or quality of a person, process, system, or physical entity. Complete documentation of performance is imperative.

Finally, constructive assessment provides management and staff with informed, expert opinion, advice, and/or recommendations on issues pertaining to the results of quality assurance monitoring, inspecting, or auditing of a cryobank. It is also the means by which the technical experts can provide opinion or advice pertaining to scientific, medical, or other technical issues on a regular or *ad hoc* basis.

The basic tenets of a quality assurance program involve a management commit-ment to a culture of quality that is cultivated and maintained for all employees. Quality is an attitude that should permeate the entire facility. Poor quality is a *symptom*, a manifestation of a much more serious and pervasive problem. The problem, not the symptom, should be treated and corrected. Management should be the example of pride in workmanship and accountability for all laboratory staff to emulate. A cryobank's (and any laboratory, for that matter) operations are only as good as its quality assurance program. The quality of a product is only as good as the weakest link in its QA program.

Important aspects of quality assurance include data collection and record main-tenance as well as personnel training and competency evaluation. Training files for laboratory staff should include their resumés, detailed job descriptions including lists of duties, documentation of training in the specific laboratory procedures during the initial training and probation period, continuing education and inservice training, proficiency evaluation, and OSHA training documentation. Annual performance reviews also reside in the personnel files. Quality assurance records include adverse experience reports, error and accident reports, and complaint files. Client feedback is essential to ensure the quality of the facility and should be solicited actively. Comments and complaints should be requested from patients and clients.

Also included in QA analysis for reproductive laboratories, specifically, are pregnancy notifications, notification of congenital anomalies, and adverse outcomes following laboratory procedures. Trend analysis investigation and correction if appropriate should be documented. At a minimum, these files will be requested by regulatory authorities during an inspection. Periodic staff QA meetings provide the forum to discuss problems as they arise. Facilities based in hospitals and medical centers may participate in hospital or departmental QA meetings, such as monthly morbidity and mortality meetings. A medical center department, hospital, or university also may have appointed QA coordinators that a laboratory and cryobank can consult.

Rochester Regional Cryobank and Andrology Laboratory has devised a quality assurance policy and procedure manual for both the andrology section and the cryopreservation section of the laboratory. One aspect of the policy is assurance of specimen integrity (i.e., chain of custody). This includes assurance of appropriate specimen collection and transport to the laboratory, as well as accurate and legible labeling of the specimen container. The policy also includes appropriate safe handling of the specimen by the laboratory staff. Documentation of any unusual occurrences with the specimens must be made on the worksheet and must be presented to the lab director.

Laboratories need accurate test and cryopreservation reports. Such records must be checked for accuracy and must be legible as they become official laboratory documents. An appropriate policy must be in place to correct errors in the report data, such as use of correction fluid, initialing of any changes on the worksheet, etc. A technician must initial or fully sign all worksheets; the laboratory director must sign final reports and records. An additional part of QA is the turn-around time for reports and data to be available for the referring physician and patient medical records. The laboratory should have a policy for the time frame for reporting lab results and cryopreservation results and records. Adherence to such a time policy should be reviewed at the periodic QA meetings and adjustments made according to the laboratory, physician, and client needs.

Assurance of patient confidentiality is also a critical part of the QA program. All patient information, including identifiers, test results, and cryopreservation records are confidential. Test results and cryopreservation records can be released only to the referring physician. Laboratories should confer with their state licensing authority to determine if results can be released by the lab staff to the patient directly. The physician could instruct the laboratory director to provide the lab results (post-thaw semen analysis, number of semen vials, embryo data) directly to the patient. However, in many cases, this results in an awkward position for the laboratory director when the patient's clinical and medical questions cannot be answered (medico-legally) by the lab personnel. Such circumstances have caused labs to change their policies regarding disclosure to patients. Lab personnel refer patients to their physicians to discuss any lab results or data. The laboratory/cryobank should have an appropriate policy in place to report results to the physicians.

The most important aspects of a quality assurance program for a cryopreservation laboratory are quality analysis of thawed specimen vials and resulting outcome of insemination/implantation (i.e., pregnancy rates). For sperm banks, a post-thaw analysis should occur for every specimen frozen. Initially, a sperm count and motility test are done prior to cryopreservation. The semen and cryopreservative mixture is placed into appropriate containers (i.e., vials, ampules, straws) and then frozen in liquid nitrogen according to laboratory procedure. Generally, one vial, containing less volume (usually 0.2 to 0.3 ml) is thawed 24 to 48 hours after initial cryopreservation. Sperm count and motility analyses are performed on this thawed semen. Based upon this analysis, the motile sperm concentration can be extrapolated to the remaining vials from that specimen on that particular date. This same protocol applies to other reproductive cells/tissues, such as epididymal aspirates and testicular biopsy tissue. An additional quality assurance method may include assessment of post-thaw motile count as vials of semen are thawed for processing and insemination. Because a 48-hour post-thaw analysis has been done already, you will have an *expected* motile count for the vial(s) from that date and an *actual* motile count when the vial is thawed for processing and insemination. This data can be collated and assessed to determine the quality of the lab procedures, survival rate, and significant trends.

Laboratories that engage in cryopreservation of embryos, oocytes, and ovarian tissue must institute an appropriate quality assurance protocol for these as well. Since such tissues, especially embryos and oocytes, would not be thawed for testing the efficacy of the procedure, the only way to determine that the procedure has worked is to assess the viability of the cells/tissue (i.e., embryos, oocytes, ovarian tissue) at the time of thaw for transfer or culture, and to QC the reagents/procedure on a mouse system (see below). For example, a laboratory can perform trend analyses, assessing the overall trends in survival of frozen-thawed embryos. Such data and assessment must be documented and accurate records maintained. Review of the data by the laboratory director with appropriate corrective actions must also be documented and maintained within the laboratory. The laboratory staff must be made aware of corrective actions and alterations in policies and procedures as appropriate.

The primary way to ensure quality in a laboratory is through audits and observations. Comprehensive audits in the laboratory should occur at least annually. These audits should be internal—conducted by the laboratory director and/or designee. Laboratory inspection checklists available through accrediting organizations (i.e., state health departments, HCFA, CAP, AATB) can be used for internal audits. Focused audits also can occur throughout the year, focusing on specific areas of the facilities operation, such as the QC protocol, procedure manual, quality assurance records, personnel records, etc. Chain of custody audits should be performed to document appropriate cell/tissue handling, storage, and disbursement. The staff member who is responsible for the specimens at each step in the procedure and for disbursement of specimens must document that he or she followed the appropriate procedures as directed by the procedure manual, policy manual, and medical director or physician authorization. Spot checks by the laboratory director and/or supervisor provide a means of keeping everyone on their toes. The whole purpose of the quality assurance program is to provide feedback to laboratory management so that assessments and corrections occur where needed.

External, independent audits comply with the FDA requirement for drug, biologic, device, and blood product QA and are also required by the AATB.[17] The AATB standards (B2.410) state that an individual familiar with, but not having performed, the specific work being reviewed shall be responsible for each QA review. The external audit, performed yearly, can identify trends and recurring problems. Focused audits help monitor critical areas and identify when problems with quality arise (AATB, K4.000). The audit should focus on the gamete/tissue collection, processing, preservation, packaging, donor and tissue testing, quarantining, labeling, storage, distribution, and records management.

Prayer for the Faithful

The QA Department is my shepherd, whether or not I want. It reviseth my SOP's. It maketh me to write down all actions and leadeth me through standards. Yea, though I walk through the shadow of an inspection, they will find few faults. For QA is with me and my procedures manual comforteth me.

The QA Department hath conducted an independent audit before me in the presence of our staff. It approveth our temperature logs and our record files brimmeth over.

Surely compliance will follow me all the days of my life; and our documentation will dwell in the archives of this tissue bank forever.

> Emmanuel K. Tayo, Ph.D., AATB
> Inspection and Compliance Officer

V. QUALITY CONTROL IN THE CRYOPRESERVATION LABORATORY

The goal of the QC program is to follow written protocols and monitor the quality of the analytical testing process of each method to assure the accuracy, precision, and reliability of test results and reports. QC is test-process oriented, while QA is test-result and patient-care outcome oriented.[13] The frequency of QC checks depends on the instrument/reagent stability, the frequency with which the test is performed, how strongly the method is technique dependent, the frequency of observed QC failure, and the experience and training needed by testing personnel (Basuray, personal communication). Components of a general QC program for all laboratories, including the cryopreservation laboratory, include a written procedures and policies manual, documentation and reporting of results, equipment maintenance, safety procedures, infection control program, staffing requirements, and documentation of suppliers and sources of chemicals and supplies.[13]

What is the difference between QA and QC? QC functions do not have to be independent of QA, and generally they are not. Quality assurance activities must represent the entire process. Quality control seeks to verify the acceptability of each individual product. Quality control activities run concurrently with the laboratory process and may not be conducted retrospectively, while QA activities proceed at all times and can occur retrospective to particular laboratory procedures and outcomes.

A. EQUIPMENT QC

The cryopreservation laboratory, as with any laboratory, must validate laboratory equipment. While some equipment may overlap between labs (general clinical labs, ART labs, cryopreservation labs), some remains unique to the cryopreservation laboratory. The laboratory director must establish a written QC protocol for each piece of equipment, which must include the procedure for QC, the frequency of QC assessment, corrective measures, and records of all QC analyses. The laboratory staff are responsible for routine QC checks that include electronic, mechanical, and operational checks necessary for proper test performance and result reporting. The equipment maintenance program involves unscheduled repairs when needed and scheduled preventive maintenance to prevent breakdown and prolong the life of equipment. It also involves the daily/weekly/monthly/quarterly equipment check that is part of the QC protocol. Table 13.2 demonstrates a regular QC checklist for an ART cryopreservation laboratory (Basuray, personal communication). University and medical center-based laboratories also may have engineering department requirements for annual equipment checks, particularly electrical equipment, electrical outlets, fire extinguishers, etc. Service contracts for other equipment as warranted must also be up-to-date. The laboratory director must document his or her review of the QC data by signature and must document corrective action where necessary. The records of the QC data must remain available to laboratory staff and to inspecting authorities. Usually, a 1 year set of QC data can be kept in a current file then archived after 1 year's time. The QC data should be reviewed at quarterly QA laboratory meetings.

TABLE 13.2
Cryopreservation Laboratory Quality Control Checklist (Selected items)

When	What	How
Day of use	pH meter	Standards pH × 3
	Osmometer	Standards × 3
Daily	Refrigerator/freezer	Temperature
	Liquid nitrogen tanks	Measure liquid levels
	Waterbath; heating block	Temperature
	Room oxygen	Oxygen level
	Room temperature	Temperature
	Lab benches	Disinfect
	Laminar flow hood	Blower gauges; disinfect
	Computer-Assisted Semen Analyzer (CASA)	Standard beads count (note, can also be done weekly/monthly)
Weekly	CASA vs. manual counts	Counting the same specimen
	Stains	
	Centrifuge	Clean
As needed	Cryopreservative (freshly made)	Mouse embryos or donor semen cryosurvival
	Media; buffers; stains (when freshly made)	Sperm survival; mouse embryo survival
Depends on tank use and status	Shipping tanks	Charge; determine if charge maintained
Quarterly or yearly	Staff	Competency
Twice yearly	External proficiency testing	Professional PT service
Monthly	In-house tech comparison	Tech-to-tech comparisons

The laboratory protocol should follow the manufacturer's suggestions for instrument operation and maintenance. Set-up, operation, and maintenance information from the manufacturer should go in a separate file or binder that is accessible to the staff member performing the QC check. Acceptable ranges for temperature controlled spaces and other equipment are indicated on the QC record sheet. Through these records and documentation, instrument stability is monitored. The observation of unusual trends should trigger documented troubleshooting procedures that include consulting with the laboratory director, contacting the company for technical assistance, removing the particular piece of equipment from use for evaluation and repair, and, in the case of a cryopreservation laboratory, possible movement of specimens/reagents/supplies to another storage area. Electrical equipment should be protected from fluctuations and interruptions in electrical currents and should be on emergency power. Back-up materials should be available for essential equipment, such as liquid nitrogen storage tanks. As with all laboratory procedures, documentation is essential.

1. Refrigerators and Freezers

Refrigerator and freezer temperature readings should be recorded daily using a thermometer that is traceable to a National Bureau of Standards (NBS) thermometer. The freezer must not be frost-free, but manual defrost. A frost-free freezer continually cycles in temperature to prevent ice build-up in the freezer compartment. The continuous cycling of temperatures causes partial thawing and refreezing of reagents which could affect the functioning of certain reagents. Temperature ranges must be established and indicated on the QC data form. It is useful to post a monthly, or even yearly, form on the refrigerator and freezer for documentation of temperature checks. Additionally, this method provides trend analysis for the laboratory director and staff doing the periodic checks of the QC data.

2. Centrifuges

Cryopreservation laboratories may use centrifugation to concentrate high volume/low count specimens, prepare IUI-ready sperm prior to freezing, or prepare thawed sperm for IUI. Centrifuges should be checked visually on a daily basis to insure proper operation. Furthermore, the centrifuges should be cleaned and disinfected weekly or monthly, depending upon the laboratory protocol. Most importantly, the centrifuge should be checked using a tachometer at least quarterly to ensure maintenance of appropriate RPMs.

3. Waterbaths and Block-Heaters

Incubators, waterbaths, and block-heaters like refrigerator/freezers should have temperature checks on a daily basis using an NBS traceable thermometer. The temperature should be recorded on the data sheet, and correction of decreasing or increasing temperature trends also should be documented.

4. Osmometer and pH Meter

The laboratory osmometer and pH meter should be checked daily and/or prior to each use. This equipment is used particularly when the laboratory prepares media for sperm processing and cryopreservation. Control solutions are tested prior to test solutions, or once at the beginning of each day to determine accuracy of readings and appropriate function of the equipment.

5. Balance

The laboratory weighing balance should be certified annually through contract with a certifying organization and should be checked monthly with a reference weight.

6. Laminar Flow Biohazard Hood

A cryopreservation laboratory, as well as any laboratory working with potentially biohazardous human materials, should have a biohazard hood under which to perform all specimen manipulations. These hoods must be checked annually by a professional certifying organization, which will check the filters, blowers, gauges, etc. to ensure proper functioning of the unit. On a daily basis, the hood should be cleaned and disinfected after use.

7. Cryopreservation Equipment

Gamete cryopreservation methods may be unique to a particular laboratory's protocol and may involve programmable freezing or manual freezing. For any method, the equipment and storage tanks must be checked to ensure proper functioning. For programmable freezers, the manufacturer's suggested QC method should be followed and should occur daily or weekly. This may include mouse embryo freezing and thawing, or donor semen freezing and thawing to test equipment function. The manual freezing method should also be verified and can be verified concurrent with QC assessment of fresh cryopreservative (see below). The liquid nitrogen storage tanks should be checked periodically (as per protocol) for liquid nitrogen levels if storing in the liquid or for temperature if storing in vapor. Because the maintenance of gametes in a frozen state is critical, and because loss of gametes due to storage tank failure can be devastating, experts recommend that storage tanks be checked daily for liquid level or temperature. The critical levels appear on the top of the data sheet. If the tank is not at the appropriate level or temperature, it should be filled manually until the desired level is reached. This holds true also for automatic fill of liquid nitrogen tanks. If a tank appears to be losing its temperature or liquid nitrogen level at a fast rate, or if condensation or ice appears on the external tank surface, the tank should be checked hourly or half-hourly to determine if the tank is failing. Appropriate remedial action should begin immediately and may involve specimen removal to a back-up tank. One must maintain the specimens in a frozen state without fluctuation in temperature, which could affect the survival of the gametes. Therefore, utmost attention should be paid to the specimens, with efforts to maintain the integrity and cryosurvival of the specimens.

8. Dry Shippers/Transport Units

Cryopreservation laboratories may transport gametes to physicians' offices or other ART laboratories. Special shippers are available such as "dry shippers" that maintain the specimens at liquid nitrogen temperature ($-196°C$). The tanks have an inner core that absorbs liquid nitrogen and can thus maintain the temperature at $-196°C$. Routine checks of the shipper tanks confirm that they maintain temperature, that is, maintenance of liquid nitrogen "charge." Tanks always should be checked for temperature maintenance following prolonged usage or prolonged transport times. Furthermore, all shipping tanks periodically should be removed from service and examined according to the manufacturer's suggested standards. Such tanks must remain continuously "charged," since tanks that are allowed to go dry may malfunction or may need to be charged with liquid nitrogen for a longer period until ready for use. Note also that such dry shipper tanks must remain upright, for, if tipped and maintained on its side, a tank will lose the liquid nitrogen charge very quickly, risking loss by thawing of enclosed specimens.

B. LABORATORY FACILITY

Laboratory work areas should be designed to minimize problems in specimen handling, examination, testing, and reporting requirements (Basuray, personal communication). This includes sufficient work bench space, desk work area, lighting, water, gas, and electrical outlets. Power fluctuations should occur seldom if ever in any laboratory setting. Environmental conditions should be appropriate for the particular laboratory and for the comfort of the lab staff. The ambient temperature and ventilation should be checked. A record sheet documenting the lab ambient temperature should be maintained. Because nitrogen gas can replace oxygen in a room, a cryopreservation laboratory that routinely uses liquid nitrogen vapor and liquid should monitor oxygen levels in the lab daily using a hand-held oxygen meter. All laboratories should have an electrical safety protocol as part of their safety manual. Electrical receptacles should never be overloaded, and each should be checked yearly by the engineering/maintenance department or building supervisor.

C. REAGENT QUALITY CONTROL

The quality of every lot number or batch of chemicals, media, and protein source, whether purchased or manufactured in-house, should be tested with an appropriate quality control system. Purchased reagents of ART laboratories usually are tested at the production site using an applicable system, but spot checks should be conducted in the end user laboratory. For example, embryology laboratories test the quality of reagents and plasticware using the mouse embryo culture system. Reagents such as culture media, cryopreservatives, and buffers used in a cryopreservation laboratory also should be tested for quality and efficacy. One method for quality control testing would use mouse embryo growth, cryopreservation, and cryosurvival. The new test reagent would be tested against an established lot of reagent previously used in the laboratory then tested against an expected survival rate. A sperm bank or andrology laboratory would test reagents and cryopreservatives using a known donor sperm specimen. With new buffers or culture media, a semen specimen can be washed, and incubated in the test solution, with motility checks periodically, perhaps up to 24 hours. The results would be compared to previously used reagents or against established expected performance results for the particular reagent. For freshly prepared cryopreservative, a donor semen specimen would be cryopreserved, then thawed at 24 to 48 hours. The post-thaw motility and count would be determined (i.e., cryosensitivity testing) and compared to previously used cryopreservative as well as previous cryosensitivity testing for that actual donor specimen. If the results of the testing of the new reagents are within the acceptable range, the reagent would be moved into general laboratory use.

Quality control of reagents and chemicals also ensures that the reagents are used prior to expiration. All reagents, chemicals, media, and cryopreservatives are labeled with the date the chemical was received or produced at the lab, the date opened, and the expiration date. The expiration date should be checked before use of each reagent. Storage requirements for each also should appear on the label, and the label should contain the initials of the person preparing the reagent and its label. Furthermore, the reagents, chemicals, and media should be checked visually for contamination at the time of use (noted by the presence of flocculent material or cloudy appearance) and color changes (for example, a pH change). The laboratory director is responsible for the QC program and must be notified of any documented exceptions to these protocols. A QC form for the preparation and testing of the reagents/media is necessary to document that the appropriate protocol was followed. This form must reside in the appropriate QC record book.

Aliquots of chemicals or culture media are not poured back into a bottle once they have been removed. Media should be aliquotted into smaller receptacles for single patient use, thus avoiding potential mix-up of reagents that may have come in to contact with patient specimens (e.g., sperm). All work is conducted in aseptic conditions, preferably under a laminar flow, biohazard hood.

D. Cryopreservation Process Quality Control

Method validation should be conducted for new methods (before their use for actual clinical testing) and for existing methods after major modifications. Tests should be evaluated using patient specimens, such as donor semen specimens or discarded patient semen specimens. In a cryopreservation laboratory, a new method for cryopreservation should be tested concurrently with the former method using the same semen specimens. In an embryology laboratory, a new method for embryo cryopreservation, for example, should be tested in the mouse embryo culture system before testing on human specimens. Mouse 2-cell embryos should be cryopreserved and thawed routinely to examine their survival rate using the current lab methodology. A survival rate of 70% is considered minimally acceptable (Basuray, personal communication). This validates continued performance of the lab method. When a new method has been validated using the mouse embryo system, it should be tested concurrently with the former method by splitting the specimens (i.e., oocytes or embryos) and processed using the two methods in comparison. The results of the validations are compiled and tabulated, then reviewed by the laboratory director who may consult with the clinical/medical director before instituting a new method. With new or modified methods, the laboratory director must ensure that the new method does not adversely affect performance specifications. The decision to initiate a new test or method is based, in part, on the accuracy, specificity, simplicity, availability, and cost of the new method. The old protocol must be removed from the manual, signed, and archived. The new procedure must be dated and signed by the lab director prior to placement in the manual. All lab staff must review the new procedure and verify their review.

E. THE PROCEDURE MANUAL AND QA/QC

The laboratory director must ensure that the procedure manual is available in the laboratory for all testing personnel. It should be easily accessible and understood so that a technologist can refer at any time to a particular procedure if needed. Each procedure should be written in clear and concise terminology using an appropriate format (usually NCCLS guidelines). The procedure manual should include every aspect of the laboratory operation, including but not limited to, specimen collection and rejection, specimen storage temperature, step by step procedures, reporting of results, labeling, normal (expected) values, and remedial action for "out of control" results. At the end of each procedure, as well as at the beginning of the procedure manual, references for the procedures should be listed. These references also should reside in the laboratory. Manufacturer's package inserts, textbooks or operator's manuals may be used in the laboratory, particularly as reference or supporting material, but never as a substitute for written protocols.

The laboratory director and designee should review all procedures yearly. Both (if applicable) should sign and date to document the protocol review. Any changes to a protocol must be reviewed by the entire lab staff. Once a procedure has been changed, the new written and signed protocol is placed in the procedure manual, while the former protocol is kept in an archive file for future reference if needed.

F. EXTERNAL AND INTERNAL QC AND PROFICIENCY TESTING (PT)

Routine (preferably twice yearly) external quality control or proficiency testing should be performed where available. Currently, no PT program exists for cryopreservation. The American Association of Bioanalysts PT program for embryology and andrology laboratories is available for sperm count, motility, viability, antisperm antibody testing, as is media for the mouse embryo culture system. A laboratory can arrange a cross-over PT program with another laboratory where the in-house manufactured cryopreservative can be tested by another laboratory in a sperm and/or mouse embryo cryopreservation survival assay. An internal PT program also can be set up by the laboratory director to assess the technologist staff ability to cryopreserve specimens using "unknown" cryopreservatives. Furthermore, an internal PT program can include all technical staff cryopreserving aliquots of the same specimen and assessment for cryosurvival. The data is then collated and analyzed by the laboratory director and documented in the QC manual. Discussion of the results can take the form of an instructional seminar for all lab staff or an in-service presentation on a particular topic so that staff can brush up on their skills. Periodic internal reviews of technical staff ability are important and routinely checked by inspecting authorities. The lab director should observe each technologist performing the daily laboratory work to determine that the procedure and protocols are followed. Such "competency evaluation" should take place at least yearly and should be documented in the staff member's personnel file.

VI. CONCLUSIONS

Quality control and quality assurance go hand in hand. These are continuous processes that ensure reliability and accuracy of laboratory procedures by competent laboratory staff. The laboratory's customers, the patients and their referring physicians, deserve quality medical laboratory care. A quality control and quality assurance program are mandated by the federal government under CLIA '88, by the College of American Pathologists (CAP) Reproductive Laboratory Accreditation Program (RLAP) program, and by a number of professional organizations and state health departments. The information presented in this chapter is intended to make laboratory personnel aware of the importance of such programs and facilitate a QC/QA program tailored to the needs of the laboratory and its particular size and procedures performed.

ACKNOWLEDGMENTS

The generous assistance of Rita Basuray, Ph.D., H.C.L.D., is gratefully acknowledged. Also, instruction and handouts provided by Emmanuel K. Tayo, Ph.D. of the American Association of Tissue Banks are greatly appreciated and acknowledged.

APPENDIX A

Andrology Laboratory—Rochester Regional Cryobank and Advanced Fertility Diagnostics University of Rochester Medical Center

ANDROLOGY QUALITY ASSURANCE MEETING MINUTES

Meeting Date: _____
Personnel Present: _____
Personnel Absent: _____
I. Old Business
    A. Review of previous quarter's meeting minutes
        1. Follow-up actions taken:

II. New Business
    A. Patient Test Management Assessment
        1. Review of criteria established for patient preparation, specimen collection, labeling, preservation, and transportation
           a. Problems identified:

           b. Corrective actions/follow-up:

        2. Review of information obtained on the laboratory's test requisition based on completeness, relevance, and the necessity for testing of the specimen
           a. ID of the 5 requisitions reviewed:
                1.   4.
                2.   5.
                3.
           b. Problems identified:

           c. Corrective actions/follow-up:

        3. Review of the use and appropriateness of the criteria established for specimen rejection
           a. Problems identified:

           b. Corrective actions/follow-up:

4. Review of test reports for the timely reporting of test results
   a. ID of the 5 test reports reviewed:
      1.   4.
      2.   5.
      3.
   b. Problems identified:

   c. Corrective actions/follow-up:

5. Review of the completeness, usefulness, and accuracy of test report
   information needed for interpretation or utilization of the results
   a. ID of the 5 test reports reviewed:
      1.   4.
      2.   5.
      3.
   b. Problems identified:

   c. Corrective actions/follow-up:

6. Review of the accuracy and reliability of the test reporting system
   a. Appropriate storage of records:

   b. Corrective action/follow-up:

7. Review of chemical expiration date log
   a. Problems identified:

   b. Corrective actions/follow-up:

8. Workload recording review
   a. Number of procedures completed this quarter:
      SA _____   SW _____   Donor cryo _____
      Pt. cryo _____   Donor vials _____
      Vials shipped _____ Antibody tests _____
      Hamster tests _____ Consults _____

   b. Problems identified:

   c. Corrective actions/follow-up:

9. Review of HTM QC records
   a. Problems identified:

   b. Corrective actions/follow-up

10. Review of HTM vs. manual microcell counts
   a. Problems identified:

   b. Corrective actions/follow-up:

11. Quality control deficiency report review
   a. Patient names chosen (5):
     1.   4.
     2.   5.
     3.
   b. Problems identified:

   c. Corrective actions/follow-up:

   d. Retrieval of test results

1. Patient names chosen (5):
  a.   d.
  b.   e.
  c.
2. Problems identified:

3. Corrective actions/follow-up:

B. Quality Control Assessment
   1. Review of equipment maintenance schedules
      a. Problems identified:

      b. Corrective actions/follow-up:

   2. Review of equipment repair logs
      a. Problems identified:

      b. Corrective actions/follow-up:

   3. Review of medium preparation records—HTF, Yolk
      a. Problems identified:

      b. Number of reports reviewed _____
      c. Corrective actions/follow-up:

      d. Revisions made to QC requirements:

   4. Error detection report review
      a. ID of the 5 test reports reviewed:
         1.   4.
         2.   5.
         3.
      b. Problems identified:

      c. Corrective actions/follow-up:

      d. Revisions made to error detection procedures:

C. Review of Inconsistencies Found Between Patient Information and Patient Test Results
   1. ID of the 5 test records reviewed:
      a.   d.
      b.   e.
      c.

2. Inconsistencies identified:

3. Corrective actions/follow-up:

D. Personnel Assessment
   1. Review of employee competence checkouts (performed at least annually for each employee)
      a. Employees evaluated this quarter:

      b. Problems identified:

      c. Corrective actions/follow-up:

      d. Revisions made to employee competence checkouts:

   2. Review of CLIA personnel competency documentation (performed at least annually for each employee)
      a. Employees evaluated this quarter:

      b. Problems identified:

      c. Corrective actions/follow-up:

   3. Review of employee use of personal protective equipment (PPE) documentation (monitored at least annually for each employee)
      a. Employees monitored this quarter:

      b. Problems identified:

      c. Corrective actions/follow-up:

E. Communication Deficiency Report Review
   1. Number of reports reviewed _____
   2. Corrective actions/follow-up:

    F. Complaint Investigation Review
        1. Number of complaints reviewed _____
        2. Corrective actions/follow-up:

    G. Quality Assurance Review with Staff
        1. Problems identified:

        2. Corrective actions/follow-up:

    H. Quality Assurance Policy Review
        1. Revisions made to QA policy:

    I. Other Topics of Interest
        1. Topics discussed:

        2. Follow-up:

Respectfully submitted by: Date:
Reviewed by: Date:

APPENDIX B

Andrology Laboratory—Rochester Regional Cryobank and Advanced Fertility Diagnostics University of Rochester Medical Center

QUALITY ASSURANCE/QUALITY IMPROVEMENT

Name:_____ Date: _____

1. Choose a recurring problem in the laboratory which you would like to improve.
2. List the symptoms that lead you to believe there is a problem.
3. What do you think the causes could be?
4. How would you determine the principle cause? What is it?
5. What changes could you make to solve the problem?
6. How could you verify the problem is solved?

REFERENCES

1. Devroey, P., Silber, S., Nagy, Z., Liu, J., Tournaye, H., Joris, H., Verheyen, G., and Van Steirteghem, A., Ongoing pregnancies and birth after intracytoplasmic sperm injection with frozen-thawed epididymal sperm, *Hum. Reprod.*, 10, 903, 1995.
2. Oates, R. D., Lobel, S. M., Harris, D. H., Pang, S., Burgess, C. M., and Carson, R. S., Efficacy of intracytoplasmic sperm injection using intentionally cryopreserved epididymal spermatozoa, *Hum. Reprod.*, 11, 133, 1996.
3. Craft, I. and Tsirigotis, M., Simplified recovery, preparation and cryopreservation of testicular spermatozoa, *Hum. Reprod.*, 10, 1623, 1995.
4. Romero, J., Remohi, J., Minguez, Y., Rubio, C., Pellicer, A., and Gil-Salom, M., Fertilization after intracytoplasmic sperm injection with cryopreserved testicular spermatozoa, *Fertil. Steril.*, 65, 877, 1996.
5. Society for Assisted Reproductive Technology and the American Society for Reproductive Medicine, Assisted reproductive technology in the United States and Canada: 1994 results generated from the American society for reproductive medicine/society for assisted reproductive technology registry, *Fertil. Steril.*, 66, 697, 1996.
6. Gunasena, K. T. and Critser, J. K., Utility of viable tissues ex vivo: banking of reproductive cells and tissues, in *Reproductive Tissue Banking, Scientific Principles*, Karow, A. M. and Critser, J. K., Academic Press, New York, 1997, ch. 1.
7. Linden, J. and Centola, G. M., New American association of tissue banks standards for semen banking, *Fertil. Steril.*, 68, 1, 1997.
8. The Food and Drug Administration, *A Proposed Approach to the Regulation of Cellular and Tissue-Based Products*, February 28, 1997.
9. Centola, G. M., Update on the use of donor gametes, sperm, and oocytes. Involvement in the FDA regulation of gamete banking—The FDA proposed rule to include reproductive cells and tissues, *ASRM News, The American Society for Reproductive Medicine*, 31, 10, 1997.
10. Code of Federal Regulations, Clinical Laboratory Improvement Amendments of 1988, *Fed. Regist.*, 53, 29590, 1988.
11. Code of Federal Regulations, Clinical Laboratory Improvement Amendments of 1988: Final Rule, *Fed. Regist.*, 57, 7002, 1992.
12. The College of American Pathologists, A summary of the major provisions of the final rules implementing the clinical laboratory improvement amendments of 1988, Northfield, IL, February, 1992.
13. Gerrity, M., Legislative efforts affecting the reproductive biology laboratory, *Curr. Opinions Obstet. Gynecol.*, 3, 623, 1993.
14. Fertility Clinic Success Rate and Certification Act of 1992. *Public Law 102–493*, 102nd Congress, October 24, 1992.
15. Clinton, T., Mandatory ART laboratory regulation: the next step, *ASRM News*, 32(4), 25, 1997.
16. Gerrity, M. Quality control and laboratory monitoring, in *In Vitro Fertilization and Embryo Transfer. A Manual of Basic Techniques*, Wolf, D. P., Bavister, B. D., Gerrity, M., and Kopf, G. S., Plenum Press, New York, 1988, 7–24.
17. American Association of Tissue Banks, *Standards for Tissue Banking*, AATB, McLean, VA, 1998.

14 Clinical Laboratory Improvement Amendments of 1988 (CLIA '88): A Review

Brooks A. Keel

CONTENTS

0-8493-1677-4/00/$0.00+$.50
© 2000 by CRC Press LLC

I. INTRODUCTION

On February 28, 1992, the Secretary of the Department of Health and Human Services (DHHS) published the final rules[1] that implemented CLIA '88. (The word "final" here is somewhat of a misnomer as several modifications of the February 28 rules have since been published.) CLIA '88 is the federal law that sets standards for almost all laboratories in this country. Although individual states and private accrediting agencies may implement clinical laboratory regulations, these rules must be at least as strict as CLIA '88 (they may in fact be more stringent than CLIA '88). CLIA '88 is specific in its definition of what constitutes a "laboratory" (see below). This chapter will provide an overview of the rules and regulations that make up CLIA '88.

II. SUBPART A—GENERAL PROVISIONS

A. DEFINITIONS AND EXCEPTIONS

CLIA defines a laboratory as "a facility for the biological, microbiological, serological, chemical, immunohematological, hematological, biophysical, cytological, pathological, or other examination of materials derived from the human body for the purpose of providing information for the diagnosis, prevention, or treatment of any disease or impairment of, or the assessment of the health of, human beings. These examinations also include procedures to determine, measure, or otherwise describe the presence or absence of various substances or organisms in the body. Facilities only collecting or preparing specimens (or both) or only serving as a mailing service and not performing testing are not considered laboratories." A few exceptions to this definition exist. These rules do not apply to components or functions of (1) any facility that performs testing only for forensic purposes; (2) research laboratories that test human specimens, but do not report patient-specific results; or (3) laboratories certified by the National Institutes on Drug Abuse (NIDA), in which drug testing is performed that meets NIDA guidelines and regulations. However, all other testing conducted by a NIDA-certified laboratory fall under this rule.

B. CATEGORIZATION AND CERTIFICATES

Laboratory tests are categorized as one of the following: (1) waived tests; (2) tests of moderate complexity, including the subcategory of Provider Performed Microscopy (PPM) procedures; or (3) tests of high complexity. Regardless of the type of testing performed, each laboratory must be either CLIA-exempt or possess one of the following CLIA certificates (valid for 2 years):

- Certificate of Registration or Registration Certificate: Required for all labs performing test procedures of moderate complexity (other than the subcategory of PPM procedures) or high complexity, or both. Laboratories performing only waived tests, PPM procedures, or any combination of these tests, are not required to obtain a registration certificate. This is given to the lab initially and applies until the lab has met the requirements for an actual Certificate of Compliance.

- Certificate of Waiver: Required for all labs performing waived tests only
- Certificate for PPM procedures: Required for all labs performing PPM tests only
- Certificate of Compliance: Required for any combination of tests categorized as high or moderate complexity or waived. This is given to labs when they have met the requirements for certification. This replaces the initial Certificate of Registration. With this certificate, your lab most likely will be inspected by your state Health Care Financing Administration (HCFA) inspectors.
- Certificate of Accreditation: Issued in lieu of the applicable certificate specified above provided the laboratory meets the standards of a private, nonprofit accreditation program approved by DHHS [e.g., College of American Pathologists (CAP), Commission on Office Laboratory Accreditation (COLA), etc.]. Really, this is the same as a Certificate of Compliance except your lab will be inspected by the private accrediting agency instead of your state HCFA inspector.

C. CERTIFICATE EXCEPTIONS

All laboratories performing tests of moderate complexity (including the subcategory of PPM) or high complexity, or any combination of these tests, must file a separate application for each laboratory location. Exceptions include the following:

- Laboratories without a fixed location, such as mobile units providing laboratory testing, health screening fairs, or other temporary testing locations, may be covered under the certificate of the designated primary site or home-base, using its address.
- Not-for-profit or federal, state, or local government laboratories that engage in limited (not more than a combination of 15 moderately complex or waived tests per certificate) public health testing may file a single application.
- Laboratories within a hospital that are located in contiguous buildings on the same campus and under common direction may file a single application or multiple applications for the laboratory sites within the same physical location or street address.

D. REPORTING CHANGES IN LABORATORY STATUS

The laboratory must report to DHHS (1) any change(s) in laboratory ownership, name, location, or director and technical supervisor within 30 days of change; (2) no later than 6 months after performing any test or examination within a specialty or subspecialty area that is not included on the laboratory's certificate of compliance; and (3) no later than 6 months after any deletions or changes in test methodologies for any test or examination included in a specialty or subspecialty, or both, for which the laboratory has been issued a certificate of compliance.

E. DEFINITION OF WAIVED TESTS

Waived tests are defined as test systems that have the following characteristics:

- Fully automated or self-contained
- Use only direct, unprocessed specimens
- Require no specimen manipulation before the analytic phase of operation
- Require no operator intervention during the analytic phase
- Provide a direct readout of results; that is, require no calculations or conversions
- Contain fail-safe mechanisms that render no result when the test system malfunctions and initiate fail-safe mechanisms rendering no test result when the result is outside the reportable range
- Require no invasive, test system troubleshooting to be performed by testing personnel and include no electronic or mechanical maintenance to be performed by testing personnel
- Test system instructions that are written at a comprehension level no higher than the seventh grade.

F. PROVIDER PERFORMED MICROSCOPY (PPM) DEFINED

PPM procedures must meet several criteria specifications. The examination must be performed personally by a physician; a midlevel practitioner, under the supervision of a physician or in independent practice only if authorized by the state; or a dentist. These procedures can be performed only during the patient's visit on a specimen obtained from his or her own patient or from a patient of a clinic, group medical practice, or other health care provider of which the practitioner is a member or an employee. The procedure must be categorized as moderately complex, and the primary instrument for performing the test must be a limited bright-field or phase-contrast microscopy. PPM specimens must be labile or delay in performing the test could compromise the accuracy of the test result. Furthermore, in order to be considered a PPM procedure, control materials are not available to monitor the entire testing process, and limited specimen handling or processing is required. Laboratories eligible to perform PPM examinations must meet the applicable requirements of proficiency testing (PT), patient test management, quality control, personnel and quality assurance, and must be subject to inspection.

Provider-performed microscopy (PPM) examinations comprise the following:

- All direct wet mount preparations for the presence or absence of bacteria, fungi, parasites, and human cellular elements
- All potassium hydroxide (KOH) preparations
- Pinworm examinations
- Fern tests
- Post-coital direct, qualitative examinations of vaginal or cervical mucus
- Urine sediment examinations
- Nasal smears for granulocytes
- Fecal leukocyte examinations
- Qualitative semen analysis (limited to the presence or absence of sperm and detection of motility)

III. SUBPART H—PARTICIPATION IN PROFICIENCY TESTING

Each laboratory must enroll in an HCFA-approved PT program. The laboratory must enroll in an approved program or programs for each of the specialties and subspecialties for which it seeks certification. The laboratory must test the samples in the same manner as patients' specimens. If the laboratory fails to participate successfully in proficiency testing for a given specialty, subspecialty, analyte, or test, or fails to take remedial action when an individual fails gynecologic cytology, sanctions will be taken.

A. PARTICIPATION IN PT AND PT SAMPLING

Laboratory personnel who routinely perform testing must test PT samples with the laboratory's regular patient workload using the laboratory's routine methods, and they must test samples the same number of times that they test patient samples. Laboratories cannot engage in any inter-laboratory communications about the results of proficiency testing sample(s) until after the date by which the laboratory must report proficiency testing results. Laboratories with multiple testing sites or separate locations must not communicate proficiency testing sample results across sites/locations until after the date by which the laboratory must report the results. PT samples or portions of samples cannot be sent to another laboratory for any analysis that it is certified to perform in its own laboratory. Any laboratory that HCFA determines intentionally referred its proficiency testing samples to another laboratory for analysis will have its certification revoked for at least 1 year. Any laboratory that receives proficiency testing samples from another laboratory for testing must notify HCFA of the receipt of those samples. The laboratory must document the handling, preparation, processing, examination, and each step in the testing and reporting of results for all proficiency testing samples and must maintain a copy of all records for a minimum of 2 years from the date of the proficiency testing event. PT is required for only the test system, assay, or examination used as the primary method for patient testing during the PT event.

B. SUCCESSFUL PARTICIPATION IN PT

For the following specialities (and subspecialties), satisfactory performance on PT testing is considered 80% correct for each analyte on which you are tested (i.e., you get four out of five right per testing event):

- Microbiology (bacteriology, mycobacteriology, mycology, parasitology, virology)
- Diagnostic immunology (syphilis serology, general immunology)
- Chemistry (routine chemistry, endocrinology, toxicology)
- Hematology (no subspecialties are defined here)

For immunohematology, minimum performance depends upon the subspecialty: ABO grouping and Rho typing, 100% correct; unexpected antibody, 80% correct; compatibility testing, 100% correct; and antibody identification, 80% correct. For the subspecialty of mycobacteriology, the number of samples and frequency of challenge is five samples per testing event and two testing events per year. For all other subspecialties listed above, the number of challenges is three times per year with five samples per testing event.

Failure to return PT results to the PT program within the time frame specified by the program is unsatisfactory performance and results in a score of zero for the testing event. The laboratory must initiate appropriate training and employ the technical assistance necessary to correct problems associated with a PT failure. Remedial action must be taken and documented, and the documentation must remain in the laboratory for 2 years. Failure to achieve an overall testing event score of satisfactory performance for two consecutive testing events or two out of three consecutive testing events is unsuccessful performance.

Under pathology, more strict criteria exist. To participate successfully in a cytology PT program for gynecologic examinations (Pap smears), each individual engaged in the examination of gynecologic preparations must test at least once a year and obtain a passing score. To ensure this annual testing of individuals, an announced or unannounced testing event will be conducted on-site in each laboratory at least once each year. The laboratory must ensure that each individual participates in an annual testing event that involves the examination of 10-slide test set. Individuals who fail this testing event are retested with another 10-slide test set. Individuals who fail this second test are subsequently retested with a 20-slide test set. Individuals receive not more than 45 minutes to complete a 10-slide test and not more than 90 minutes to complete a 20-slide test. An individual's unexcused failure to appear for a retest will result in test failure. An individual is determined to have failed the annual testing event if he or she scores less than 90% on a 10-slide test set. For an individual who fails an annual PT event, the laboratory must schedule a retesting event which must take place within 45 days after receipt of the failure notification. An individual is determined to have failed the second testing event if he or she scores less than 90% on a 10-slide test set. For an individual who fails a second testing event, the laboratory must provide him or her with documented, remedial training and education in the area of failure and must assure that all gynecologic slides evaluated subsequent to the notice of failure are reexamined until the individual is again retested with a 20-slide test set and scores at least 90%. Reexamination of slides must be documented. An individual is determined to have failed the third testing event if he or she scores less than 90% on a 20-slide test set. An individual who fails the third testing event must cease examining gynecologic slide preparations immediately upon notification of test failure and may not resume examining gynecologic slides until the laboratory assures that the individual obtains at least 35 hours of documented, formally structured, continuing education in diagnostic cytopathology that focuses on the examination of gynecologic preparations, and until he or she is retested with a 20-slide test set and scores at least 90%. If a laboratory fails to ensure that individuals are tested or those who fail a testing event are retested, or fails to take required remedial actions, HCFA will initiate intermediate sanctions or limit the laboratory's certificate to exclude gynecologic cytology testing under CLIA, and, if applicable, suspend the laboratory's Medicare and Medicaid payments for gynecologic cytology testing.

IV. SUBPART J—PATIENT TEST MANAGEMENT

Each laboratory performing moderate complexity (including the subcategory of PPM), or high complexity testing, or any combination of these tests, must employ and maintain a system that provides for proper patient preparation; proper specimen collection, identification, preservation, transportation, and processing; and accurate result reporting. This system must assure optimum patient specimen integrity and positive identification throughout the preanalytic (pre-testing), analytic (testing), and postanalytic (post-testing) processes and must meet the standards of this subpart as they apply to the testing performed.

A. SPECIMEN SUBMISSION AND HANDLING

The laboratory must have written policies and procedures for each of the following, if applicable: (1) methods used for the preparation of patients; (2) specimen collection; (3) specimen labeling; (4) specimen preservation; (5) conditions for specimen transportation; and (6) specimen processing. Such policies and procedures must assure positive identification and optimum integrity of the patient specimens from the time the specimens are collected until testing has been completed and the results reported. If the laboratory accepts referral specimens, written instructions must be available to clients and must include, as appropriate, the information specified above. Oral explanation of instructions to patients for specimen collection, including patient preparation, may serve as a supplement to written instructions where applicable.

B. TEST REQUISITION

The laboratory must perform tests only at the written or electronic request of an authorized person. Oral requests for laboratory tests are honored only if the laboratory subsequently requests written authorization for testing within 30 days. The laboratory must maintain the written authorization or documentation of efforts made to obtain a written authorization. Records of test requisitions or test authorizations must be retained for a minimum of 2 years. The patient's chart or medical record, if used as the test requisition, must be retained for a minimum of 2 years and must be available to the laboratory at the time of testing and available to DHHS upon request.

The laboratory must assure that the requisition or test authorization includes: (1) the patient's name or other unique identifier; (2) the name and address of the authorized person requesting the test and, if appropriate, the individual responsible for utilizing the test results or the name and address of the laboratory submitting the specimen, including, as applicable, a contact person to enable the reporting of imminent life-threatening laboratory results or panic values; (3) the test(s) to be performed; and (4) the date of specimen collection. For Pap smears, the patient's last menstrual period, age or date of birth, and indication of whether the patient had a previous abnormal report, treatment, or biopsy also must be included. Any additional information relevant and necessary to a specific test to assure accurate and timely testing and reporting of results must be on the requisition as well.

C. Test Records

The laboratory must maintain a record system for reliable identification of patient specimens as they are processed and tested to assure that accurate test results are reported. Records of patient testing, including, if applicable, instrument printouts, must be retained for at least 2 years. Immunohematology records and transfusion records must be retained for 5 years. Records of blood and blood product testing must be maintained for 5 years after processing records have been completed, or 6 months after the latest expiration date, whichever is the later date. The record system must provide documentation of information specified above and include (1) the patient identification number, accession number, or other unique identification of the specimen; (2) the date and time of specimen receipt into the laboratory; (3) the condition and disposition of specimens that do not meet the laboratory's criteria for specimen acceptability; and (4) the records and dates of all specimen testing, including the identity of the personnel who performed the test(s), which are necessary to assure proper identification and accurate reporting of patient test results.

D. Test Report

The laboratory report must be sent promptly to the authorized person, the individual responsible for using the test results, or the laboratory that initially requested the test. The original report or an exact duplicate of each test report, including final and preliminary report, must remain in the testing laboratory for a period of at least 2 years after the date of reporting. Immunohematology reports and transfusion records must be retained by the laboratory for a period of no less than 5 years. Records of blood and blood product testing must be maintained for a period not less than 5 years after processing records have been completed, or 6 months after the latest expiration date, whichever is the later. For pathology, test reports must be retained for a period of at least 10 years after the date of reporting. This information may be maintained as part of the patient's chart or medical record which must be readily available to the laboratory and to DHHS upon request. The laboratory must have adequate systems in place to report results in a timely, accurate, reliable, and confidential manner and ensure patient confidentiality throughout those parts of the testing process that are under the laboratory's control.

The test report must indicate the name and address of the laboratory location at which the test was performed, the test performed, the test result, and, if applicable, the units of measurement. The laboratory must indicate on the test report any information regarding the condition and disposition of specimens that do not meet the laboratory's criteria for acceptability. Pertinent "reference" or "normal" ranges, as determined by the laboratory performing the tests, must be available to the authorized person who ordered the tests or the individual responsible for utilizing the test results. The results or transcripts of laboratory tests or examinations must be released only to authorized persons or to the individual responsible for utilizing the test results. The laboratory must develop and follow written procedures for reporting imminent life-threatening laboratory results or panic values. In addition, the laboratory must immediately alert the entity requesting the test or the individual responsible for utilizing the test results when any test result indicates an imminent life-threatening condition. The laboratory must, upon request, provide to clients a list of the laboratory's test methods and the performance specifications of each method used to test patient specimens. In addition, information that may affect the interpretation of test results, such as test interferences, must be provided upon request. Pertinent updates on testing information must be provided to clients whenever changes occur that affect the test results or interpretation of test results. The original report or exact duplicates of test reports must be maintained by the laboratory in a manner that permits ready identification and timely accessibility.

E. REFERRAL OF SPECIMENS

A laboratory must refer specimens for testing only to a laboratory possessing a valid certificate authorizing the performance of testing in the specialty or subspecialty of service for the level of complexity in which the referred test is categorized. The referring laboratory must not revise results or information directly related to the interpretation of results provided by the testing laboratory. The referring laboratory may permit each testing laboratory to send the test result directly to the authorized person who initially requested the test. The referring laboratory must retain or be able to produce an exact duplicate of each testing laboratory's report. The authorized person who orders a test or procedure must be notified by the referring laboratory of the name and address of each laboratory location at which a test was performed.

V. SUBPART K—QUALITY CONTROL

The laboratory must establish and follow written quality control procedures for monitoring and evaluating the quality of the analytical testing process of each method to assure the accuracy and reliability of patient test results and reports, unless an alternative procedure specified in the manufacturer's protocol has been cleared by the Food and Drug Administration (FDA) as meeting certain CLIA requirements for quality control or DHHS approves an equivalent procedure.

A. LABORATORY GENERAL REQUIREMENTS

The laboratory must (1) follow the manufacturer's instructions for instrument or test system operation and test performance; (2) have a procedure manual describing the processes for testing and reporting patient test results; (3) perform and document calibration procedures or check calibration at least once every six months; (4) perform and document control procedures using at least two levels of control materials each day of testing; (5) perform and document applicable specialty and subspecialty control procedures; (6) perform and document that remedial action occurred when problems or errors are identified; and (7) maintain records of all quality control activities for 2 years. Quality control records for immunohematology and blood and blood products must be maintained for 5 years.

B. FACILITIES

The laboratory must be constructed, arranged, and maintained to ensure the space, ventilation, and utilities necessary for conducting all phases of testing, including the preanalytic (pre-testing), analytic (testing), and postanalytic (post-testing) phases. Safety precautions must be established, posted, and observed to ensure protection from physical, chemical, biochemical, and electrical hazards, and biohazardous materials.

C. TEST METHODS, EQUIPMENT, INSTRUMENTATION, REAGENTS, MATERIALS, AND SUPPLIES

Test methodologies and equipment must be selected and testing performed in a manner that provides test results within the laboratory's stated performance specifications for each test method. The laboratory must have appropriate and sufficient equipment, instruments, reagents, materials, and supplies for the type and volume of testing performed and for the maintenance of quality during the preanalytic, analytic, and postanalytic phases of testing. The laboratory must define criteria for those conditions that are essential for proper reagent and specimen storage, and accurate and reliable test system operation and test result reporting. These conditions include, if applicable, water quality, temperature, humidity, and protection of equipment and instrumentation from fluctuations and interruptions in electrical current that adversely affect patient test results and test reports. Remedial actions taken to correct conditions that fail to meet the criteria specified above must be documented.

Reagents, solutions, culture media, control materials, calibration materials, and other supplies, as appropriate, must be labeled to indicate (1) identity and, when significant, titer, strength, or concentration; (2) recommended storage requirements; (3) preparation and expiration date; and (4) other pertinent information required for proper use. Reagents, solutions, culture media, control materials, calibration materials, and other supplies must be prepared, stored, and handled to ensure that the reagents are not used when they have exceeded their expiration date, have deteriorated, or are of substandard quality. The laboratory must comply with the FDA product dating requirements for blood products and other biologicals, and labeling requirements for all other *in vitro* diagnostics. Components of reagent kits of different lot numbers cannot be interchanged unless otherwise specified by the manufacturer.

D. PROCEDURE MANUAL

A written procedure manual for the performance of all analytical methods used by the laboratory must be readily available and followed by laboratory personnel. Textbooks may supplement these written descriptions, but may not replace the laboratory's written procedures for testing or examining specimens. The procedure manual must include, when applicable to the test procedure, the following:

- Requirements for specimen collection and processing, and criteria for specimen rejection

- Procedures for microscopic examinations, including the detection of inadequately prepared slides
- Step-by-step performance of the procedure, including test calculations and interpretation of results
- Preparation of slides, solutions, calibrators, controls, reagents, stains, and other materials used in testing
- Calibration and calibration verification procedures
- The reportable range for patient test results as established or verified
- Control procedures
- Remedial action to be taken when calibration or control results fail to meet the laboratory's criteria for acceptability
- Limitations in methodologies, including interfering substances
- Reference range (normal values)
- Imminent life-threatening laboratory results or panic values
- Pertinent literature references
- Appropriate criteria for specimen storage and preservation to ensure specimen integrity until testing is completed
- The laboratory's system for reporting patient results including, when appropriate, the protocol for reporting panic values
- Description of the course of action to be taken in the event that a test system becomes inoperable
- Criteria for the referral of specimens including procedures for specimen submission and handling

Manufacturers' package inserts or operator manuals may be used, when applicable, to meet the requirements of this section. Any of the items of this section not provided by the manufacturer must be provided by the laboratory. The laboratory director must approve, sign, and date procedures. If the directorship of the laboratory changes, procedures must be re-approved, signed, and dated. Each change in a procedure must be approved, signed, and dated by the current director of the laboratory. The laboratory must maintain a copy of each procedure with the dates of initial use and discontinuance. Discontinued procedures should be filed separate from active procedures. These records must be retained for 2 years after a procedure has been discontinued.

E. ESTABLISHMENT AND VERIFICATION OF METHOD PERFORMANCE SPECIFICATIONS

Prior to reporting patient test results, the laboratory must verify or establish, for each method, the performance specifications for the following performance characteristics: (1) accuracy and precision; (2) analytical sensitivity and specificity, if applicable; (3) the reportable range of patient test results; (4) the reference range(s) (normal values); and (5) any other applicable performance characteristic. Laboratories are not required to verify or establish performance specifications for any test method of moderate or high complexity in use prior to September 1, 1992.

Each laboratory that introduces a new procedure for patient testing using a device (instrument, kit, or test system) cleared by the FDA as meeting certain CLIA requirements for quality control, must demonstrate, prior to reporting patient test results, that it can obtain the performance specifications for accuracy, precision, and reportable range of patient test results comparable to those established by the manufacturer. The laboratory must also verify that the manufacturer's reference range is appropriate for the laboratory's patient population. Each laboratory that introduces a new method or device must, prior to reporting patient test results, have documentation of the verification or establishment of all applicable test performance specifications and verify or establish for each method the performance specifications for the following performance characteristics, as applicable: accuracy, precision, analytical sensitivity, analytical specificity to include interfering substances, reportable range of patient test results, reference range(s), and any other performance characteristic required for test performance.

F. EQUIPMENT MAINTENANCE AND FUNCTION CHECKS

The laboratory must perform equipment maintenance and function checks that include electronic, mechanical, and operational checks necessary for the proper test performance and test result reporting of equipment, instruments, and test systems, to assure accurate and reliable test results and reports. The laboratory must perform maintenance as defined by the manufacturer, with at least the frequency specified by the manufacturer, and document all maintenance performed.

G. CALIBRATION AND CALIBRATION VERIFICATION

Calibration and calibration verification procedures substantiate the continued accuracy of the test method throughout the laboratory's reportable range for patient test results. *Calibration* is the process of testing and adjusting an instrument, kit, or test system to provide a known relationship between the measurement response and the value of the substance that is being measured by the test procedure. *Calibration verification* is the assaying of calibration materials in the same manner as patient samples to confirm that the calibration of the instrument, kit, or test system has remained stable throughout the laboratory's reportable range for patient test results. The *reportable range of patient test results* is the range of test result values over which the laboratory can establish or verify the accuracy of the instrument, kit, or test system measurement response.

For laboratory test procedures that are performed using instruments, kits, or test systems that have been cleared by the FDA as meeting certain CLIA requirements for quality control, the laboratory must, at a minimum, follow the manufacturer's instructions for calibration and calibration verification procedures using calibration materials specified by the manufacturer. To verify the laboratory's established reportable range of patient test results, the lab must include at least a minimal (or zero) value, a mid-point value, and a maximum value at the upper limit of that range.

The laboratory must perform calibration verification procedures at least once every 6 months and whenever any of the following occur: (1) a complete change of reagents for a procedure is introduced, unless the laboratory can demonstrate that changing reagent lot numbers does not affect the range used to report patient test results or control values. (Note: If all of the reagents for a test are packaged together, the laboratory is not required to perform calibration verification for each package of reagents, provided the packages of reagents arrived in the same shipment and contain the same lot number.); (2) major preventive maintenance or replacement of critical parts occurs that may influence test performance; (3) controls reflect an unusual trend or shift or are outside of the laboratory's acceptable limits and other means of assessing and correcting unacceptable control values have failed to identify and correct the problem; or (4) the laboratory's established schedule for verifying the reportable range for patient test results requires more frequent calibration verification.

H. CONTROL PROCEDURES

Control procedures are performed on a routine basis to monitor the stability of the method or test system. Control and calibration materials provide a means to indirectly assess the accuracy and precision of patient test results. The laboratory must, at a minimum, follow the manufacturer's instructions for control procedures. The laboratory must evaluate instrument and reagent stability and operator variance in determining the number, type, and frequency of testing calibration or control materials and establish criteria for acceptability used to monitor test performance during a run of patient specimen(s). A run is an interval within which the accuracy and precision of a testing system is expected to be stable, but cannot be greater than 24 hours or less than the frequency recommended by the manufacturer. For each procedure, the laboratory must monitor test performance using calibration materials or control materials or a combination thereof.

For qualitative tests, the laboratory must include a positive and negative control with each run of patient specimens. For quantitative tests, the laboratory must include at least two samples of different concentrations of either calibration materials, control materials, or a combination thereof with the frequency of not less than once each run of patient specimens. For electrophoretic determinations, at least one control sample must be used in each electrophoretic cell, and the control sample must contain fractions representative of those routinely reported in patient specimens.

Each day of use, the laboratory must evaluate the detection phase of direct antigen systems using an appropriate positive and negative control material (organism or antigen extract). When direct antigen systems include an extraction phase, the system must be checked each day of use using a positive organism. If calibration materials and control materials are not available, the laboratory must have an alternative mechanism to assure the validity of patient test results.

Control samples must be tested in the same manner as patient specimens. When calibration or control materials are used, statistical parameters (e.g., mean and standard deviation) for each lot number of calibration material and each lot of control material must be determined through repetitive testing. The stated values of an assayed control material may be used as the target values provided the stated values correspond to the methodology and instrumentation employed by the laboratory and are verified by the laboratory. The laboratory must establish statistical parameters for unassayed materials over time through concurrent testing with calibration materials or control materials with previously determined statistical parameters. Control results must meet the laboratory's criteria for acceptability prior to reporting patient test results.

The laboratory must check each batch or shipment of reagents, discs, stains, antisera, and identification systems (systems using two or more substrates) when prepared or opened for positive and negative reactivity, as well as graded reactivity if applicable. Each day of use, the laboratory must test staining materials for intended reactivity to ensure predictable staining characteristics. The laboratory must check fluorescent stains for positive and negative reactivity each time of use.

The laboratory must check each batch or shipment of media for sterility if it is intended to be sterile and sterility is required for testing. Media must also be checked for its ability to support growth, and as appropriate, selectivity/inhibition and/or biochemical response. The laboratory may use manufacturer's media control checks provided the manufacturer's product insert specifies that their quality control checks meet the National Committee for Clinical Laboratory Standards (NCCLS) for media quality control. The laboratory must document that the physical characteristics of the media are not compromised and report any deterioration in the media to the manufacturer. The laboratory must follow the manufacturer's specifications for using the media and must be responsible for the test results. CLIA '88 indicates that a batch of media (solid, semi-solid, or liquid) consists of all tubes, plates, or containers of the same medium prepared at the same time and in the same laboratory; or, if received from an outside source or commercial supplier, consists of all of the plates, tubes, or containers of the same medium that have the same lot numbers and are received in a single shipment.

I. REMEDIAL ACTION

Remedial action policies and procedures must be established by the laboratory and applied as necessary to maintain the laboratory's operation for testing patient specimens in a manner that assures accurate and reliable patient test results and reports. The laboratory must document all remedial actions taken when test systems do not meet the laboratory's established performance specifications. Such instances include, but are not limited to, equipment or methodologies that perform outside of established operating parameters or performance specifications, patient test values that are outside of the laboratory's reportable range of patient test results, or the determination that the laboratory's reference range for a test procedure is inappropriate for the laboratory's patient population. Remedial action also must be documented when results of control and calibration materials fail to meet the laboratory's established criteria for acceptability. All patient test results obtained in the unacceptable test run or since the last acceptable test run must be evaluated to determine if patient test results have been adversely affected, and the laboratory must take the remedial action necessary to ensure the reporting of accurate and reliable patient test results. If the laboratory cannot report patient test results within its established time frames, remedial action must be documented. The laboratory must determine, based on the urgency of the patient test(s) requested, the need to notify the appropriate individual of the delayed testing.

Remedial action also must occur when errors in the reported patient test results are detected. The laboratory must promptly notify the authorized person ordering or individual utilizing the test results of reporting errors and must issue corrected reports promptly. The laboratory must maintain exact duplicates of the original report as well as the corrected report for 2 years.

J. QUALITY CONTROL RECORDS

The laboratory must document and maintain records of all quality control activities specified above and retain records for at least 2 years. Immunohematology quality control records must be maintained for a period of no less than 5 years. In addition, quality control records for blood and blood products must be maintained for a period not less than 5 years after processing records have been completed, or 6 months after the latest expiration date, whichever is the later date.

VI. SUBPART M—PERSONNEL, PPM

A. PPM PERSONNEL AND QUALIFICATIONS

Laboratories performing PPM testing procedures are required to have a qualified director and testing personnel. The director must possess a state license as a laboratory director if the licensing is required, and be a physician, a state-authorized midlevel practitioner, or a dentist. In order to qualify as testing personnel, the individual must possess a state license if the licensing is required and be a physician, a state-authorized midlevel practitioner under the supervision of a physician or in independent practice if authorized by the state, or a dentist.

B. PPM DIRECTOR RESPONSIBILITIES

The laboratory director is responsible for the overall operation and administration of the laboratory, including the prompt, accurate, and proficient reporting of test results. The laboratory director must direct no more than five laboratories and must ensure that any PPM procedure is performed by a qualified individual in accordance with applicable requirements.

C. PPM TESTING PERSONNEL RESPONSIBILITIES

The testing personnel are responsible for specimen processing, test performance, and test results reporting. Any PPM procedure must be (1) personally performed by a physician, a supervised midlevel practiontioner or a dentist; (2) performed during the patient's visit on a specimen obtained from his or her own patient or from the patient of a clinic, group medical practice, or other health care provider, in which the physician, midlevel practitioner, or dentist is a member or an employee; and (3) performed using a bright-field or a phrase-contrast microscope.

VII. SUBPART M—PERSONNEL, MODERATE COMPLEXITY

A. MODERATE COMPLEXITY PERSONNEL REQUIRED

Laboratories performing moderate complexity testing procedures are required to have a qualified director, technical consultant, clinical consultant, and testing personnel. One or more individuals, if qualified, can assume multiple positions in the laboratory.

B. MODERATE COMPLEXITY DIRECTOR QUALIFICATIONS

In order to meet the CLIA '88 qualifications for directing moderate complexity testing, an individual must meet one of the following five requirements:

1. Licensed and board certified pathologists; or
2. Licensed physician and have
   - 1-year-experience directing or supervising nonwaived tests, or
   - 20 continuing education units (CEUs) in laboratory practice, or
   - Clinical laboratory training during residency; or
3. Hold an earned doctoral degree in a chemical, physical, biological, or clinical laboratory science from an accredited institution; and
   - Be certified by the American Board of Medical Microbiology, the American Board of Clinical Chemistry, the American Board of Bio-analysis, or the American Board of Medical Laboratory Immunology; or
   - Have had at least 1 year experience directing or supervising nonwaived laboratory testing; or
4. Have earned a master's degree in a chemical, physical, biological, or clinical laboratory science or medical technology from an accredited institution; and
   - Have at least 1 year of laboratory training or experience, or both in nonwaived testing; and
   - In addition, have at least 1 year of supervisory laboratory experience in nonwaived testing; or
5. Have earned a bachelor's degree in a chemical, physical, or biological science or medical technology from an accredited institution; and
   - Have at least 2 years of laboratory training or experience, or both in nonwaived testing; and
   - In addition, have at least 2 years of supervisory laboratory experience in nonwaived testing.

C. MODERATE COMPLEXITY DIRECTOR RESPONSIBILITIES

The laboratory director is responsible for the overall operation and administration of the laboratory, including the employment of personnel who are competent to perform test procedures, and record and report test results promptly, accurately, and proficiently. The laboratory director also assures compliance with the applicable regulations. The laboratory director, if qualified, may perform the duties of the technical consultant, clinical consultant, and testing personnel, or delegate these responsibilities to personnel meeting the qualifications of these positions. If the laboratory director reapportions performance of his or her responsibilities, he or she remains responsible for ensuring that all duties are properly performed. The laboratory director must be accessible to the laboratory to provide on-site, telephone, or electronic consultation as needed. Each individual may direct no more than five laboratories.

The director of moderate complexity testing has many responsibilities. The director must perform the following:

- Ensure that testing systems developed for each of the tests performed in the laboratory provide quality laboratory services for all aspects of test performance, which includes the preanalytic, analytic, and postanalytic phases of testing
- Ensure that the physical plant and environmental conditions of the laboratory are appropriate for the testing performed and provide a safe environment in which employees are protected from physical, chemical, and biological hazards
- Ensure that the test methodologies selected have the capability of providing the quality of results required for patient care, that verification procedures used are adequate to determine the accuracy, precision, and other pertinent performance characteristics of the method, and that laboratory personnel are performing the test methods as required for accurate and reliable results
- Ensure that the laboratory is enrolled in a DHHS-approved proficiency testing program for the testing performed and that (1) the proficiency testing samples are tested as required under subpart H of this part; (2) the results are returned within the time frames established by the proficiency testing program; (3) all proficiency testing reports received are reviewed by the appropriate staff to evaluate the laboratory's performance and to identify any problems that require corrective action; and (4) an approved corrective action plan is followed when any proficiency testing results are deemed unacceptable or unsatisfactory
- Ensure that the quality control and quality assurance programs are established and maintained and to identify failures in quality as they occur
- Ensure the establishment and maintenance of acceptable levels of analytical performance for each test system
- Ensure that all necessary remedial actions are taken and documented whenever significant deviations from the laboratory's established performance specifications occur and that patient test results are reported only when the system functions properly
- Ensure that reports of test results include pertinent information required for interpretation
- Ensure that consultation is available to the laboratory's clients on matters relating to the quality of the test results reported and their interpretation concerning specific patient conditions

- Employ a sufficient number of laboratory personnel with the appropriate education and experience or training to consult, to supervise and perform tests accurately, and to report test results in accordance with the personnel responsibilities described in this subpart
- Ensure that prior to testing patients' specimens, all personnel hold appropriate education and experience, receive the appropriate training for the type and complexity of the services offered, and demonstrate that they can perform all testing operations reliably to provide and report accurate results
- Ensure that policies and procedures are established for monitoring individuals who conduct preanalytical, analytical, and postanalytical phases of testing to assure that they are competent and maintain their competency to process specimens, perform test procedures, and report test results promptly and proficiently, and whenever necessary, identify needs for remedial training or continuing education to improve skills
- Ensure that an approved procedure manual is available to all personnel responsible for any aspect of the testing process
- Specify, in writing, the responsibilities and duties of each consultant and each person engaged in the performance of the preanalytic, analytic, and postanalytic phases of testing and identify which examinations and procedures each individual is authorized to perform, whether supervision is required for specimen processing, test performance, or results reporting, and whether consultant or director review is required prior to reporting patient test results

D. MODERATE COMPLEXITY TECHNICAL CONSULTANT QUALIFICATIONS

The laboratory must employ one or more individuals who are qualified by education and training or experience to provide technical consultation for each of the specialties and subspecialties of service in which the laboratory performs moderate complexity tests or procedures. The director of a laboratory performing moderate complexity testing may function as the technical consultant provided he or she meets the qualifications specified in this section. The technical consultant must possess a state license if required. The technical consultant must be:

- Licensed and board-certified pathologist; or
- Licensed physician or hold an earned doctoral or master's degree in a chemical, physical, biological, or clinical laboratory science or medical technology from an accredited institution and have at least 1 year of laboratory training or experience, or both, in nonwaived testing, in the designated specialty or subspecialty areas of service for which the technical consultant is responsible; or
- Recipient of a bachelor's degree in a chemical, physical, or biological science or medical technology from an accredited institution; and have at least 2 years of laboratory training or experience, or both in nonwaived testing, in the designated specialty or subspecialty areas of service for which the technical consultant is responsible.

The technical consultant requirements for "laboratory training or experience, or both" in each specialty or subspecialty may be acquired concurrently in more than one of the specialties or subspecialties of service, excluding waived tests. For example, an individual who has a bachelor's degree in biology and 2 years of documented work experience performing tests of moderate complexity in all specialties and subspecialties of service would be qualified as a technical consultant in a laboratory performing moderate complexity testing in all specialties and subspecialties of service.

E. MODERATE COMPLEXITY TECHNICAL CONSULTANT RESPONSIBILITIES

The technical consultant must be accessible to the laboratory to provide on-site, telephone, or electronic consultation. The technical consultant has the following responsibilities:

- Selecting test methodology appropriate for the clinical use of the test results
- Verifying the test procedures performed and establishing the laboratory's test performance characteristics, including the precision and accuracy of each test and test system
- Enrolling and participating in a DHHS approved PT program commensurate with the services offered
- Establishing a quality control program appropriate for the testing performed; establishing the parameters for acceptable levels of analytic performance; ensuring that these levels are maintained throughout the entire testing process from the initial receipt of the specimen through sample analysis and reporting of test results
- Resolving technical problems and ensuring that remedial actions ensue whenever test systems deviate from the laboratory's established performance specifications
- Ensuring that patient test results are not reported until all corrective actions have been taken and the test system is functioning properly
- Identifying training needs and assuring that each individual performing tests receives regular in-service training and education appropriate for the type and complexity of the laboratory services performed
- Evaluating the competency of all testing personnel and assuring that the staff maintain their competency to perform test procedures and report test results promptly, accurately, and proficiently. The procedures for evaluation of the competency of the staff must include, but are not limited to (1) direct observations of routine patient test performance, including patient preparation, if applicable, specimen handling, processing, and testing; (2) monitoring the recording and reporting of test results; (3) review of intermediate test results or worksheets, quality control records, proficiency testing results, and preventive maintenance records; (4) direct observation of instrument maintenance and function checks;

(5) assessment of test performance through testing previously analyzed specimens, internal blind testing samples, or external proficiency testing samples; and (6) assessment of problem solving skills

- Evaluating and documenting the performance of individuals responsible for moderate complexity testing at least semiannually during the first year the individual tests patient specimens. Thereafter, evaluations must occur at least annually unless test methodology or instrumentation changes, in which case, prior to reporting patient test results, the individual's performance must be reevaluated to include the use of the new test methodology or instrumentation

F. MODERATE COMPLEXITY CLINICAL CONSULTANT QUALIFICATIONS AND RESPONSIBILITIES

The moderate complexity clinical consultant must be either a qualified laboratory director or a licensed physician. The clinical consultant must (1) be available to provide clinical consultation to the laboratory's clients and to assist the laboratory's clients in ensuring that appropriate tests are ordered to meet the clinical expectations; (2) ensure that reports of test results include pertinent information required for specific patient interpretation; and (3) ensure that consultation is available and communicated to the laboratory's clients on matters related to the quality of the test results reported and their interpretation concerning specific patient conditions.

G. MODERATE COMPLEXITY TESTING PERSONNEL QUALIFICATIONS

In order to qualify for moderate complexity testing, an individual must possess a state license, if required, and meet one of the following four requirements:

1. Be a licensed physician or have earned a doctoral, master's, or bachelor's degree in a chemical, physical, biological, or clinical laboratory science or medical technology from an accredited institution; or
2. Have earned an associate's degree in a chemical, physical, or biological science or medical technology from an accredited institution; or
3. Be a high school graduate or equivalent and have successfully completed an official military medical laboratory procedures course of at least 50 weeks duration and have held the military enlisted occupational specialty of medical laboratory specialist (laboratory technician); or
4. Have earned an high school diploma or equivalent and have documentation of training appropriate for the testing performed prior to analyzing patient specimens. Such training must ensure that the individual has (1) the skills required for proper specimen collection, including patient preparation, if applicable, labeling, handling, preservation or fixation, processing or preparation, transportation and storage of specimens; (2) the skills required for implementing all standard laboratory procedures; (3) the skills required for performing each test method and for proper instrument use; (4) the skills required for performing preventive maintenance, troubleshooting,

and calibration procedures related to each test performed; (5) a working knowledge of reagent stability and storage; (6) the skills required to implement the quality control policies and procedures of the laboratory; (7) an awareness of the factors that influence test results; and (8) the skills required to assess and verify the validity of patient test results through the evaluation of quality control sample values prior to reporting patient test results.

H. MODERATE COMPLEXITY TESTING PERSONNEL RESPONSIBILITIES

Testing personnel in the moderate complexity laboratory are responsible for (1) following the laboratory's procedures for specimen handling and processing, test analyses, and records reporting and maintenance; (2) maintaining records that demonstrate that PT samples are tested in the same manner as patient samples; (3) adhering to the laboratory's quality control policies, documenting all quality control activities, instrument and procedural calibrations, and maintenance performed; (4) following the laboratory's established corrective action policies and procedures whenever test systems fall outside the laboratory's established acceptable levels of performance; (5) identifying problems that may adversely affect test performance or test results and either correcting the problems or immediately notifying the technical consultant, clinical consultant, or director; and (6) documenting all corrective actions taken when test systems deviate from the laboratory's established performance specifications.

VIII. SUBPART M—PERSONNEL, HIGH COMPLEXITY

A. PERSONNEL REQUIRED

Laboratories performing high complexity testing procedures are required to have a qualified director, clinical consultant, technical consultant, general supervisor, and testing personnel. One or more individuals, if qualified, can assume multiple positions in the laboratory.

B. HIGH COMPLEXITY DIRECTOR QUALIFICATIONS

In order to direct a high complexity laboratory, an individual must be a

- Licensed and board-certified pathologist; or
- Doctor of medicine, doctor of osteopathy, or doctor of podiatric medicine licensed to practice medicine, osteopathy, or podiatry in the state in which the laboratory is located, and have at least 1 year of laboratory training during medical residency or at least 2 years of experience directing or supervising high complexity testing; or
- Recipient of a doctoral degree in a chemical, physical, biological, or clinical laboratory science from an accredited institution and certified by the American Board of Medical Microbiology, the American Board of Clinical Chemistry, the American Board of Bioanalysis, the American

Board of Medical Laboratory Immunology, or other board deemed comparable by DHHS; or (until December 31, 2000) have at least 2 years of clinical laboratory training or experience and at least 2 years directing or supervising high complexity testing (i.e., 4 years total clinical laboratory experience) and (after December 31, 2000) be board certified; or

- Laboratory director who previously qualified or could have qualified as a laboratory director under regulations at 42 CFR 493.1415, published March 14, 1990 at 55 FR 9538, on or before February 28, 1992; or
- On or before February 28, 1992, an individual qualified under state law to direct a laboratory in the state; or
- For the subspecialty of oral pathology, an individual certified by the American Board of Oral Pathology, American Board of Pathology, the American Osteopathic Board of Pathology, or possessing qualifications that are equivalent to those required for certification.

C. High Complexity Director Responsibilities

The laboratory director, if qualified, may perform the duties of the technical supervisor, clinical consultant, general supervisor, and testing personnel, or delegate these responsibilities to personnel meeting the qualifications. If the laboratory director reapportions performance of his or her responsibilities, he or she remains responsible for ensuring that all duties are properly performed. The laboratory director must be accessible to the laboratory to provide on-site, telephone, or electronic consultation as needed. Each individual may direct no more than five laboratories.

The laboratory director has a number of responsibilities. The director must perform the following:

- Ensure that testing systems provide quality laboratory services for all aspects of test performance
- Ensure that the facilities are safe
- Ensure that test methodologies are verified as being accurate and precise
- Ensure that the laboratory enrolls in and appropriately performs approved proficiency testing
- Ensure that quality control and assurance programs are established and followed
- Ensure that acceptable analytical performance parameters are established and maintained
- Ensure that remedial action is taken and documented when testing performance characteristics deviate from normal
- Ensure that test result reports include pertinent information required for clinical interpretation
- Ensure that clinical consultation is available for quality of test reports and clinical interpretation
- Ensure that a sufficient number of appropriately trained personnel are employed

- Ensure that all personnel have demonstrated proficiency in testing before reporting results
- Ensure that all personnel maintain their competency and identify remedial training needs
- Ensure that an approved procedure manual is available to all testing personnel
- Ensure that the authorization, responsibilities, and duties of all personnel are specified in writing

D. High Complexity Technical Supervisor Qualifications

In order for an individual to qualify as a technical supervisor of high complexity testing the individual must be a

1. Licensed and board-certified pathologist; or
2. Licensed physician or hold an earned doctoral degree in a chemical, physical, biological, or clinical laboratory science or medical technology from an accredited institution and have 1 year clinical laboratory training or experience, or both, in high complexity testing within the speciality; or
3. Recipient of a master's degree in a chemical, physical, biological, or clinical laboratory science or medical technology from an accredited institution and have 2 years clinical laboratory training or experience, or both, in high complexity testing within the speciality; or
4. Recipient of a bachelor's degree in a chemical, physical, biological, or clinical laboratory science or medical technology from an accredited institution and 4 years clinical laboratory training or experience, or both, in high complexity testing within the speciality.

In addition, the individual also must have 6 months of experience in high complexity testing within the subspecialty. This 6-month-experience within the subspecialty is not required for the specialities of chemistry, diagnostic immunology, and hematology. The specialties and subspecialties of cytology, histopathology, oral pathology, histocompatibility, clinical cytogenetics, and immunohematology have stricter qualifications for technical supervisor.

E. High Complexity Technical Supervisor Responsibilities

The technical supervisor must be accessible to the laboratory to provide on-site, telephone, or electronic consultation. The technical supervisor is responsible for

- Selecting the test methodology that is appropriate for the clinical use of the test results;
- Verifying the test procedures performed and establishing the laboratory's test performance characteristics, including the precision and accuracy of each test and test system;

- Enrolling and participating in a DHHS-approved PT program commensurate with the services offered;
- Establishing a quality control program appropriate for the testing performed; establishing the parameters for acceptable levels of analytic performance; ensuring that these levels are maintained throughout the entire testing process from the initial receipt of the specimen through sample analysis and reporting of test results;
- Resolving technical problems and ensuring that remedial actions ensue whenever test systems deviate from the laboratory's established performance specifications;
- Ensuring that patient test results are not reported until all corrective actions have been taken and the test system is functioning properly;
- Identifying training needs and assuring that each individual performing tests receives regular in-service training and education appropriate for the type and complexity of the laboratory services performed;
- Evaluating the competency of all testing personnel and assuring that the staff maintain their competency to perform test procedures and report test results promptly, accurately, and proficiently. The procedures for staff evaluation must include, but are not limited to (1) direct observations of routine patient test performance, including patient preparation, specimen handling, processing, and testing; (2) monitoring the recording and reporting of test results; (3) review of intermediate test results or worksheets, quality control records, proficiency testing results, and preventive maintenance records; (4) direct observation of instrument maintenance and function checks; (5) assessment of test performance through testing previously analyzed specimens, internal blind testing samples, or external proficiency testing samples; and (6) assessment of problem solving skills
- Evaluating and documenting the performance of individuals responsible for high complexity testing at least semiannually during the first year the individual tests patient specimens. Thereafter, evaluations must occur at least annually unless test methodology or instrumentation changes, in which case, prior to reporting patient test results, the individual's performance must be reevaluated to include the use of the new test methodology or instrumentation

In cytology, the technical supervisor or the qualified individual (1) may perform the duties of the cytology general supervisor and the cytotechnologist; (2) must establish the workload limit for each individual examining slides; (3) must reassess the workload limit for each individual examining slides at least every 6 months and adjust as necessary; (4) must perform the functions specified above; (5) must ensure that each individual examining gynecologic preparations participates in a DHHS-approved cytology proficiency testing program and achieves a passing score; and (6) if responsible for screening cytology slide preparations, must document the number of cytology slides screened in 24 hours and the number of hours devoted during each 24-hour period to screening cytology slides.

F. HIGH COMPLEXITY CLINICAL CONSULTANT QUALIFICATIONS AND RESPONSIBILITIES

The clinical consultant in the high complexity laboratory must be qualified either as a laboratory director or a licensed physician. The clinical consultant must (1) be available to provide consultation to the laboratory's clients; (2) be available to assist the laboratory's clients in ensuring that appropriate tests are ordered to meet the clinical expectations; (3) ensure that reports of test results include pertinent information required for specific patient interpretation; and (4) ensure that consultation is available and communicated to the laboratory's clients on matters related to the quality of the test results reported and their interpretation concerning specific patient conditions.

G. HIGH COMPLEXITY GENERAL SUPERVISOR QUALIFICATIONS AND RESPONSIBILITIES

In order to qualify as a general supervisor of a high complexity laboratory, the individual must (1) possess a state license, if required, and qualify as a high complexity director or technical supervisor as defined above; or (2) be a licensed physician or have earned a doctoral, master's, or bachelor's degree in a chemical, physical, biological, or clinical laboratory science or medical technology from an accredited institution and have at least 1 year of laboratory training or experience, or both, in high complexity testing.

The responsibilities of the general supervisor include the following:

*   Must be accessible to testing personnel at all times testing is performed to provide on-site, telephone, or electronic consultation to resolve technical problems in accordance with policies and procedures established either by the laboratory director or technical supervisor
*   Is responsible for providing day-to-day supervision of high complexity test performance by testing qualified personnel
*   Is responsible for monitoring test analyses and specimen examinations to ensure that acceptable levels of analytic performance are maintained
*   The director or technical supervisor may delegate to the general supervisor the responsibility for (1) assuring that all remedial actions occur whenever test systems deviate from the laboratory's established performance specifications; (2) ensuring that patient test results are not reported until all corrective actions have been taken and the test system is properly functioning; (3) providing orientation to all testing personnel; and (4) annually evaluating and documenting the performance of all testing personnel

H. HIGH COMPLEXITY TESTING PERSONNEL QUALIFICATIONS

In order to meet the CLIA '88 qualifications for performing testing in a high complexity laboratory, an individual must meet one of the following five requirements:

1. Be a licensed physician or have earned a doctoral, master's, or bachelor's degree in a chemical, physical, biological, or clinical laboratory science or medical technology from an accredited institution; or
2. Have earned an associates degree in lab science or medical technology or equivalent education and training; or
3. On or before April 24, 1995, be a high school graduate and have specific clinical laboratory training; or
4. Until September 1, 1997, have a high school diploma and have specific clinical laboratory experience; or
5. After September 1, 1997, obtain an associate's degree.

I. HIGH COMPLEXITY TESTING PERSONNEL RESPONSIBILITIES

Testing personnel in the high complexity laboratory are responsible for

- Following the laboratory's procedures for handling and processing specimens, analyzing tests, and reporting and maintaining records of patient test results
- Maintaining records that demonstrate that PT samples are tested in the same manner as patient specimens
- Adhering to the laboratory's quality control policies, documenting all quality control activities, instrument and procedural calibrations, and maintenance performed
- Following the laboratory's established policies and procedures whenever test systems fall outside the laboratory's established acceptable levels of performance
- Identifying problems that may adversely affect test performance or test results and either correcting the problems or immediately notifying the general supervisor, technical supervisor, clinical consultant, or director
- Documenting all corrective actions taken when test systems deviate from the laboratory's established performance specifications
- Performing high complexity testing only under the on-site, direct supervision of a qualified general supervisor. *Exception*: For individuals who were performing high complexity testing on or before January 19, 1993, the requirements of this section do not apply, provided that all high complexity testing performed by the individual in the absence of a general supervisor is reviewed within 24 hours by a general supervisor

IX. SUBPART P—QUALITY ASSURANCE

Each laboratory performing moderate complexity (including the PPM subcategory) or high complexity testing, or any combination of these tests, must establish and follow written policies and procedures for a comprehensive quality assurance (QA) program that is designed to monitor and evaluate the ongoing and overall quality of the total testing process (preanalytic, analytic, postanalytic). The laboratory's quality assurance program must evaluate the effectiveness of its policies and procedures;

identify and correct problems; assure the accurate, reliable, and prompt reporting of test results; and assure the adequacy and competency of the staff. As necessary, the laboratory must revise policies and procedures based upon the results of those evaluations. The laboratory must meet the standards as they apply to the services offered, complexity of tests and results, and the unique practices of each testing entity. All quality assurance activities must be documented.

A. PATIENT TEST MANAGEMENT

The laboratory must monitor, evaluate, and revise the following, based on the results of its evaluations:

- The criteria established for patient preparation, specimen collection, labeling, preservation, and transportation
- The information solicited and obtained on the laboratory's test requisition for its completeness, relevance, and necessity for the testing of patient specimens
- The use and appropriateness of the criteria established for specimen rejection
- The completeness, usefulness, and accuracy of the test report information necessary for the interpretation or utilization of test results
- The timely reporting of test results based on testing priorities (STAT, routine, etc.)
- The accuracy and reliability of test reporting systems, appropriate storage of records, and retrieval of test results

B. QUALITY CONTROL ASSESSMENT AND PT

The laboratory must have an ongoing mechanism to evaluate the corrective actions taken under remedial actions. Ineffective policies and procedures must be revised based on the outcome of the evaluation. The mechanism must evaluate and review the effectiveness of corrective actions taken for (1) problems identified during the evaluation of calibration and control data for each test method; (2) problems identified during the evaluation of patient test values for the purpose of verifying the reference range of a test method; and (3) errors detected in reported results. The corrective actions taken for any unacceptable, unsatisfactory, or unsuccessful PT result(s) must also be evaluated for effectiveness.

C. COMPARISON OF TEST RESULTS

If a laboratory performs the same test using different methodologies or instruments, or performs the same test at multiple testing sites, the laboratory must have a system that twice a year evaluates and defines the relationship between test results using the different methodologies, instruments, or testing sites. If a laboratory performs tests that are not included under PT programs, the laboratory must have a system for verifying the accuracy of its test results at least twice a year.

D. RELATIONSHIP OF PATIENT INFORMATION TO PATIENT TEST RESULTS

For internal quality assurance, the laboratory must have a mechanism to identify and evaluate patient test results that appear inconsistent with relevant criteria such as (1) patient age and sex; (2) diagnosis or pertinent clinical data, when provided; (3) distribution of patient test results when available; and (4) relationship with other test parameters, when available within the laboratory.

E. PERSONNEL ASSESSMENT

The laboratory must have an ongoing mechanism to evaluate the effectiveness of its policies and procedures for assuring employee competence and, if applicable, consultant competence.

F. COMMUNICATIONS

The laboratory must have a system in place to document problems that occur as a result of breakdowns in communication between the laboratory and the authorized individual who orders or receives the results of test procedures or examinations. Corrective actions must be taken, as necessary, to resolve the problems and minimize communication breakdowns.

G. COMPLAINT INVESTIGATIONS

The laboratory must have a system in place to ensure that all complaints and problems reported to the laboratory are documented. When appropriate, it must investigate complaints and institute corrective actions.

H. QUALITY ASSURANCE REVIEW WITH STAFF

The laboratory must have a mechanism for documenting and assessing problems identified during quality assurance reviews and discussing them with the staff. The laboratory must take corrective actions necessary to prevent recurrences. This mechanism of review is typically in the form of periodic (i.e., monthly or quarterly) QA meetings. QA meetings are essential for effective physician-lab relationships, especially in large clinical programs with multiple players. The reader is referred to Chapters 12 and 13 for more a more detailed discussion of the QA process and to Chapter 15 for the importance of effective physician-laboratory relationships.

I. QUALITY ASSURANCE RECORDS

The laboratory must maintain documentation of all quality assurance activities including problems identified and corrective actions taken. All quality assurance records must be available to DHHS and maintained for a period of 2 years.

X. SUBPART Q—INSPECTION

DHHS or its designee may conduct announced or unannounced inspections of any laboratory at any time during its hours of operation to assess compliance with the applicable requirements in order to (1) determine that testing proceeds or the laboratory operates in a manner that does not constitute an imminent and serious risk to public health; (2) evaluate complaints from the public; (3) determine whether the laboratory performs tests beyond the procedures for which the lab is certified; and (4) determine whether the laboratory performs tests in accordance with the manufacturer's or producer's instructions.

The laboratory may be required as part of this inspection to (1) permit DHHS or its designee to interview all laboratory employees concerning the laboratory's compliance with the applicable requirements; (2) permit DHHS or its designee access to all areas of the facility including specimen procurement and processing areas, storage facilities for specimens, reagents, supplies, records, reports, and testing and reporting areas; (3) permit employees to be observed performing tests, data analysis, and reporting; and (4) provide copies to DHHS or its designee of all records and data that the agency requires under these regulations.

The laboratory must provide, upon reasonable request, all information and data needed by DHHS or its designee to make a determination of compliance with the requirements of CLIA. Failure to permit an inspection under this subsection will result in the suspension of Medicare and Medicaid payments to the laboratory or termination of the laboratory's participation in Medicare and Medicaid and suspension of or action to revoke the laboratory's CLIA certificate. DHHS or its designee may conduct unannounced or announced, random, validation inspections of any accredited or CLIA-exempt laboratory at any time during its hours of operation.

XI. SUBPART R—ENFORCEMENT PROCEDURES

One of the strengths of CLIA '88 is that its participation is not voluntary; it is mandatory. It covers all laboratories, regardless of size, test volume, location, or type of testing performed. CLIA '88 provides for intermediate sanctions on laboratories that perform clinical diagnostic tests on human specimens when those laboratories are found to be out of compliance and requires the Secretary of DHHS to develop and implement a range of such sanctions. These sanctions may include suspension, limitation or revocation of the laboratory's certificate, civil suit against the laboratory, or imprisonment or fine for any person convicted of intentional violation of CLIA '88 requirements. Fines can range from $50 to $10,000 per day. In addition, the Secretary of DHHS is required to publish annually a list of all laboratories that have been sanctioned during the preceding year.

XII. SUBPART T—CONSULTATIONS

DHHS established a Clinical Laboratory Improvement Advisory Committee to advise and make recommendations on technical and scientific aspects of CLIA. The Clinical Laboratory Improvement Advisory Committee is comprised of individuals involved in the provision of laboratory services, utilization of laboratory services, development of laboratory testing or methodology, and others as approved by DHHS. DHHS designates specialized subcommittees as necessary. The Clinical Laboratory Improvement Advisory Committee or any designated subcommittees meets as needed, but not less than once each year.

The Clinical Laboratory Improvement Advisory Committee or subcommittee, at the request of DHHS, reviews and makes recommendations concerning (1) criteria for categorizing tests and examinations of moderate complexity (including the subcategory) and high complexity; (2) determination of waived tests; (3) personnel standards; (4) patient test management, quality control, quality assurance standards; (5) PT standards; (6) applicability to the standards of new technology; and (7) other issues relevant to part 493, if requested by DHHS.

XIII. DATES AND PUBLICATION OF CLIA '88 REGULATIONS

Federal Register, Vol. 57, No. 40, Friday, February 28, 1992, p. 7002
Federal Register, Vol. 57, No. 148, Friday, July 31, 1992, p. 33992
Federal Register, Vol. 57, No. 155, Tuesday, August 11, 1992, p. 35760
Federal Register, Vol. 58, No. 11, Tuesday, January 19, 1993, p. 5215
Federal Register, Vol. 58, No. 139, Thursday, July 22, 1993, p. 39154
Federal Register, Vol. 59, No. 233, Tuesday, December 6, 1994, p. 62605
Federal Register, Vol. 60, No. 78, Monday, April 24, 1995, p. 20036
Federal Register, Vol. 60, No. 177, Wednesday, September 13, 1995, p. 47540
Federal Register, Vol. 60, No. 230, Thursday, November 30, 1995, p. 61509

REFERENCES

1. Clinical Laboratory Improvement Amendments of 1988: Final Rule. *Federal Register* 57, 7002, 1992.

15 The Physician-Laboratory Relationship

Brooks A. Keel

CONTENTS

I. INTRODUCTION

The practice of clinical laboratory medicine dates back to Hippocrates, Galen, and Maimonedes, who first mentioned the use of urine tests (uroscopy) in the diagnosis of disease. Later, in the 17th century, Robert Boyle published some of his chemical analyses on urine as on blood. In a 1848 lecture to medical students, the British physician Arthur Garrod stated, "How imperfect our knowledge must be both of the healthy and diseased condition of the body if we do not call in the aid of chemistry to elucidate the phenomena."

Until the beginning of this century, the physician usually performed "laboratory" tests on the urine at the bedside of the patient as a part of the clinical assessment of the patient's condition. The texture, color, volume, and *taste* (note these were the pre-OSHA days) of the urine served as indicators of numerous ailments including kidney and blood diseases and diabetes.

With the advent of phlebotomy in the early 1900s, a wide assortment of chemical analyses became available. Initially the physician performed these tests. However, as time went on, the physician found himself less able to remain up-to-date on the developing chemical methodologies and more dependent on the capabilities of the scientists who specialized in the practice of clinical laboratory medicine. As a result, laboratory activity moved away from the physician at the bedside and came to the realm of the laboratory professional who, more often than not, came from the sciences and not from the medical field. Unfortunately, over time this move created some misconceptions about who is doing the tests (the "lab people") and who is ordering the tests (the "docs"). Moreover, problems related to *why* some laboratory procedures are ordered not only have led to misunderstandings between laboratorian and clinician but have raised issues of improper and, in some cases, unethical use of laboratory testing. Because the laboratory director ultimately is responsible for the function of the lab, he or she faces the dilemma of performing, reporting, and billing laboratory tests when the medical necessity of the order is in question. The director must then decide whether to perform the test as ordered (or in some cases "just do as you are told") or discuss the clinical relevance of the order with the physician. This discussion should be one between two colleagues, during which the laboratorian and the clinician learn from each other and collaborate to improve health care for the patient. However, many times this discussion never happens or results in bruised egos, or worse, the threat of job security. Either way, the laboratory must be the one to initiate the discussion.

What role should the lab play in proper patient care management? What is the actual responsibility of the lab in maintaining communications with the ordering physician? Should lab orders or procedures be challenged when the medical necessity is in question? Does the lab have a responsibility to report obvious unethical laboratory ordering practices? Can a lab director's job be placed in jeopardy by questioning the laboratory orders of physicians? This chapter will attempt to answer these questions in the following sections while providing some suggestions for improved relationships between the lab and the physician.

II. CLIA '88 AND THE PHYSICIAN-LABORATORY RELATIONSHIP

A detailed description of the rules and regulations of the Clinical Laboratory Improvement Amendments of 1988 (CLIA '88) can be found in Chapter 14. The reader should become familiar with these rules. The discussion below will concentrate on those parts of CLIA '88 that deal specifically with the relationships between the laboratory and the referring physician.

A. LAB DIRECTOR RESPONSIBILITY

CLIA '88 spells out the responsibility of the director clearly. As stated (section 493.1445), the "laboratory director is responsible for the overall operation and administration of the Laboratory ... and for assuring compliance with the applicable regulations." In other words, the director is ultimately responsible for everything that takes place in the lab. If the laboratory has more than one individual qualifying as director, the laboratory is required to designate one individual who has ultimate responsibility for overall operation and administration of the laboratory. The requirement that a laboratory must function under the direction of a qualified person is not met automatically simply because the director meets the education and experience requirements. The lab must demonstrate that the individual does, in fact, provide effective direction over the operation of the laboratory. No grey areas can exist regarding who is in charge.

CLIA '88 also charges that directors provide consultation to the laboratory's clients (i.e., the ordering physician) on matters relating to the quality of the test results reported and their interpretation concerning specific patient conditions. This responsibility includes being available to assist the ordering physician in ensuring that appropriate tests are ordered to meet the clinical expectations. This may be the actual responsibility of the director, or he or she may delegate this responsibility to the clinical consultant.

B. PATIENT TEST MANAGEMENT

CLIA '88 has specific requirements regarding the receipt and processing of specimens (Section 493.1101). The laboratory must perform tests only at the *written or electronic* request of an authorized person. Oral requests for laboratory tests are permitted only if the laboratory subsequently obtains written authorization for testing within 30 days, and these written requests must reside in the laboratory for at least 2 years. For embryo labs, the test requisition is often the patient's chart. If the patient's chart or medical record is used as the test requisition, it must be available to the personnel performing the test at the time of testing or prior to reporting results and to the Department of Health and Human Services (DHHS) upon request. In other words, you have the right to refuse testing if a proper requisition is not made available. In fact, you will be in violation of CLIA '88 if you do not have these records. Note, however, that you are required to have a written mechanism for obtaining these written records. If the laboratory attempts to obtain written authorization for oral test requests within 30 days, the requirement is met.

Although not required by CLIA '88, you should check each chart to be sure that all the appropriate informed consent documents are signed and witnessed before you perform any ART procedures. Do not rely on someone else telling you everything is in order. Instruct your ordering physicians that CLIA '88 requires that you must have access to the patient's chart before performing any procedures.

You can only accept specimens for testing from an *authorized person*. CLIA '88 defines this person as an individual authorized under state law to order tests or receive results, or both. This usually refers to a physician or his or her nurse acting on behalf of the physician. However, in some states this may not be true, and the patient may order a test on him or herself and may request to receive the test results directly. Find out from your state department of health who is authorized to order tests and refuse to accept orders from those who are not authorized. In my lab, we consider test orders the same as drug prescriptions. Your laboratory should never "fill" the order without the "prescription," which must be signed by a physician.

The laboratory also must assure that the requisition contains the patient's name or other identifier, the name and address of the authorized ordering person, the test to be performed, the date of specimen collection, and any information relevant and necessary to a specific test to assure accurate and timely testing and reporting of results. If any specimen information other than the patient name or unique identifier is missing from the test requisition or patient chart, the *laboratory* determines whether to test the specimen. Laboratories either should obtain missing information or should indicate on the test report or chart that any limitations of test results stem from the omission of patient information. However, if the lab determines that the missing information is essential to the provision of accurate results, it must be obtained before testing. If the requisition has designated areas for obtaining information, and the laboratory provides instructions to its clients specifying that these items must be completed, the laboratory has demonstrated compliance with the requirement. Attempts to gain the necessary information must be documented.

The laboratory test report must be sent promptly to the authorized person, the individual responsible for using the test results, or laboratory that initially requested the test. The laboratory must have adequate systems in place (i.e., written policies) to report results in a timely, accurate, reliable, and confidential manner and to ensure patient confidentiality throughout those parts of the testing process that are under the lab's control. The results must be released only to authorized persons or the individual utilizing the test results. You should not release information to patients unless you have written authorization from the ordering physician or your state allows such a release. Regardless, your laboratory should have written policies in place that detail how this should be handled.

C. QUALITY ASSURANCE

CLIA '88 requires each lab to establish and follow written policies and procedures for a comprehensive quality assurance (QA) program designed to monitor and evaluate the ongoing and overall quality of the total testing process. This is usually met by a periodic (e.g., monthly) QA meeting that includes the laboratory personnel and, if possible, the ordering physician and his or her staff. This is particularly important in ART programs where a team approach between the clinicians and the laboratorian is common. This meeting is where the relationship between the lab and the physician is defined clearly from the beginning and refined continually. Specifically, CLIA '88 requires you to address several functions:

- The laboratory must have ongoing mechanisms for monitoring all aspects of patient test management mentioned above, including criteria established for patient preparation, sample collection, quality control, test requisition, and test reporting.
- The laboratory must have a system in place to document problems that occur as a result of breakdowns in communication between the laboratory and the authorized individual who orders or receives the results of test procedures. Furthermore, corrective actions taken to resolve the problems and minimize communications breakdowns must be documented.
- The laboratory must have a system in place to assure that all complaints and problems reported to the laboratory are documented. Investigations of complaints must be made, when appropriate, and corrective actions instituted, with ongoing monitoring to minimize reoccurrences.
- The laboratory must maintain documentation of all QA activities including problems identified and corrective actions taken.

The Reproductive Medicine Laboratories in Wichita, KS uses a QA checklist (modified from Hutchinson, see Appendix at the end of this chapter) that covers each topic required by CLIA '88. We have further modified this checklist to cover discussion topics, for example, protocol criteria. The checklist can be printed with ample space between each topic, and the review process and discussions on any problems from the past month can be handwritten on the forms. If no problems have occurred, then enter "NTR" (nothing to report). The beauty of this checklist is twofold: first, it reminds (forces) you to cover each topic; second, it serves as your documentation (i.e., minutes) for the QA meeting. You should have the various directors of the various laboratories/clinics sign the finished document and provide everyone in attendance copies. The minutes from the previous meeting are also used as a guide for the next meeting, where remedial actions and other items can be discussed.

QA meetings are essential for effective physician-lab relationships, especially in large programs with many employees. If properly performed, the QA meeting opens lines of communication, addresses problems and solutions in a positive way, keeps everyone informed, and eliminates the behind the scenes complaining that can occur between the lab and the clinic. These meetings should be constructive and objective, pointing out problems that need attention rather than laying blame. QA meetings also are required by CLIA '88 and by the College of American Pathologists (CAP). If you meet with resistance (very few people want another meeting), explain that the meetings are not a matter of choice. Then use these meetings as a forum for increased communication.

III. SUMMARY

What are your legal rights as a lab director? What can you do if you think laboratory procedures are being ordered when they are not medically necessary or ethical? The following are points to remember:

- As director, you are responsible for everything in the lab, and for all test results reported.
- You are required legally to accept orders only from authorized individuals. You are not required, however, to perform tests if you do not want to. You can refuse to do testing regardless of who orders it.
- There can be only one director. The physician in your group may be the "medical director" of the program and the unquestioned boss, but if you are the named lab director, then you are responsible for the lab, and no one else.
- You are required to document that you have attempted to obtain written test requisitions. Put it in writing. If you get no response, then you have at least documented your attempt.
- Ordering inappropriate laboratory tests and then charging the patient for the test is fraud. Make no mistake about it. The government (not to mention insurance companies) takes a dim view of this activity. If you know of fraudulent activity, make an anonymous phone call and report it.
- It is your responsibility to consult with the ordering physician. For example, write him/her a nice letter to inform him or her that ordering routine seminal fructose determinations is not indicated on normospermic specimens, even though third party payers may be willing to reimburse for

this test (this actually has happened). You may not change the ordering practice, but you have documented your attempt at "consulting."

- Although you will not find any mention in CLIA '88 about informed consent, you should confirm personally that patient consent for your procedures is documented. Remind your ordering physician that CLIA '88 requires you to have the patient's chart in the lab before you can do the procedure. Check for yourself. As director, you may be held responsible.
- Take advantage of regularly scheduled QA meetings and involve the entire staff. Such involvement improves communication dramatically.

APPENDIX

GENERAL OPERATING PROCEDURE

TITLE: QUALITY ASSURANCE CHECKLIST

Date:_____ _____

Attendance:

_____ _____

_____ _____

_____ _____

_____ _____

_____ _____

_____ _____

_____ _____

_____ _____

_____ _____

I. Laboratory
   A. Pre-Analytic Testing Standards
      1. Patient preparation, specimen collection, labeling, preservation, transportation, and chain of custody
      2. The laboratory test requisition requirements
      3. The criteria used for specimen rejection
      4. The organization of the test report forms
      5. The timely reporting of test results
   B. Analytical Component Standards
      1. Analytical processes as follows
         a. The evaluation of quality control data for each test method
         b. The evaluation of ART fertilization and pregnancy rates
         c. Errors in reported test results
      2. Proficiency testing review and assessment, including remediation associated with unsuccessful performance
   C. The Post-Analytical Component
      1. Personnel assessment
         The effectiveness of the laboratory's ongoing policies and procedures for assuring employee competence, or the competence of other laboratory employees such as consultants is also reviewed.
      2. Communication
         The Committee reviews, confirms, and documents all communication problems between the labs and the Center.

      3. Complaint investigation

      The Committee investigates any complaint that the laboratory or Center receives. It also reflects any remediation accompanying this investigation.

II. Procedure Criteria

  A. Criteria for ICSI

  B. Criteria for Hatching

  C. Criteria for Heavy Insemination

  D. Criteria for Donor, ART

  E. Criteria for IVF

  F. Criteria for GIFT

  G. Criteria for FET

  H. Criteria for Donor, AI

  I. Other Procedure Criteria

  J. Patient Scheduling

    1. Criteria

    2. Problems

III. Quality Assurance Review

The Center Committee reviews problems identified above and subsequently reviews them with the laboratory or Center staff. System improvements installed as a result of problem solving are also reviewed with the staff. The process is documented in the lab or Center staff meeting minutes.

  A. Quality Assurance Records

    1. All records of Quality Assurance activities are maintained in the Center for a period of two years following the last use of the procedure. All records are available for DHHS inspection.

    2. I certify that the above listed items were reviewed during the meeting which occurred this date and any support or reference documentation is attached to this form. The documentation summarizes the minutes of the meeting as well as any action taken, subcommittee activity begun, or remedial activity either in process or completed.

Signed:

_____   _____

Center Director   Date

_____   _____

Andrology Lab Director   Date

_____   _____

ART Lab Director   Date

(Modified from Hutchison, D., *Total Quality Management in the Clinical Laboratory*, ASQC, Quality Press, Milwaukee, WI, 1994.)

16 Ethics and the Assisted Reproductive Technologies

Christopher J. De Jonge

CONTENTS

I. INTRODUCTION

As I was leafing through the newspaper I was struck by a headline that read, "2nd Twin Born 8 Years Later." At first glance the story seemed the fodder of tabloid news, but as I read further I soon learned that the story was factual and that assisted reproductive technologies facilitated this rather curious set of events. Ironically, it was 20 years earlier, in 1978, that the first "test tube" baby was conceived and born as a result of assisted reproductive technologies (ART). These two remarkable events caused me to think about some of the changes that have occurred in ART over the past two decades, for example, controlled ovarian hyperstimulation, gamete donation, surrogacy, and preimplantation genetic diagnosis. I wondered whether the placement of the news story, appearing not on the first page in bold headlines but rather late in the paper, was somehow significant. For example, could we, as a society, be at a place in time where a news story harking the birth of twins born 8 years apart is viewed as pedestrian or less-than-significant news? Does, for example, the formation of unique family structure(s), heretofore unattainable, require less consideration today than 20 years ago? Is society more permissive or accepting of ART practices and its sometimes unique outcomes? The answers to these and the many other questions that percolate as a result of ART are not answered easily.

Today, after the birth of thousands of babies, ART has become an integral part of the healthcare industry throughout the world. The ARTs encompass many aspects of reproductive medicine, from the rather simple intrauterine insemination (IUI) to the more advanced intracytoplasmic sperm injection (ICSI) and preimplantation genetics screening (PGS). In as much as many of the infertility therapies involve laboratory technologies we can state unequivocally that the ART laboratory is an equal partner with its clinical colleague in providing infertility services, and as such shares in the responsibilities of all treatment-associated sequelae, both good and bad. Sequelae from infertility treatment comes in many forms, for example, from treatment failure to excessive success. Evidence of treatment outcome, particularly the more dramatic, can be found all too frequently by reading newspapers or watching the nightly news. Indeed, perhaps the most recent and paradoxically astounding report was the birth of septuplets to a couple in Iowa, U.S. I should imagine that this fantastic event must have sent shudders through the collective conscience of all infertility practitioners because clearly this was an undesirable and excessive success. A consequence of this and other related stories is the stimulation of discussion, and in particular, ethical discussion, concerning the practice(s) of ART. It is the latter, i.e., ethics as it relates to ARTs, that will be the focus of this chapter.

First, let me be clear in stating that the purpose of this chapter is not to serve as an instructional, how-to-do-it manual. I am not an ethicist, but rather a reproductive scientist who has a tangential and an admittedly incomplete appreciation of the field of ethics. However, I do have a basic foundation of the field and I feel confident that I am competent to write on the topic of "Ethics and the Assisted Reproductive Technologies." My intended goal is to stimulate readers to investigate further into the relationship/association between ethics and ART. And, equally important, I hope to stimulate readers to engage in formal open discussion about the "ART" we practice and the ethical issues that coexist.

This chapter is structured in essentially four parts. The first part will characterize what is meant by the term *ethics*. The second part will provide representative examples of ethical theory. The third part, and in many ways tied to the previous, will review some legal aspects specific to reproduction. The fourth and final part will review the co-evolution of ethics and ART, with some representative examples provided. Finally, the resources section consists of review and/or consensus articles from which the reader can obtain a plethora of diverse additional resources on related topics.

II. THE ETHICAL FRAMEWORK

Former U.S. Supreme Court Chief Justice Earl Warren said on the issue of ethics and society that, "Society would come to grief without ethics, which is unenforceable in the courts, and cannot be made part of the law." Ethics, in its simplest form, takes an academic, typically nonlegal, view of what is right and wrong. Morality, on the other hand, takes a less formal view of the same issues and typically is learned from family, early schools, and the church. Ordinary citizens have ethical responsibilities that typically are expressed in moral terms. Professionals, e.g., physicians, scientists, and litigators, on the other hand, have ethical responsibilities that extend beyond those of the lay person. Thus, the professional must be vigilant about shunning participation in deception, avoiding conflicts of interest with other obligations, and remaining faithful agents for their customers' interests. A recent and notorious example of a gross failure to uphold the ethical responsibilities of the professional is found in the case of a notable group of physicians at the University of California-Irvine who provided oocytes and embryos to recipients without the knowledge or consent of the donor.

How do ethics come to bear within a technical profession? As an example, the scientist might ask the technical question of whether a certain procedure can be done. In so doing, he or she, if operating according to the ethical responsibilities of a professional, will seek the opinion of peers as represented in a body with a name such as *Institutional Review Board* (IRB). The IRB makes determinations concerning whether a project fulfills the criteria outlined above for professional and ethical conduct. The question might be then, how are questions of ethics addressed and how might they possibly be resolved? The answer lies, in part, within ethical theory.

III. ETHICAL THEORY

Ethical theory provides the framework to approach the underlying rationale of a situation, which then facilitates the classification and enhanced understanding of the arguments, resulting ultimately (at least in many situations) in the ability to defend conclusions about right and wrong for that situation. However, more than one ethical theory exists for addressing a question or issue. Some theories try to be prescriptive, e.g., what must, should, ought to be done, while others are descriptive. Some representative examples of ethical theory are described briefly below.

Deontology is perhaps the *purest* form of ethical theory. Stemming from the work of Immanual Kant (1724–1804), this form of ethical theory deals with duty and moral obligation. It is somewhat independent of life's realities in that the goodness or value of the motives and the ends of the act are minimally important. The act itself is of prime importance. From a societal viewpoint, deontological theory rejects acts that harm minorities and/or individuals.

Utilitarianism is a distinct rival to deontology in that it focuses on the consequences and not the acts. Put simply, to determine good one must ask whether the ends justify the means. Utilitarianism requires that *good* be prospectively defined and ultimately quantified. A final contrast of utilitarianism to deontology is that the welfare of minorities and individuals is sacrificed for the majority. The goal is to achieve the greatest good for the greatest number.

The last theory to be presented is called **Ethical Relativism**, and it might be considered to have a more modern foundation than the previous theories in that it stresses cultural diversity. Indeed, this theory stems from the recognition and acknowledgment that many differences exist among individuals and groups. Therefore, what is deemed ethical depends on the individual, the group, the culture, etc. In many ways, this theory argues against requiring universal obedience to a rule or action.

To outline other forms of ethical theory is beyond the scope of this chapter. However, this section does strive to help the reader appreciate some of the more common forms of ethical theory and begin to view ART in their light. At the beginning of these sections on ethics, a quote from a legal expert was offered in which he stated that "ethics ... cannot be made part of the law." However, we should consider legal aspects of reproduction in parallel with ethics. In so doing, we (professionals and society) might resolve or move towards resolution of some of the issues, practices, and perceived problems that have or will become a part of ART.

IV. U.S. LAW AND REPRODUCTION

In 1978, the United Nations formally declared that it is a right of "men and women of full age ... to marry and found a family," and in the same year the first IVF baby was born. In recent times the U.S. Supreme Court has concluded, through dicta, that if the issue of "right to procreate" arose, they would recognize that as a right to reproduce, at least for married persons.

Reproduction has been linked to several clauses in the 14th Amendment of the U.S. Constitution. In so doing, the constitution and government have formally provided for the protection of the rights of its citizens in regards to family formation via reproduction. Specifically, in 1972 the right to reproduce was linked to the due process clause of the 14th Amendment as evidenced in the following excerpt:

> "If the right of privacy means anything, it is the right of the individual, married or single, to be free of unwarranted governmental intrusion into matters so fundamentally affecting a person as the decision whether to bear or beget a child."

Thus, the fundamental right of privacy that is afforded and protected by the due process clause became functionally linked to "family, marriage, motherhood, procreation, and child rearing."

Another significant addition to the 14th Amendment is the equal protection clause, which provides for the "equal application" of laws to all persons. This clause is considered to be an important protector of civil rights. Thus, by virtue of the due process and the equal protection clauses, protection of individual autonomy in matters of family relationships and formation, i.e., procreation, is protected for all citizens.

In conclusion, procreative liberty is specifically guaranteed under the 14th amendment to the U.S. constitution and is highlighted philosophically in the following statement issued by the U.S. Supreme Court: "the Constitution protects the sanctity of the family precisely because the institution of the family is deeply rooted in this Nation's history and tradition." However, the court's statements were made before the implementation of IVF techniques. Protection of noncoital reproduction was not included in any of the statements released by this nation's highest court. However, the general assumption is made that the right to reproduce would also be protected for the couple who can make a family only through noncoital methods, i.e., through ARTs.

V. INFORMED CONSENT

The process of informed consent is a means to protect the patient's right to make autonomous decisions. It is further meant to protect the patient from any potential coercion by the healthcare professional. Informed consent is required by law for all clinical circumstances. By definition, informed consent means that a patient is given sufficient information so that he or she understands (1) the nature of his or her condition and the purpose of the proposed procedure or treatment; 2) the risks, consequences, and probability of success of the proposed procedure or treatment; (3) alternatives; and (4) prognosis if the procedure is not performed or any treatment given.

ART encompasses all procedures used in conjunction with the medical diagnosis and therapeutic treatment of the subfertile couple. Appropriate therapy requires adequate and thorough diagnostic testing for both male and female partners, such as blood chemistries, ovulation detection, determination of competent anatomical structures, semen analysis, and other relevant tests. Some common therapies (and the pathologies being treated) are intrauterine insemination (cervical factor, unexplained infertility, male factor infertility), *in vitro* fertilization (ovarian dysfunction, male factor, tubal pathology), gamete intrafallopian tubal transfer (unexplained fertility, endometriosis), intracytoplasmic sperm injection (severe male factor infertility), assisted hatching (implantation failure, advanced maternal age), and surrogacy (absent or malformed uterus).

Typically, informed consent is provided as testing and or procedures are initiated, meaning that it is a progressive process and not done in one lump sum. Thus, the prospective patients should, and indeed must, be informed of the many issues/factors that relate to their impending treatment. Some of the pertinent issues can be itemized. First, what are the qualifications of the infertility team, what are the success rates for that clinic in treating infertility, and what is the estimated financial burden? Second, patients should know of treatment-associated risks, such as (1) risk of side effects from hormone therapy, e.g., increased risk of certain cancers; (2) risk of sequelae from surgical procedures to treat pathology, e.g., adhesions; (3) risk from intrauterine insemination, e.g., multiple gestation, antisperm antibody formation; (4) risk from *in vitro* fertilization, e.g., infection, blood loss, multiple gestation; (5) psychological consequences, e.g., failure; and (6) out-of-control motivation resulting in overwhelming debt.

By virtue of the organization at most ART centers, the physician is responsible for ensuring that the patient has received adequate informed consent. As an aside, perhaps the term adequate is one that should be defined as some minimal standard(s) set forth by formal peer-group consensus. (See for example the American Society for Reproductive Medicine Practice Committee Report entitled, "Elements to be considered in obtaining informed consent for ART.") If the couple agrees to accept the risk then they will be asked to sign a document that states they have received information, weighed the risks/consequences against their desires, motivation, and future health, and accept all the above.

VI. ETHICS AND ART

Can *in vitro* fertilization, which arises by noncoital methods, be considered in the same or similar context as coital reproduction? Coital reproduction is protected not for the coitus, but for what the coitus makes possible: it enables the couple to unite egg and sperm for the possibility of rearing a child of their own. Thus, the use of noncoital techniques, such as IVF or IUI, to unite sperm and egg, necessitated by the couple's infertility, also should be protected.

I will offer as an aside that some couples, while having the legal freedom to make a choice of *in vitro* fertilization are limited by their moral convictions. An example could be the devout Catholic couple. A traditional Catholic view is that the unitive and procreative should be combined in one act, thus making the separation of sex and reproduction wrong. Interestingly, a couple such as this can try to achieve pregnancy through GIFT, and often under the provision that coitus occur at the peri-GIFT time. If one accepts that noncoital reproduction is a part of our *procreative liberty* (right to reproduce) then under what conditions can its application be considered appropriate or inappropriate, and how much technological intervention is acceptable?

The ARTs contain numerous aspects that question whether something should be done and, if so, for whom. One prominent example is ICSI. ICSI burst on to the ART stage in the early 1990s. This advanced form of ART appeared to be a piece of the infertility treatment puzzle that had long been prized. With this technique a whole new spectrum of patient/pathology was effectively addressed (I intentionally refrain from using the term *treated* because the condition causing the male subfertility is not being treated per se). Couples for whom the male partner had severely diminished sperm counts, motility, or even aspermia now had the option of using genetic material from within their intimate relationship rather than foreign genetic material derived from a known or unknown sperm donor. Despite the redeeming qualities associated with application of ICSI the question must still be asked, "Should this technique be used?"

Based on countless discussions and numerous meetings, the consensus would be that ICSI should be used to facilitate conception for subfertile couples. However, the ability to raise this question comes, somewhat, at the heels of implementation of the technology. The *a priori* opportunity to determine (based on scientific testing and statistical analyses of results) whether ICSI, as a technique, can and should be included in the clinical armamentarium of infertility treatment never occurred. Thus, in my opinion, the cart has preceded the horse. As a consequence, the field faces questions about the male population for whom ICSI is best suited and, more importantly, the safety of ICSI for the putative offspring.

Based on current data, ICSI does not appear to induce congenital abnormalities in the offspring. Sex chromosome abnormalities are increased. The ability to make conclusions about both of the previous issues is difficult and largely because of epidemiological reasons. Also unresolved is whether the offspring are developmentally or mentally compromised. In contrast, evidence is mounting that under certain circumstances, e.g., nonobstructive azoospermia resulting from microdeletions on the Y-chromosome, that the father's subfertility will be passed along to male offspring thus obligating the son to seek ART assistance when family building becomes desirable. Only time will reveal the potential limitations of the male offspring's reproductive capacity. These issues present themselves as, somewhat, ethical dilemmas. As a result the question can again be asked, "Is it ethical to offer ICSI as a treatment for male subfertility, particularly when we do not have answers to some basic and important questions?" I cannot provide a conclusive answer to this question. Suffice it to say that the human ICSI experiment continues daily, and as a result new information streams forth about the consequences of ICSI.

Because a part of the definition of infertility includes the word *disease*, I think that we might agree that, for medical reasons, the use of ARTs to help a couple start a family is permissible and even facilitated (by insurance coverage). When a medical condition exists, e.g., endometriosis, ovulation dysfunction, varicocele, the physician is carrying out his or her oath "to honorably treat (using ART) and heal the patient (either by treatment or by facilitating a pregnancy)." However, examples abound in which no medical condition, i.e., pathology, existed yet the patient was treated as an infertility patient. The following stories, obtained principally through the media, raise questions about the ethics (consciously shunning participation in deception, avoiding conflicts of interest with other obligations, and remaining faithful agents for their customers' interests) of some of the professionals who practice ART and who help to perpetuate the sensationalism and suspicion often associated with ARTs.

1. A 63-year-old woman gave birth to a baby after having undergone ART. I cannot ascertain any medical indication in this woman that could be termed *disease* and thus necessitate ART treatment. Based solely on suspicion, I would speculate that this post-menopausal woman and her husband (never described) simply wanted a baby.
2. A 50⁺-year-old woman in Italy gave birth after using ARTs. Her reason for wanting conception was because her only son was killed in an auto accident.
3. A common, nonmedical example includes the couple, regardless of present fertility status, who want a baby of a specific gender because they have enough of the opposite gender.
4. A woman wanted a gestational surrogate so she could avoid stretch marks. Another woman wanted a surrogate because she was too busy in her business life to take "time out" to gestate a baby.

These are only a few examples derived from the lay press that cast aspersion on ART, and rightfully so. However, standing in stark contrast are an overwhelming number of ethically legitimate and positively motivated ART stories. Unfortunately, these stories do not appear often in the lay press. My guess (and perhaps jaded) is that these latter stories do not appear simply because they are not spectacular and thus do not sell papers or capture viewing audiences.

At the risk of assigning blame, the media has, in part, contributed to the commercialization/commodification of ART. One consequence is that ART programs have become very competitive. Physicians and their patients want the positive outcome of a pregnancy, and sometimes that motivation supercedes thoughtful consideration of risk. Evidence for this assertion comes from the Society for Assisted Reproduction Technologies IVF Registry where the percentages of multiple gestations resulting from IVF exceed those by coitus.

The appropriate number of embryos for transfer is at present a contentious issue in the U.S. In the U.K., Australia, and many European countries, laws address embryo maxima for transfer. As a consequence these countries tend to have reduced multiple gestation rates, particularly in regards to higher order gestations (≥3 conceptuses), compared to the U.S. In the U.S. no laws exist presently that restrict the number of embryos that can be transferred. As a result, physicians and patients may feel motivated, driven by a "Smith vs. Jones" mentality, to transfer an embryo number that not only increases the likelihood for pregnancy but that increases the chance of a multiple gestation (e.g., see De Jonge and Wolf). A negative consequence of multiple gestations are the potentially serious medical situations, e.g., prematurity and preeclampsia, that can arise. When such sequelae do occur, hospitalization is often required and sometimes mandates heroic efforts to address the health issue.

Although it stands as one of the more extreme examples, the hospital costs for the recently born septuplets probably approached or exceeded $1 million U.S. Clearly the financial burden is not assumed solely by the parents, but rather by insurance companies. Thus, we can speculate that because ARTs contribute to higher order gestations, and often result in hospitalization, insurance carriers are less likely to offer infertility coverage, and if they do the guidelines become so restrictive as to make the financial reimbursement trivial (relative to patient outlay). Bearing this in mind, we find that a fair proportion of individuals who seek treatment for infertility do not have a means of paying for these services other than out of their own pocket. Situations all too frequently arise in which couples take out second and third mortgages on homes and property in order to pay for their IVF cycle(s). When viewed in total, ART can be criticized for being available only to a select few, i.e., middle to upper classes, and thus failing to satisfy various ethical theories. As a result, this issue recurs as part of ethical discussions about ARTs.

Other ethical issues have evolved as a result of ARTs. Some of the more notable and widely discussed issues include patient age, marital status, sexual orientation, posthumous sperm collection, surrogacy, gamete and embryo donation (e.g., intrafamilial gamete donation, anonymity, and payment), preimplantation genetic screening, and cloning. While critically important and relevant, coverage of these topics is beyond the scope of this single chapter, and the reader is directed to one or more of the reviews listed in the resource section. However, I will close this section by citing a recent scientific abstract in which the authors posed and tested the question: "Are biologically dead sperm reproductively dead?" The investigators subjected sperm to various treatments to induce death at cellular and molecular levels prior to ICSI. Based on their results they concluded that dead sperm (in patients with necrospermia) can be used successfully to make babies.

Equally as significant as the aforementioned are issues related laboratory function. The most notable example of a breakdown in laboratory function, i.e., quality control and assurance (QC/QA), is the case of the white Dutch couple who, via ART, gave birth to both a white and black child. The cause was attributed to a contaminated pipette. In an attempt to avoid or at least diminish the potential for laboratory errors, ART laboratories are subjected to inspection processes where they must demonstrate that rigorous QC/QA programs are in place. If they pass inspection successfully, then the laboratory is certified as complying with established policies and procedures. Paradoxically, the same is not true for the clinical arm of the ART practice, at least in the U.S.

VII. DISCUSSION

Can quality and integrity of character be regulated by law? The answer is a resounding no. We attempt to do so, but diversity in individuals precludes success. Every day on the evening news we are deluged by stories involving poor character and lack of integrity, some examples being murder, child abandonment, or perjury. The field of ART is no different than the field of common life. But because our field is so intimately tied to the essence of humanity, life, and spirituality, infractions due to poor quality in character or lack of integrity are the stuff of high drama—a physician using his own semen to inseminate tens of women, another physician selling drugs used in ART for paper bags filled with money to support personal gain, the nonconsented donation of embryos to unsuspecting recipients, or perhaps even more dramatic, the simultaneous birth of a black and white child to a white couple who required ART service. All stand as cases of quality standards and basic operating procedures gone ignored. Society as a whole does not ignore such incidences, but rather focuses its magnifying glass. The result is often outrage, suspicion, and condemnation.

Currently, the constitutional status of procreative liberty requires that the legal system, except possibly for surrogacy, leave ART decisions largely to the discretion of the physicians, patients, and institutions involved. My hope is that the field will move toward self-regulation and, as a consequence, that many positive results will occur such that ART is seen in a more tempered and favorable light, with decreased suspicion by the public and insurance providers.

In conclusion, I find it significant that the National Advisory Board on Ethics in Reproduction (NABER) has closed its doors. The reason given was lack of funding. So with the demise of NABER I am left wondering, anxiously, where the societal collective conscience for reproductive technologies will reside now that the only independent show in town has closed its doors. I guess the answer to this question must wait until the onset of the next millennium.

VIII. RESOURCES

PEER-REVIEWED ARTICLES

Andrews, L., Elster, N., Gatter, R. et al., ART into science: regulation of fertility techniques, *Science*, 281, 651–2, 1998.

Callahan, T. L., Hall, J. E., Ettner, S. L., Christiansen, C. L., Greene, M. F., and Crowley, W. F., Jr., The economic impact of multiple-gestation pregnancies and the contribution of assisted-reproduction techniques to their incidence, *N. Engl. J. Med.*, 331, 244–9, 1994.

De Jonge, C. J. and Wolf, D. P., Opinion—Embryo number for transfer should be regulated, *Fertil. Steril.*, 68, 784–6, 1997.

De Jonge, C. J. and Pierce, J., Intracytoplasmic sperm injection—What kind of reproduction is being assisted?, *Hum. Reprod.*, 10, 2518–20, 1995.

Djerassi, C., Sex in an age of mechanical reproduction, *Science*, 285, 53–4, 1999.

Edwards, R. G. and Sharpe, D. J., Social values and research in human embryology, *Nature*, 231, 87–91, 1971.

Edwards, R. G., Fertilization of human eggs *in vitro*: morals, ethics and the law, *Q. Rev. Biol.*, 49, 3–26, 1974.

Garel, M., Stark, C., Blondel, B., Lefebvre, G., Vauthier-Brouzes, D., and Zorn, J. R., Psychological reactions after multifetal pregnancy reduction: a 2-year follow-up study, *Hum. Reprod.*, 12, 617–22, 1997.

Garel, M., Salobir, C., and Blondel, B., Psychological consequences of having triplets: a 4-year follow-up study, *Fertil. Steril.*, 67, 1162–5, 1997.

Jewell, S. E. and Yip, R., Increasing trends in plural births in the United States, *Obstet. Gynecol.*, 85, 229–32, 1995.

Jones, H. W., Jr. and Toner, J. P., The infertile couple, *N. Engl. J. Med.*, 329, 1710–1715, 1993.

Pierce, J., Reitemeier, P. J., Jameton, A., Maclin, V. M., and De Jonge, C. J., Should gamete donation between family members be restricted?, *Hum. Reprod.*, 10, 1330–2, 1995.

Tognoni, G. and Geraci, Approaches to informed consent, *Controlled Clinical Trials*, 18, 621–627, 1997.

Luke, B., The changing pattern of multiple births in the United States: maternal and infant characteristics, 1973 and 1990, *Obstet. Gynecol.*, 84, 101–6, 1994.

Lancaster, P. A. L., Registers of *in vitro* fertilization and assisted conception, in *Genetics and Assisted Human Conception. Human Reproduction*, Vol. 11 (Suppl 4), Van Steirteghem, A., Devroey, P., and Liebaers, I., Eds., Oxford University Press, 1996, 89–104.

McKinney, M., Downey, J., and Timor-Tritsch, I., The psychological effects of multifetal pregnancy reduction, *Fertil. Steril.*, 64, 51–61, 1995.

Page, D. C., Silber, S., and Brown, L. G., Men with infertility caused by *AZFc* deletion can produce sons by intracytoplasmic sperm injection, but are likely to transmit the deletion and infertility, *Hum. Reprod.*, 14, 1722–1726, 1999.

Society for Assisted Reproductive Technology and The American Society for Reproductive Medicine, Assisted reproductive technology in the United States and Canada: 1994 results generated from the American Society for Reproductive Medicine/Society for Assisted Reproductive Technology Registry, *Fertil. Steril.*, 66, 697–704, 1996.

BOOKS AND REPORTS

Eggs, Embryos and Ethics: A New Era in Reproductive Technology, Stanford Law and Policy Review, 1995, Vol. 6, No. 2, www.stanford.edu/group/SLPR/sixtwo.html.

Shenfield, F. and Sureau, C., Eds., *Ethical Dilemmas in Assisted Reproduction, Studies in Profertility Series*, Vol 7, Parthenon Publishing Group, New York, 1997.

The Ethics Committee of the American Fertility Society, Ethical considerations of assisted reproductive technologies, *Fertil. Steril.*, 62, Suppl. 1, 1994.

Human Fertilization and Embryology Act 1990, Her Majesty's Stationery Office, London, UK.

Human Fertilization and Embryo Authority Annual Reports. Human Fertilization and Embryo Authority, Paxton House, 30 Artillery Lane, London E1 7LS, England.

Englert, Y., Ed., Gamete donation: current ethics in the European union, *Hum. Reprod.*, 13(Suppl 2), 1998.

NABER, The Work of the National Advisory Board on Ethics in Reproduction, The National Advisory Board on Ethics in Reproduction, 1995, Vol. 1, No. 1.

NABER, Is Assisted Reproduction a Process Ripe for Regulation?, The National Advisory Board on Ethics in Reproduction, 1995, Vol. 1, No. 3.

The New York State Task Force on Life and the Law, Assisted Reproductive Technologies: Analysis and Recommendations for Public Policy, 1998.

17 Managed Care and ART

Norbert Gleicher

CONTENTS

I. INTRODUCTION

Assisted reproductive technologies (ART) in all but a handful of states are not considered covered services by most health plans. Consequently, ART exists in most part of the country outside of traditional healthcare in a strict, fee-for-service environment. Why then should the topic of "Managed Care and ART" be subject of discussion in this volume at all?

The answer to this question lies not only in the foresight of the editors of this book, but in what will happen over the next decade to the fertility industry. While we cannot predict precisely where healthcare trends are going, a few developments seem obvious and practically unavoidable. For example, the current fertility market will shrink unless the profession finds ways to grow the market beyond its current level. As baby boomers age out of fertility care, only an expansion of fertility services to new patient populations, which currently do not receive such services, can make up for the loss. This is possible.

Currently, only approximately one quarter of couples who require fertility care receive treatment. Many who do not enter treatment do so based on personal considerations. In fact, even among couples who see an infertility specialist, approximately one third will choose to discontinue treatment for other than economic reasons.[1] However, a majority of couples who need, but do not receive, care never enter treatment because they cannot afford it. Market expansion, therefore, depends to a great extent on making fertility services affordable.

Improving affordability must be achieved. If it is not, infertility care will be a miserable area to practice in, involving cut-throat competition in a rapidly shrinking marketplace. More simply stated, fertility services must expand from Bloomindales to Sears, from a service to the rich to a treatment open to everybody.

In practical terms this means that we as providers must rethink our fee structures, reconsider how we provide infertility care and, most importantly, better understand what represents cost-effective, high-quality infertility care. These steps must occur whether we believe that insurance coverage for fertility services will expand or not. Independent of insurance coverage, the cost of fertility services in the years to come will determine how large a market we will serve.

II. ART IS NOT INFERTILITY

ART has made incredible progress over the last decade. As pregnancy rates have improved,[2] new treatment modalities have allowed new patient populations to achieve parenthood,[3] and ART use has increased dramatically world-wide. In fact, among laypeople, ART is frequently equated with fertility care as a whole. Clearly, ART represents the most visible part of infertility treatment. Barely a day passes when an ART-related topic does not catch the fancy of the media, whether for positive or negative reasons.

ART, however, should not obtain a similarly exaggerated position within the community of providers of fertility services. One is tempted to perform ART procedures earlier within algorithms of fertility care as pregnancy rates with ART improve. National statistics leave no doubt that the average ART cycle yields a higher pregnancy rate than the average ovulation induction cycle. This, however, does not suggest that ART should replace the cheaper and less invasive ovulation induction cycle. In fact, in a prospectively randomized study, we recently demonstrated that ART as a first-line treatment approach was highly cost-inefficient.[4] In other words, ART represents an outstanding treatment option at the end of a standard treatment algorithm. If ART is advanced prematurely, cost will be dramatically higher with no obvious benefit in pregnancy rates.

III. WHAT IS A PROPER FERTILITY ALGORITHM?

The appropriate question is not where ART falls in fertility therapy, but what is the proper fertility algorithm for a particular patient at a particular point in time. The time reference is important because circumstances change constantly. As the efficacy of treatment options improves (or deteriorates) in relation to each other, treatment algorithms must be reevaluated. This is the reason why healthcare, just as every other industrial process, conducts ongoing review. What makes sense today may not tomorrow because of new scientific discoveries, e.g., intracytoplasmic sperm insertion (ICSI) has dramatically affected the treatment algorithm for male infertility.[3] Everybody who still follows the pre-ICSI treatment approach to very low semen counts would be scientifically and clinically out of touch. Embryo selection has impacted the *in vitro* fertilization (IVF) process in general.[5] Laboratories that do not select embryos will uniformly lag in pregnancy as well as implantation rates.

In short, only a constant clinical re-engineering process will at any given point provide for the most effective and cost-efficient clinical algorithm. Where ART will stand within such an algorithm will vary over time. We must recognize, however, that ART represents only a small piece of total fertility care. Its principal function is to be part of the process that allows most couples to achieve pregnancy at the lowest possible cost. ART is not a specialty on its own, nor is it a panacea for all infertility.

IV. COST-EFFECTIVE CARE

The smart consumer and/or insurance carrier should not be interested in a fertility center's ART-related pregnancy rates. Table 17.1 outlines the questions that really should be asked. As this table demonstrates, the term ART does not even appear in the questionnaire and, yet, a fertility center that offered answers to the four questions posed in the table would be more transparent in its quality of care than any combination of ART statistics could ever offer.

TABLE 17.1
Important Questions for an Infertility Center

1. What is the percentage of couples who are pregnant (deliver) after 3, 6, 9, or 12 months of care?
2. What is the cost per pregnancy (delivery)?
3. What is the percentage of multiples (twins, triplets, etc.) among pregnancies achieved?
4. What is the patient drop-out rate from treatment among couples who do not conceive after 3, 6, 9, or 12 months of treatment?

The truth of the matter is that neither patient nor insurance carrier cares how pregnancies are achieved as long as they are achieved rapidly, at minimal cost, and with patient satisfaction. Therefore, the question "What are your ART pregnancy rates?" is irrelevant. The relevant question should address how many patients conceive in what time interval.

Similarly, we should not be concerned with the costs for one ART cycle, but with how much it will cost to ahieve a pregnancy (or reach delivery) by whatever method. The incidence of multiple gestations plays an important role in this consideration. Fertility practitioners are well aware that pregnancy rates can be driven up (and not only in ART) by increasing in parallel the risk of multiple births. The cost of such an approach can be staggering, whether in traditional fertility therapies or with ART.[6]

Finally, none of our services has real economic value unless we have a satisfied customer. Patient satisfaction can be measured in many ways. Short of complex patient questionnaires or telephone satisfaction surveys, we have noted a direct correlation between patient drop-out rates from treatment and patient satisfaction.[1,7] This is the reason for the fourth question in Table 17.1. Any other mode of assessing patient satisfaction could be equally effective.

To summarize, the ART-provider must recognize that ART represents only one component in a rather complex array of treatment options. The successful ART provider, whether clinical or embryologist, will recognize this fact and will position the ART program accordingly within a fully integrated fertility center.

V. THE INSURANCE CARRIER

As noted earlier, most health plans, whether managed or not, do not perceive themselves as providing coverage for infertility services. This is obviously a misconception since we all know that intentional miscoding in such cases covers at least a limited amount of fertility services.[8] What this "underground economy" really achieves is, in fact, highly inefficient. Expensive repeat surgeries will be paid for, while more effective treatments will not. Under the disguise of organic disease, a patient may have repeated tubal surgeries with practically zero pregnancy chance; she, however, will not be covered for even one ART cycle.

Smart insurance carriers are starting to recognize this fact. While no definite data have been published so far, the insurance community is currently examining approximately $6.00 per member per year, which is rendered in inefficient care to their patients who do not have specific coverage for infertility services. This represents approximately $.50 per member per month (PMPM), which does not cover a full fertility capitation but could pay for a significant portion of it.

As the insurance industry recognizes that lack of insurance coverage for fertility services costs them significant dollars and that their dollars subsidize inefficient care, they also recognize that it is in their interest to turn the "underground economy" of fertility services inside-out. This can only be done by offering fertility benefits.

It is, therefore, this author's opinion that insurance coverage for fertility services will continue to increase. Such voluntary insurance coverage already is increasingly offered on both coasts. The rest of the country will follow, driven by a tight job market that will require employers to offer improved benefits packages. The speed of the expansion in insurance coverage will, however, depend on the overall cost of this new benefit. If we maintain fertility services at their current cost structure, the process will be slow and tedious. Similarly, if we continue to make media headlines about multiple births, insurance coverage will remain an uphill battle.

The choices seem obvious: as a profession we owe it to the public to offer our services to the largest possible recipient pool. We are not only providers to the rich. Poor people also deserve children if they suffer from infertility. If we want infertility to be considered like other "diseases," we have to treat the "disease" in everybody.

VI. THE PROVIDER

Many of my friends in the specialty do not like insurance coverage and I cannot blame them. They have successful practices in markets without insurance coverage. Their services are paid for in cash, often ahead of time and with considerable margins. Why should they advocate a change in the system?

The answer is twofold: first, because it is the right thing to do since we do not want to be seen as only providing to the affluent; second, because a change toward insurance coverage is inevitable.

Once a provider of significant market prominence offers coverage, other providers usually have no choice but to follow suit. Oxford has announced limited coverage in the New York/New Jersey/Connecticut area. There can be no doubt competitors will have to follow. Kaiser is taking a similarly leading role on the west coast. Others will follow there as well.

Once a market moves toward coverage, two developments usually reshape the provider scene: first, the cost structure for fertility services drops dramatically. Since only volume can make up for decreasing unit prices, provider networks arise that can do bulk contracting.

Both of these developments may hurt the passive and currently content provider. Because this author sees an increasing market penetration by insurance products as inevitable, it would seem prudent for providers in still unaffected markets to prepare for the inevitable. This is one circumstance where being wrong in a prediction will not harm this author's standing with his peers. Being right, however, and having contributed to their preparedness may help protect their livelihood.

VII. THE INSURANCE CONTRACT

The complexities of contracting fall outside the scope of this chapter. For that purpose, the reader is referred to a recent monograph by this author and others that discusses contracting in reproductive medicine.[9] Suffice it to say, contracting in reproductive endocinology and infertility is a complex process. Whether contracts with insurance carriers are on a fee-for-service, case-rate, or capitation basis, providers had better know what they are doing when they sign a (usually discounted) contract.

As in other matters, certain megatrends are apparent in contracting. Two deserve special attention: first, contracts increasingly will go to those who are willing to share risk; second, because the ability to assume risk goes hand-in-hand with size and proper capitalization, contracts will go to larger provider groups. The implications for the small provider seem obvious.

VIII. SUMMARY AND CONFLICT STATEMENT

This chapter offers a view of the world that may not be shared by all or even most of my colleagues. It is based on many years of experience in dealing with insurance companies as both an advisor and a provider. As a provider, I hope that many of my opinions and predictions will turn out to be wrong. As a scientifically trained individual, I must go where the facts lead me.

It is important to note that I am an executive of a for-profit commercial entity (GynCor, Inc.) that actively pursues commercial goals within our specialty of reproductive medicine. Because I am also a shareholder in GynCor, Inc., it is possible, if not probable, that my position and/or ownership may affect my judgments. The reader is advised to consider this fact in assessing the content of this chapter.

REFERENCES

1. Gleicher, N., VanderLaan, B., Karande, V., Morris, R., Nadherney, K., and Pratt, D., Infertility treatment dropout and insurance coverage, *Obstet. Gynecol.*, 88, 289–293, 1996.
2. Jones, H. W. and Touer, J. P., The infertile couple, *N. Engl. J. Med.*, 329, 1710–1715, 1993.
3. Palermo, G., Devroey, J. H., and Van Steirteghem, A. C., Pregnancies after intracytoplasmic injection of single spermatozoan into an oocyte, *Lancet*, 340, 17–18, 1992.
4. Karande, V., Korn, A., Morris, R., Rao, R., Balin, M., Rinehart, J., Dohn, K., VanderLaan, B., and Gleicher, N., A prospective randomized trial assessing outcome and cost of *in vitro* fertilization versus a traditional infertility treatment algorithm, *Fertil. Steril.*, 71, 468–475, 1999.
5. Bongso, A., Fong, C. Y., Ng, S. C., Kumar, J., and Trounson, A. O., Improving the success of human IVF through day 5 and day 6 transfer: the use of improved *in vitro* systems, *J. Assist. Reprod. Genet.*, 14(s), 13s(abstract), 1997.
6. Callahan, T. I., Hall, J. E., Etner, S. L., Christiansen, C. L., Greene, M. F., and Crowley, W. F., Jr., The economic impact of multiple gestation pregnancies and the contribution of assisted reproductive techniques to their incidence, *N. Engl. J. Med.*, 331, 244–249, 1994.
7. VanderLaan, B., Karande, V., Krohm, C., Morris, R., Pratt, D., and Gleicher, N., Cost considerations with infertility therapy: outcome and cost comparison between HMO and PPO care based on physician and facility cost, *Hum. Reprod.*, 13, 1200–1205, 1998.
8. Cain, J. M., Is deception for reimbursement in obstetrics and gynecology justified?, *Obstet. Gynecol.*, 82, 475–478, 1993.
9. Gleicher, N., Ed., *Managed Care, Infertility and Reproductive Medicine Clinics of North America*, Vol. 9:1, January 1998.

Index

A

Milton Keynes UK
Ingram Content Group UK Ltd.
UKHW021826071024
449327UK00021B/1450